PRECISION NUTRITION AND ENDOCRINE HEALTH

From Pregnancy to Chronic Diseases

PRECISION NUTRITION AND ENDOCRINE HEALTH

From Pregnancy to Chronic Diseases

Thakur Gurjeet Singh, PhD
Sanjana Mehta, PhD
Editors

AAP | APPLE ACADEMIC PRESS

First edition published 2026

Apple Academic Press Inc.
1265 Goldenrod Circle, NE,
Palm Bay, FL 32905 USA

760 Laurentian Drive, Unit 19,
Burlington, ON L7N 0A4, Canada

CRC Press
2385 NW Executive Center Drive,
Suite 320, Boca Raton FL 33431

4 Park Square, Milton Park,
Abingdon, Oxon, OX14 4RN, UK

Library and Archives Canada Cataloguing in Publication

CIP data on file with Canada Library and Archives

Library of Congress Cataloging-in-Publication Data

CIP data on file with US Library of Congress

ISBN: 978-1-998511-86-0 (hbk)
ISBN: 978-1-998511-87-7 (ebk)
DOI: 10.1201/9781998511877

About the Editors

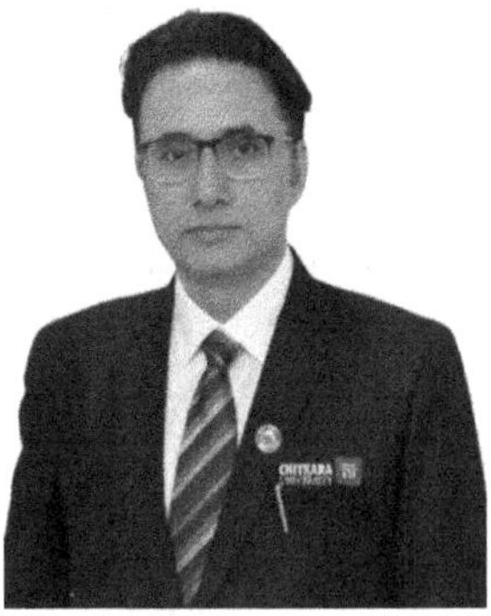

Prof. (Dr.) Thakur Gurjeet Singh
Dean, Chitkara College of Pharmacy, Chitkara University, Punjab, India

Thakur Gurjeet Singh, PhD, brings to the forefront a wealth of expertise and leadership cultivated through his role as Dean at Chitkara College of Pharmacy, Chitkara University, Punjab. Dr. Singh is globally recognized researcher consecutively for last three years as one of the top 2% of scientists, an honor bestowed by Stanford University.

Spanning over 17 years, his academic and industrial experience is distinguished by more than 470 published papers, accruing an impressive 7923 citations, reflecting his significant scholarly impact, characterized by an H-Index surpassing 47 and an i10 Index of 164. Notably, his contributions are underscored by an impact factor of 1190.5 and an RG Score of 1598.

With a doctoral specialization in pharmacology and a prolific career focused on neuropharmacology, substance dependence, pharmacological preconditioning, and drug discovery, Dr. Singh has mentored more than 22 PhD scholars and over 108 postgraduate research candidates, contributing significantly to translational science in neurodegenerative and metabolic disorders. His expertise spans both preclinical and clinical research, with deep insights into animal modeling, behavioral pharmacology, and experimental therapeutics.

Under his visionary leadership, the Chitkara College of Pharmacy became the first institute in Punjab to establish the Indian Pharmaceutical Association–Students' Forum's (IPA-SF) Punjab State Chapter, fostering professional engagement and national-level visibility for student pharmacists. He also serve as Faculty Advisor at ISPOR–The Professional Society for Health Economics and Outcomes Research Student Chapter at the Chitkara College of Pharmacy, empowering students to explore health economics, outcomes research, and value-based healthcare practices. In his role as the National Vice President of the Society of Clinical Research and Medical Professionals (SCRMP–International), he contributes to advancing global standards in clinical research, education, and professional excellence.

An editorial board member and editor of the *Journal of Pharmaceutical Technology, Research and Management*, Dr. Singh is a recognized contributor to scholarly publishing. His academic footprint includes numerous book chapters published by global leaders such as Elsevier, Springer Nature, Taylor & Francis, and Apple Academic Press, in areas ranging from nanotechnology and diabetes management to pharmacoeconomics and clinical therapeutics. He also serves as Director, Quality Management System at the Herbal and Ayush Product Testing and Standardization Lab (HAPTSL) at Chitkara University's College of Pharmacy, where he leads efforts to ensure global regulatory compliance through advanced instrumentation and a multidisciplinary team committed to excellence in Ayurvedic product standardization.

He has received multiple prestigious awards, including the outstanding researcher award, teacher's excellence awards, and accolades for innovation, patent filings, and research consultancy. Dr. Singh's enduring commitment to academic excellence, scientific inquiry, and institutional growth continues to elevate Chitkara College of Pharmacy as a hub of innovation, regulatory alignment, and interdisciplinary research in India's pharmaceutical landscape.

Dr. Singh has an MPharm (Pharmaceutical Sciences—Pharmacology), PDCR (Clinical Research & PCPV (Pharmacovigilance), and PhD (Pharmaceutical Sciences), Punjab, India.

ORCID ID: 0000-0003-2979-1590,
Scopus ID: 27667828700,
Google Scholar ID: puCyockAAAAJ&hl,
Vidwan ID: 383169

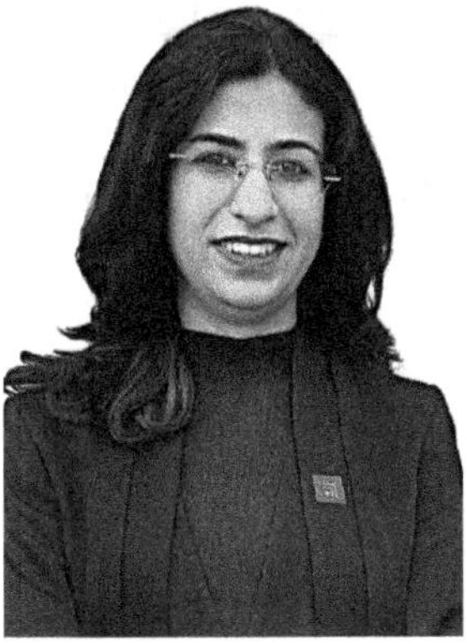

Dr. Sanjana Mehta, PharmD, PhD
Assistant Professor, HOD (PharmD), Chitkara College of Pharmacy, Chitkara University, Punjab, India
Researcher, Educator, Innovation Catalyst, and Clinical Pharmacology Expert

Sanjana Mehta, PhD, is a dedicated academician, researcher, and innovation mentor with PharmD and PhD degrees in Pharmaceutical Sciences. Currently serving as Assistant Professor and HOD (PharmD) at the Chitkara College of Pharmacy, Chitkara University (Punjab), she brings over five years of experience in academic leadership, clinical pharmacology, and translational research.

She actively coordinates the Institutional Innovation Cell (IIC) where she fosters a vibrant ecosystem for student-led innovation, start-up incubation, and interdisciplinary research. In her roles as Education Officer of the ISPOR–The Professional Society for Health Economics and Outcomes Research Student Chapter, Faculty Coordinator for Indian Pharmaceutical Association–Students' Forum's (IPA-SF) Punjab State Chapter, and Faculty Adviser at Society of Clinical Research and Medical Professionals (SCRMP) Student Forum Punjab State Chapter (Pharmacy Wing), Dr. Mehta empowers students to engage with global trends in pharmacoeconomics, public health policy, and community pharmacy practice.

Beyond research, she is a trained professional in vaccine administration and basic life support (BLS) under the prestigious Indian Pharmaceutical Association and the International Pharmaceutical Federation (IPA-FIP) collaborative "Train the Trainer" program, equipped with hands-on expertise in vaccine delivery, CPR, AED use, and ethical emergency response protocols. This training further enhances her role in healthcare education and community outreach.

She continues to mentor PharmD, MPharm, and PhD scholars in innovative, patient-centered research. Her research focus lies in advanced pharmacotherapeutics, metabolic disorders, and patient-centric innovations, with several patents and funded projects to her credit.

She also has a registered Copyright (L-110308/2022) to her credit, the DN-22 QoL Questionnaire (Diabetic Neuropathy Quality of Life Questionnaire).

Recognized with awards including the Best PhD Award, Dr. Mehta is known for her academic rigor, mentoring excellence, and commitment to public health advancement.

ORCID ID: 0000-0002-5517-4273
Scopus ID: 57213267102
Google Scholar ID: V3hUwOgAAAAJ
Vidwan ID: 381413

Contents

Contributors

Sapna Ahuja
Chitkara College of Pharmacy, Chitkara University, Punjab, India

Ebele Joan Ajagun
Bioresources Development Center, National Biotechnology Development Agency, Ogbomoso, Oyo, Nigeria

Athrv Arora
Chitkara College of Pharmacy, Chitkara University, Punjab, India

Abraham Olufemi Asuku
Bioresources Development Center, National Biotechnology Development Agency, Ogbomoso, Oyo, Nigeria; Department of Physiology, Faculty of Basic Medical Sciences, College of Health Sciences, University of Ilorin, Ilorin, Kwara, Nigeria

Saheli Banerjee
Department of Chemistry and Chemical Biology,
Indian Institute of Technology (Indian School of Mines), Dhanbad, Jharkhand, India

Shubham Singh Bartwal
National Institute of Pharmaceutical Education and Research (NIPER), Hyderabad, Telangana, India

Alok Bhatt
School of Pharmacy, Graphic Era Hill University, Dehradun, Uttarakhand, India

Teeshyo Bhattacharya
National Institute of Pharmaceutical Education and Research (NIPER), Kolkata, West Bengal, India

Subhash Chander
Amity Institute of Phytochemistry and Phytomedicine (AIP&P), Amity University Uttar Pradesh, Noida, Uttar Pradesh, India

Balakumar Chandrasekaran
Faculty of Pharmacy, Philadelphia University, Amman, Jordan

Samrat Chauhan
Chitkara College of Pharmacy, Chitkara University, Punjab, India

Dinesh Kumar Chellappan
School of Pharmacy, International Medical University, Bukit Jalil, Kuala Lumpur, Malaysia

Nitin Chitranshi
Faculty of Medicine, Health and Human Sciences, Macquarie University, North Ryde,
New South Wales, Australia

Sushma Devi
Chitkara College of Pharmacy, Chitkara University, Punjab, India

Anuvab Dey
Department of Biosciences and Bioengineering, Indian Institute of Technology Guwahati, Assam, India

Sanchit Dhankhar
Chitkara College of Pharmacy, Chitkara University, Punjab, India

Bhavesh Dharmani
Chitkara College of Pharmacy, Chitkara University, Punjab, India

Sayed Mohammed Firdous
P.G. Institute of Medical Sciences, Dhurabila, Dhamkuria, Paschim Medinipur, West Bengal, India

Madhukar Garg
Chitkara College of Pharmacy, Chitkara University, Punjab, India

Nidhi Garg
Department of Health and Family Welfare, Punjab, India

Nitika Garg
Chitkara College of Pharmacy, Chitkara University, Punjab, India

Tirath Garg
Gian Sagar Dental College and Hospital, Punjab, India

Subhrojyoti Ghosh
Department of Biotechnology, Indian Institute of Technology Madras, Chennai, Tamil Nadu, India

Anirban Hait
Department of Biotechnology, Heritage Institute of Technology, Kolkata, West Bengal, India

Neelparna Indu
Department of Biotechnology, Heritage Institute of Technology, Kolkata, West Bengal, India

Deepika Joshi
Siddhartha Institute of Pharmacy, Dehradun, Uttarakhand, India

Divya Kanwar
Chitkara College of Pharmacy, Chitkara University, Punjab, India

Gurpreet Kaur
Department of Pharmacology,
Amar Shaheed Baba Ajit Singh Jujhar Singh Memorial College of Pharmacy, Bela, Ropar, Punjab, India; I. K. Gujral Punjab Technical University, Kapurthala, Jalandhar, Punjab, India

Loveleen Kaur
Chitkara College of Pharmacy, Chitkara University, Punjab, India

Rajwinder Kaur
Chitkara College of Pharmacy, Chitkara University, Punjab, India

Rupinder Kaur
Chitkara College of Pharmacy, Chitkara University, Punjab, India

Ujjwal Kaushik
Chitkara College of Pharmacy, Chitkara University, Punjab, India

Sofia Kokkinis
Discipline of Pharmacy, Graduate School of Health, University of Technology Sydney, Sydney, New South Wales, Australia; Faculty of Health, Australian Research Center in Complementary and Integrative Medicine, University of Technology Sydney, Ultimo, New South Wales, Australia

Yogesh A. Kulkarni
Shobhaben Pratapbhai Patel School of Pharmacy and Technology Management, SVKM's Narsee Monjee Institute of Management Studies (NMIMS) Deemed to Be University, Mumbai, Maharashtra, India

Ajay Singh Kushwah
Department of Pharmacology,
Amar Shaheed Baba Ajit Singh Jujhar Singh Memorial College of Pharmacy, Bela, Ropar, Punjab, India

Atharva Anand Mahajan
Tata Memorial Center, Advanced Center for Treatment, Research and Education, Mumbai, Maharashtra, India

Raniya Malik
Discipline of Pharmacy, Graduate School of Health, University of Technology Sydney, Sydney, New South Wales, Australia; Faculty of Health, Australian Research Center in Complementary and Integrative Medicine, University of Technology Sydney, Ultimo, New South Wales, Australia

Sakshi Malik
Acute and General Medicine, Hull University Teaching Hospitals NHS Trust, Hull, United Kingdom

Bikash Manandhar
Discipline of Pharmacy, Graduate School of Health, University of Technology Sydney, Sydney, New South Wales, Australia; Faculty of Health, Australian Research Center in Complementary and Integrative Medicine, University of Technology Sydney, Ultimo, New South Wales, Australia

Samir Mehndiratta
Discipline of Pharmacy, Graduate School of Health, University of Technology Sydney, Sydney, New South Wales, Australia; Faculty of Health, Australian Research Center in Complementary and Integrative Medicine, University of Technology Sydney, Ultimo, New South Wales, Australia

Sanjana Mehta
Chitkara College of Pharmacy, Chitkara University, Punjab, India

Showkat R. Mir
School of Pharmaceutical Education and Research, Jamia Hamdard, New Delhi, India

Chanchal Mittal
National Institute of Pharmaceutical Education and Research (NIPER), Kolkata, West Bengal, India

Pooja Mittal
Chitkara College of Pharmacy, Chitkara University, Punjab, India

Vishnu Mittal
Guru Gobind Singh College of Pharmacy, Haryana, India

Ranit Mondal
Department of Pharmaceutical Technology, Jadavpur University, Kolkata, West Bengal, India

Dania Mughal
Pediatric Diabetes, North Lincolnshire and Goole NHS Trust, Grimsby, United Kingdom

Srinivas Nammi
School of Science, Western Sydney University, Penrith, New South Wales, Australia

Ejeatuluchukwu-alo Obi
Toxicology Unit, Department of Pharmacology, College of Health Science, Nnamdi Azikiwe University, Nnewi, Anambra, Nigeria

Gbonjubola Oyinlola Ogungbangbe
Department of Physiology, Faculty of Basic Medical Sciences, College of Health Sciences, University of Ilorin, Ilorin, Kwara, Nigeria

Tobiloba Samuel Olajide
Laboratory for Experimental and Translational Neurobiology, University of Medical Sciences, Ondo, Nigeria

Brian G. Oliver
School of Life Sciences, University of Technology Sydney, Sydney, New South Wales, Australia; Woolcock Institute of Medical Research, University of Sydney, Sydney, New South Wales, Australia

Toheeb O. Oyerinde
Laboratory for Experimental and Translational Neurobiology, University of Medical Sciences, Ondo, Nigeria

Sourav Pal
Department of Pharmacology, Calcutta Institute of Pharmaceutical Technology and AHS, Uluberia, Howrah, West Bengal, India

Terezinha de Jesus Andreoli Pinto
Department of Pharmacy, Faculty of Pharmaceutical Sciences, University of São Paulo, São Paulo, Brazil

Pankaj Popli
Chitkara College of Pharmacy, Chitkara University, Punjab, India; Department of Pharmacy, Jagannath University, Bahadurgarh, Haryana, India

Deepika Raina
School of Pharmacy, Graphic Era Hill University, Dehradun, Uttarakhand, India

Nidhi Rani
Chitkara College of Pharmacy, Chitkara University, Punjab, India

Haroon Riasat
Diabetes and Endocrinology, Hull University Teaching Hospitals NHS Trust, Hull, United Kingdom

Monika Saini
MM College of Pharmacy, Maharishi Markandeshwar (Deemed to be University), Mullana, Ambala, Haryana, India

Komal Sall
Chitkara College of Pharmacy, Chitkara University, Punjab, India

K. A. Shaima
Shambhunath Institute of Pharmacy, Jhalwa, Prayagraj, Uttar Pradesh, India

Akhil Sharma
Chitkara College of Pharmacy, Chitkara University, Punjab, India

Himanshu Sharma
Chitkara College of Pharmacy, Chitkara University, Punjab, India

Bhavana Singh
School of Pharmacy, Sharda University, Greater Noida, Uttar Pradesh, India

Pargat Singh
Chitkara College of Pharmacy, Chitkara University, Punjab, India

Sima Singh
Department of Pharmacy, University of Naples Federico II, Naples, Italy

Thakur Gurjeet Singh
Chitkara College of Pharmacy, Chitkara University, Punjab, India

Parul Sood
School of Pharmacy, Chitkara University, Solan, Himachal Pradesh, India

Rajan Swami
Chitkara College of Pharmacy, Chitkara University, Punjab, India

Henaroop Tiwana
Discipline of Pharmacy, Graduate School of Health, University of Technology Sydney, Sydney, New South Wales, Australia

Lavish Vaid
Chitkara College of Pharmacy, Chitkara University, Punjab, India

Amisha Vora
Shobhaben Pratapbhai Patel School of Pharmacy and Technology Management,
SVKM's Narsee Monjee Institute of Management Studies (NMIMS) Deemed to Be University,
Mumbai, Maharashtra, India

Pranali B. Yeram
Shobhaben Pratapbhai Patel School of Pharmacy and Technology Management,
SVKM's Narsee Monjee Institute of Management Studies (NMIMS) Deemed to Be University,
Mumbai, Maharashtra, India

Abbreviations

ABCA1	ATP-binding cassette transporter 1
ACL	ATP citrate lyase
ACOG	American College of Obstetricians and Gynecologists
ADA	American Diabetes Association
ALDH	aldehyde dehydrogenases
AMPK	adenosine-monophosphate-activated protein kinase
AMPK	AMP-activated protein kinase
APMAP	adipocyte plasma membrane-associated protein
AR	androgen receptor
AS-IV	astragaloside IV
ATP	adenosine triphosphate
ATPIII	adult treatment panel-III
AX	arabinoxylans
AXOS	arabinoxylan-oligosaccharides
BAT	brown adipose tissue
BCA	bradford or bicinchoninic acid
BMI	body mass index
CAT	catalase
CDG	congenital disorders of glycosylation
CDK5	cyclin-dependent kinase 5
CDKAL1	cyclin-dependent kinase five regulatory subunit-associated protein 1-like 1
CEE	conjugated equine oestrogens
CKD	chronic kidney disease
COX	cyclooxygenase
CRC	colorectal cancer
CRP	C-reactive protein
CS	cushing's syndrome
CVD	cardiovascular disease
DAEC	diffusely adherent E. Coli
DASH	dietary approach to stop hypertension
DBS	dried blood spot
DHEA	dehydroepiandrosterone
DM	diabetes mellitus
DN	diabetic nephropathy
DNMTs	DNA methyltransferases

DP	degrees of polymerization
DPP4	dipeptidyl peptidase-4
DR	diabetic retinopathy
DRI	dietary reference intakes
ECM	excessive extracellular matrix
EGCG	epigallocatechin gallate
EMT	epithelial-mesenchymal transition
ESRD	end-stage renal disease
ETBF	enterotoxigenic bacteroides fragilis
FG	fasting glucose
FMT	fecal microbiota transplants
FSGS	focal segmental glomerulosclerosis
FSH	follicle-stimulating hormone
FTO	fat mass and obesity-associated protein
GA	glycyrrhizic acid
GCK	glucokinase
GCKR	glucokinase regulatory protein
GDM	gestational diabetes mellitus
GE	geniposide
GF	comparing germ-free
GFR	glomerular filtration rate
GH	growth hormone
GIT	gastrointestinal tract
GLUT4	glucose transporter 4
GN	glomerulonephritis
GWAS	genome-wide association studies
HATs	histone acetyltransferases
HDACs	histone deacetylases
HDL	high-density lipoprotein
HFD	high-fat diet
HG	high glucose
HPLC	high-performance liquid chromatography
HRT	hormone replacement treatment
IDF	international diabetes federation
IECs	ileal epithelial cells
IEF	isoelectric focusing
IEM	inborn errors of metabolism
IFN	interferon
IGF-I	insulin-like growth factor
INS-1 cells	insulinoma cell line
INSIG1	insulin-induced gene 1
IPG	immobilized ph gradient
IRS1	insulin receptor substrate 1

IT	insulin therapy
IV	intravenously
LATs	lysine acetyltransferases
LDH	layer double hydroxide
LOH	low androgen levels
LOX1	lipoxygenase-1
LPL	lipoprotein lipase
MCP	mother-child protection
MCP-1	monocyte chemotactic protein 1
MCR4	melanocortin receptor 4
MDA	malondialdehyde
MDA	myeloperoxidase
MDPA	medroxyprogesterone acetate
MF	mangiferin
MMPs	matrix metalloproteinases
MNT	medical nutrition therapy
MS	metabolic syndrome
MS	multiple sclerosis
MSUD	maple syrup urine disease
MTNR1B	melatonin receptor 1B
NADPH	nicotinamide adenine dinucleotide phosphate
NAFLD	non-alcoholic fatty liver disease
NAG	N-acetylgucosaminidase
NDDG	National Diabetes Data Group
NE	nanoemulsion
NEC	neonatal necrotizing enterocolitis
NO	nitric oxide
NPY	neuropeptide Y
OGTT	oral glucose tolerance test
OH	overt hypothyroidism
OS	oxidative stress
OW	overweight
PAGE	polyacrylamide gel electrophoresis
PAK1	p21-activated kinase 1
PC	phospholipidated curcumin
PCNA	proliferating cell nuclear antigens
PCOS	polycystic ovarian syndrome
PDK1	protein kinase 1
PET	positron emission tomography
PGE2	prostaglandin E2
PI3K	phosphatidylinositol 3-kinase
PKC	protein kinase C
POMC	pro-opiomelanocortin

POR	pooled odds ratio
PPAR-δ	peroxisome proliferator-activated receptor δ
PPPM	predictive, preventive, personalized medicine
PRRs	pattern recognition receptors
PTM	post-translational modifications
PTP1B	protein tyrosine phosphatase 1B
RAAS	renin-angiotensin-aldosterone system
RCTs	randomized controlled trials
RIPA	radioimmunoprecipitation assay
RNS	reactive nitrogen species
ROS	reactive oxygen species
SAM	s-adenyl methionine
SCFAs	short-chain fatty acids
SCH	subclinical classifications
SD	sprague dawley
SDS	sodium dodecyl sulphate
SDS-PAGE	sulfate-polyacrylamide gel electrophoresis
SERMs	selective oestrogen receptor modulators
SERT	serotonin transporter
SFA	saturated fatty acids
SLNs	solid lipid nps
SNP	sodium nitroprusside
SOD	superoxide dismutase
STAT3	signal transducer and activator of transcription 3
TC	total cholesterol
TG	triglycerides
TH1	type 1 t helper
THs	thyroid hormones
TLRs	toll-like receptors
TSH	thyroid-stimulating hormone
TSHR	thyroid-stimulating hormone receptor
TTF-1	thyroid transcription factor 1
UC	unformulated curcumin
UTRs	untranslated regions
VEGF	vascular endothelial growth factor
VLDL-C	very low-density lipoprotein cholesterol
VMS	vasomotor symptoms
WAT	white adipose tissue
WHI	women's health initiative
WHO	world health organization
XOS	xylo-oligosaccharides
ZO-1	zonulin

Foreword

In an era where chronic diseases are on the rise and personalized medicine is gaining traction, *Precision Nutrition and Endocrine Health: From Pregnancy to Chronic Diseases* serves as a crucial resource for healthcare professionals and researchers. This book emerges as an influential work that not only bridges the gap between these two critical domains but also sets the stage for a transformative approach to health and wellness across the lifespan.

From the moment of conception, nutrition plays a vital role in shaping endocrine health, which in turn influences growth, development, and long-term health outcomes. One of the book's standout features is its holistic perspective. It addresses the continuum of endocrine health, beginning with prenatal nutrition and maternal health and extending to the prevention and management of chronic diseases such as diabetes, thyroid disorders, and metabolic syndrome. Each chapter meticulously explores how nutritional interventions can influence endocrine function and overall health, backed by the latest scientific evidence and clinical best practices.

The authors present cutting-edge research and practical insights that highlight the importance of personalized nutrition strategies in optimizing endocrine health by focusing on individual genetic, environmental, and lifestyle factors. This book equips the reader with the knowledge and tools needed to implement effective nutritional strategies that support endocrine health and mitigate the risk of chronic diseases. Moreover, it empowers readers to make informed decisions about their health, fostering a proactive approach to wellness that is grounded in science.

I commend the editors and contributors for their dedication and expertise in compiling this invaluable resource. Their collective efforts have resulted in a book that will undoubtedly inform and inspire advancements in the fields of endocrinology and metabolism. It is my hope that the insights and strategies presented herein will serve as a guiding light for healthcare professionals as they strive to improve the lives of individuals affected by these challenging conditions.

—Mahender Bishnoi, PhD
Scientist E,
National Agri-Food Biotechnology Institute

Foreword

It is with great pleasure that I introduce *Precision Nutrition and Endocrine Health: From Pregnancy to Chronic Diseases.* This exceptional book is a landmark achievement in the field of nutrition, offering an in-depth analysis of how personalized dietary approaches can profoundly influence endocrine health.

The concept of precision nutrition is transforming our understanding of diet and health. By tailoring nutritional interventions to the specific needs of individuals, we can achieve better health outcomes and more effectively manage endocrine disorders. This book delves into these topics, providing a comprehensive guide to the latest research and practical applications of precision nutrition in the context of endocrine health.

The authors have expertly navigated the complex relationships between nutrition, hormonal balance, and metabolic health. From the pivotal role of nutrition during pregnancy, influencing both maternal and fetal health, to addressing chronic conditions such as diabetes and metabolic syndrome, this book covers a wide spectrum of issues. Each chapter offers evidence-based recommendations and practical strategies, making it a valuable resource for healthcare professionals seeking to implement precision nutrition in their practice.

I applaud the authors for their commitment to this pioneering work. Their detailed exploration of the science behind precision nutrition and its application to endocrine health is both informative and inspiring. This book is poised to become an essential reference for clinicians, researchers, and students dedicated to advancing the field of nutrition and improving patient outcomes.

Precision Nutrition and Endocrine Health: From Pregnancy to Chronic Diseases is a testament to the authors' expertise and vision. It provides a thorough understanding of how individualized nutritional strategies can optimize endocrine function and promote better health across the lifespan.

—Nirmal Singh, PhD
Professor and Former Head,
Department of Pharmaceutical Sciences and Drug Research,
Punjabi University, Patiala, Punjab, India

Preface

The book *Precision Nutrition and Endocrine Health: From Pregnancy to Chronic Diseases* serves as a beacon of knowledge, uniting the latest insights and research from esteemed experts worldwide. It offers a comprehensive exploration of the pivotal relationship between nutrition and endocrine health, recognizing the profound impact of nutrition from the earliest stages of life onward. This understanding is fundamental to enhancing health interventions and outcomes globally.

Our team of distinguished experts in nutrition, endocrinology, and related fields presents cutting-edge research and practical strategies within these pages. From prenatal nutrition to the management of chronic diseases like diabetes and metabolic syndrome, each chapter provides a clinical perspective backed by the latest scientific evidence and best clinical practices. To ensure accessibility, we've crafted the text in clear, straightforward language, complemented by numerous figures and tables.

We aspire for *Precision Nutrition and Endocrine Health: From Pregnancy to Chronic Diseases* to serve as an invaluable reference, advancing knowledge and improving patient care. By offering insights into these complex conditions, we aim to contribute to better health outcomes for individuals worldwide affected by endocrine and metabolic diseases.

We extend our deepest gratitude to the authors who generously shared their expertise and insights, contributing significantly to this endeavor. Their dedication has been instrumental in creating a resource that will benefit healthcare professionals, researchers, and students. Additionally, we express our appreciation to Apple Academic Press and their team for the opportunity to publish this volume. Lastly, we acknowledge the unwavering support of our family members, whose love, encouragement, and patience have sustained us throughout this journey.

—Editors

CHAPTER 1

Genetic and Epigenetic Insights into Gestational Diabetes Mellitus: Implications for Early Diagnosis and Management

SOURAV PAL,[1] SAYED MOHAMMED FIRDOUS,[2,*] and EJEATULUCHUKWU-ALO OBI[3]

[1]*Department of Pharmacology, Calcutta Institute of Pharmaceutical Technology and AHS, Uluberia, Howrah, West Bengal, India*

[2]*P. G. Institute of Medical Sciences, Dhurabila, Dhamkuria, Paschim Medinipur, West Bengal, India*

[3]*Toxicology Unit, Department of Pharmacology, College of Health Science, Nnamdi Azikiwe University, Nnewi, Anambra, Nigeria*

*Corresponding author

ABSTRACT

Gestational diabetes mellitus is a disorder that affects both women and their unborn children, and it is characterized by poor glucose tolerance throughout pregnancy. People with several SNPs are more likely to develop type 2 diabetes at some point in their lives. The various genetic variants associated with an increased risk of developing GDM are examined in this comprehensive review. SNPs in transcription factors like TCF7L2 and MTNR1B affect insulin synthesis and secretion. When membrane proteins like GNB3 and KCNQ1 undergo alterations, insulin signaling and transport are negatively impacted. SNPs in genes encoding enzymes like DIO2 and FTO disrupt metabolism and increase insulin resistance.

Precision Nutrition and Endocrine Health: Synthesis, Characterization, and Applications.
Thakur Gurjeet Singh and Sanjana Mehta (Eds.)

DOI: 10.1201/9781998511877-1

Variations in VEGFA and MIF polymorphisms affect protein expression, leading to endothelial dysfunction and increased pro-inflammatory cytokines—two hallmarks of T2DM. This review seeks to enhance health outcomes for women and infants by raising awareness of these genetic variants' potential implications on GDM predisposition and promoting their role in early detection and therapy. Pregnancy-related GDM can harm the mother and child. Epigenetic changes may explain metabolic anomalies in fetal programming. In unknown ways, the *FTO* gene impacts metabolic parameters via epigenetic mechanisms. This study investigates whether GDM is linked to epigenetic modifications in placental DNA at FTO promoter CpG sites. Metabolic parameters and placenta *FTO* gene methylation are examined between GDM and non-GDM mothers. These findings may reveal GDM's epigenetic processes and effects on maternal metabolic health. In conclusion, GDM is complex and affected by hereditary and nonhereditary factors. Knowledge of GDM's genetic and epigenetic aspects can enhance early diagnosis, prevention, and management.

1.1 INTRODUCTION

Diabetes mellitus (DM) pertains to an oscillation of common metabolic illnesses characterized by high glucose levels in the blood (hyperglycemia) and the resulting acute and chronic consequences (Moini et al., 2022). Four different forms of DM are identified: Type 1 DM, an autoimmune illness that causes the loss of pancreatic cells responsible for producing insulin (Roep et al., 2021), and Type 2 DM (T2DM), characterized by a gradual resistance to insulin resulting in reduced insulin output (Blaslov et al., 2018). The third category includes a range of illnesses in which DM is a recognized cause, such as monogenic disorders (e.g., maturity-onset diabetes of the young) and endocrine imbalances (e.g., Cushing's syndrome) (Venyo et al., 2023). Gestational diabetes mellitus (GDM), which is the fourth subtype, affects around 7% of pregnancies. Annually, gestational diabetes impacts between 2% to 10% of pregnancies in the United States (Powe et al., 2022). The incidence of GDM in India exhibits variability, with documented estimates ranging from 7% to approximately 16%. During a ten-year study at a tertiary care research facility, it was discovered that 29.47% of pregnant women were diagnosed with GDM during the first trimester, 52.42% during the second trimester, and 18.11%

during the third trimester (Panaitescu et al., 2016). The occurrence of gestational diabetes in India has been documented to vary from 3.8% to as high as 41% in different areas. These discrepancies are believed to be influenced by variations in the age and socioeconomic status of pregnant women in different locations (Unnikrishnan et al., 2020). The diagnosis is established by assessing fasting glucose levels, doing oral glucose tolerance tests, and evaluating symptoms of hyperglycemia. Common risk factors for GDM include a familial predisposition to T2DM, being of an older age during pregnancy, having polycystic ovarian syndrome, having previously experienced GDM, or having a history of delivering babies weighing above 4 kg (Li et al., 2020). Specific risk factors, such as elevated BMI, inactive way of life, and pre-existing hypertension, can be reduced.

In a typical pregnancy, a woman's body changes, such as weight gain, placenta growth, and metabolism shifts. Reduced insulin sensitivity allows the body to absorb and store glucose for use later in pregnancy, which is a significant metabolic change (Stern et al., 2021). Nevertheless, insulin resistance becomes more pronounced in the second part of pregnancy (about 20 to 24 weeks). It may be influenced by placental hormones (hPG, hPL, cortisol, estrogen, and progesterone) and inflammatory cytokines such as TNF-α (Figure 1.1). To make up for the insulin resistance in the mother, this causes the pancreatic β cells to enlarge and become more active. GDM can occur when this adjustment causes β-cell malfunction or insufficient compensation for glucose loads in specific instances. Factors that increase the likelihood of gestational diabetes include being overweight, having T2DM, having a family history of GDM, being a mother who is 35 years old or older, and having polycystic ovarian syndrome (PCOS) (Pirotta et al., 2020).

GDM must be discriminated from T2DM either prior to or during pregnancy. GDM is diagnosed based on specific criteria, which include fasting glucose levels of 92 mg/dl, glucose levels of ≥180 mg/dl in the 60th minute of the oral glucose tolerance test (OGTT), or glucose levels of ≥153 mg/dl in the 120th Minute of OGTT. Undiagnosed GDM can result in severe complications, including pre-eclampsia, macrosomia (excessive fetal growth), fetal hyperinsulinemia, anoxia, heart failure, birth abnormalities, and polyhydramnios (Choudhury et al., 2021). Following childbirth, women who have had GDM are at a heightened risk of having either T2DM or type 1 DM. Particles, genes, and epigenetic cascades associated

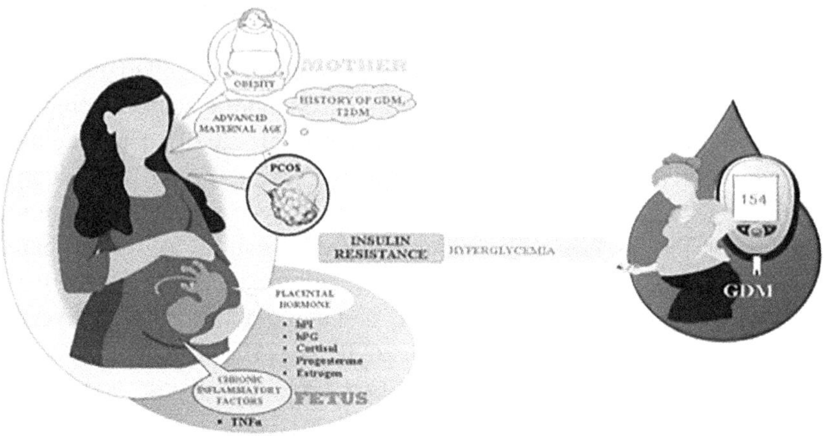

FIGURE 1.1 Predisposing factors for GDM.

with T2DM are now being investigated for their role in developing GDM. The chances of getting GDM may be increased by genes like *TCF7L2*, *KCNJ11*, glucokinase (GCK), and glucokinase regulatory protein (GCKR), which are related to β-cell activity and insulin secretion (Jääskeläinen et al., 2022). Another risk factor for GDM is changes in proteins that control the proper secretion of insulin (Nair et al., 2021). Despite the strong connection observed with other genes, the relationship between CDKAL1, fat mass and obesity-associated protein (FTO), insulin receptor substrate 1 (IRS1), and GDM is still poorly understood. This review emphasizes the importance of early screening for GDM, discusses well-established risk factors, and investigates novel genetic and epigenetic factors, offering significant insights into prospective directions for future study.

1.2 GENETIC PREDISPOSITION TO GDM

Throughout pregnancy, a range of physiological changes occur, specifically in how the mother's body processes glucose, which is crucial for the growth and development of the fetus. In the later stages of pregnancy, there is an increase in catabolic processes, which leads to higher levels of glycemia, insulinemia, and fatty acids (Ziętek et al., 2021). Mechanisms such as the adjustments made by pancreatic β-cells and the glucose production by the liver play an imperative role in sustaining optimal glucose levels despite the decrease in maternal insulin sensitivity. The rising occurrence of GDM, a significant metabolic condition during pregnancy, is associated with increasing rates of obesity, older maternal age, and sedentary behaviors. The etiology of GDM is multifaceted and involves a complicated interaction between environmental, genetic, and epigenetic variables (Shankar et al., 2023; Singhet al., 2020). Comp compelling evidence suggests a significant genetic link to GDM, which tends to reoccur in consecutive pregnancies. There are noticeable differences in health outcomes based on ethnicity, with Southeast Asian groups having the highest risk, which is approximately 25%. A correlation between GDM and T2DM has been discovered, in which specific genetic variations related to the production of insulin, insulin resistance, and the metabolism of glucose increase the likelihood of developing GDM. Postpartum diabetes is seven times more prevalent in women with a family history of GDM. Comprehending the complex genetic links between GDM and T2DM is essential, considering their everyday basis of insulin resistance (Li et al., 2020; Sharma et al., 2020; Singh et al., 2020). These findings emphasize the importance of thorough genetic evaluations, particularly for high-risk groups, to improve strategies for preventing, detecting, and managing GDM and future diabetes (Sharma et al., 2020).

Although candidate gene screening has successfully identified loci associated with T2DM, many of these loci lacked a sufficiently robust connection to warrant further investigation (Lake et al., 2021). Although there were links, they did not consistently imply an increased probability of getting GDM. Potential reasons for these findings may be the limited sample numbers and the narrow range of genetic Polymorphisms considered, focusing on glycemic characteristics rather than disease-related factors in screening potential genes. Genome-wide association Studies have identified over 70 loci linked to T2DM (Ekta et al., 2020; Garg et al., 2021; Kodama et al., 2018). However, which specific genes play the most significant role in predicting the probability of getting GDM remains uncertain. This emphasizes the significance of conducting more extensive research to comprehend the genetic complexities of GDM and its potential distinctions from T2DM. Several techniques, including animal model studies, positional cloning, genome-wide association studies, and next-generation sequencing, are used to discover potential genes based on their biological viability and existing understanding of gene function (Sahu et al., 2020; Singh and Singh, 2021) A recent extensive analysis found

83 potential genes associated with *GDM. TCF7L2, KCNQ1, CDKAL1, IRS1*, and *MTNR1B* have been extensively investigated due to their high connection with GDM (Zhang et al., 2018). These findings emphasize the complex genetic foundations of GDM, providing insight into possible treatment targets and the joint genetic base of GDM and T2DM.

1.2.1 *TCF7L2* AND GDM

TCF7L2, a transcription factor found on chromosome 10q25, plays a crucial role in the development of GDM. *TCF7L2* exhibits high expression levels in adipose tissue, the pancreas, and several other tissues. It significantly affects glucose regulation and is the most notable hereditary factor linked to T2DM (del Bosque-Plata et al., 2021; Vishwakarma et al., 2022). Adipokines, such as leptin and adiponectin, are signaling hormones secreted by adipocytes and are regulated by *TCF7L2* (Al-Mansoori et al., 2022; Singh et al., 2021). The regulation of hunger and energy expenditure are both affected by these hormones. Higher levels of leptin are detected in cases of GDM, which may contribute to macrosomia (Bernea et al., 2022). Conversely, lower levels of adiponectin are linked to insulin resistance. While the exact processes by which *TCF7L2* contributes to T2DM are not yet fully understood, certain studies indicate its role in adipocyte formation. Furthermore, *TCF7L2* might function in the PI3K/AKT cascade, which is essential for transmitting insulin signaling and maintaining glucose balance. The *TCF7L2* gene produces a transcription factor that has an HMG domain (Li et al., 2021). The WNT signal activates this transcription factor and combines with β-catenin in the cytoplasm to create a transcriptional complex. The *TCF7L2* gene polymorphism rs7903146 is linked to reduced insulin production and an elevated risk of GDM. Individuals who carry the T allele of TCF7L2 rs7903146 have been demonstrated to exhibit impaired glucose and lipid metabolism in GDM. The TCF7L2 gene polymorphism rs290487 has been linked to an increased incidence of GDM in the Chinese Han population. This study identifies seven *TCF7L2* genetic variations positively linked to GDM, suggesting a common genetic foundation between GDM and T2DM (Zhang et al., 2022). TCF7L2 polymorphisms, established as dependable indicators of T2DM, have been discovered to elevate the likelihood of GDM. Hypotheses provide a probable situation in which abnormal Wnt signaling, which may be caused by *TCF7L2* dysfunction, could affect both the transcription of genes specific to β cells and the structural stability of KATP channels (Figure 1.2). This dual phenomenon may contribute to the impaired insulin secretion found in GDM. Additional study is necessary to examine the complicated molecular pathways that connect Wnt signaling, *TCF7L2* expression, and the physiological processes that regulate insulin production.

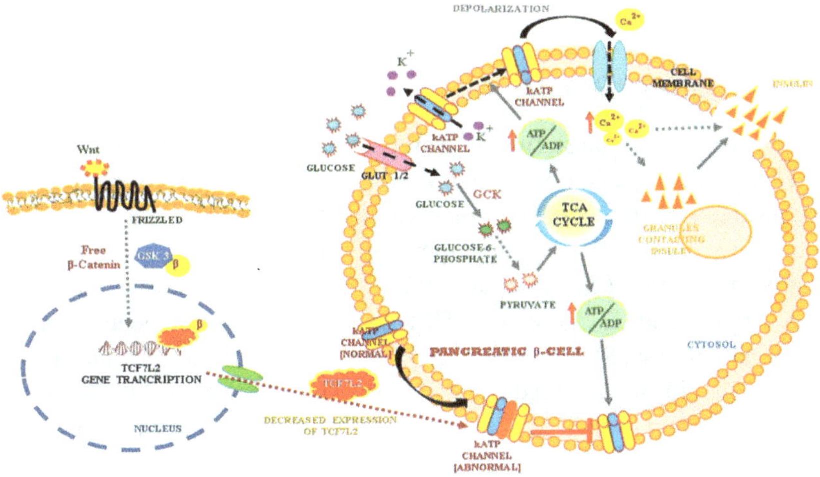

FIGURE 1.2 Correlation of GDM and improperly expressing TCF7L2 Wnt signaling via Frizzled receptors and GSK-β induces TCF7L2 transcription. Reduced TCF7L2 expression alters KATP channel formation, hindering calcium influx and insulin secretion. This highlights potential links between Wnt signaling, TCF7L2 dysregulation, and impaired insulin release, shedding light on GDM pathophysiology.

1.2.2 KCNJ11 AND GDM

The significance of the *KCNJ11* gene in GDM is emphasized because it plays a crucial role in controlling insulin secretion through the K-ATP channel (Rosik et al., 2020). The *KCNJ11* gene polymorphism rs5219 has been found to have a slight connection with GDM (Lenin et al., 2018). Genetic mutations and diseases can cause disruptions in the insulin secretion mechanism, resulting in the premature termination of insulin synthesis. This leads to a scarcity of insulin in both T2DM and GDM. *KCNQ1* is on chromosome 11p15 and is expressed in vital tissues, including the kidney, brain, heart, and pancreatic islets. The choice of *KCNQ1* as a potential gene for GDM is based on its known connection with T2DM, which makes it a suitable option for studying the genetic causes of GDM. The presence of the *KCNQ1* gene polymorphism rs2237895 has been linked to a higher susceptibility to GDM in women from Pakistan (Benny et al., 2021). *KCNQ1* gene polymorphisms are believed to impact glucose metabolism and insulin production, potentially compromising β cell function. This can exacerbate pre-diabetic symptoms. The candidate-gene technique has been instrumental in examining several SNPs in the *KCNQ1* gene for their possible association with GDM (Cao et al., 2020).

1.2.3 CDKAL1 AND GDM

Cyclin-dependent kinase five regulatory subunit-associated protein 1-like 1 (*CDKAL1*) is located on chromosome 6q22.3. It has an essential effect on insulin secretion and the functioning of β-cells. *CDKAL1* acts as a negative regulator of cyclin-dependent kinase 5 (CDK5) and inhibits insulin production (Ghosh et al., 2022). Case-control research involving 316 controls and 321 cases of GDM revealed that certain genetic variations, namely rs9295478, rs6935599, and rs7747752, were found to be associated with an increased risk of GDM (Abu Samra et al., 2022). Moreover, a meta-analysis encompassing five studies conducted on various populations demonstrated that rs7754840 and rs7756992 were linked to a heightened risk of GDM in both Asian and Caucasian groups (Amin et al., 2022). *CDKAL1* suppresses CDK5 activity, impacting β cell function and insulin sensitivity during glucose stimulation. Significantly, it is involved in abnormalities associated with the conversion of proinsulin and the insulin response, emphasizing its importance in the complex regulatory system of maintaining glucose balance.

1.2.4 IRS1 AND GDM

IRS1, situated on chromosome 2q36.3, is a crucial element of the insulin receptor. It is mainly found in insulin-sensitive tissues and is vital in the insulin signaling cascade. Evidence shows that the rs1801278 (G972R) genetic mutation increases insulin resistance and inhibits IRS1 function (Mehta et al., 2022; Omar et al., 2021). This polymorphism has been examined in several populations, such as Saudi Arabians, Greeks, Scandinavians, and Russians, and has attracted attention due to its probable link with insulin resistance (Rasool et al., 2022). Ten case-control studies conducted from 2005 to 2014 examined the association between genetic variations in IRS1 and melatonin receptor 1B (MTNR1B) with the development and progression of GDM (Rosik et al., 2020). IRS1 is essential for the movement of GLUT4 and serves as a critical mediator in conveying signals from insulin and IGF-1 receptors to proteins inside the cell. Disruptions in cascades associated with IRS1 can result in insulin resistance, affecting blood glucose regulation. The rs1801278 polymorphism was also examined concerning GDM; this variant is linked to decreased insulin production and an increased risk of T2DM (Figure 1.3). In addition, women with GDM showed elevated baseline phosphorylation of serine 312 on IRS-1, suggesting an increase in the production of inhibitory serine kinases (Capurso et al., 2018; Mehta et al., 2022). In women with GDM, administering insulin during a glucose load decreased the tyrosine phosphorylation of IRS-1 (Li et al., 2022). This finding corresponds to the observed rise in the expression of inhibitory serine kinase. The results emphasize the complex connection between IRS1 genetic variations, insulin resistance, and the occurrence of GDM, providing significant knowledge for focused interventions and individualized management approaches.

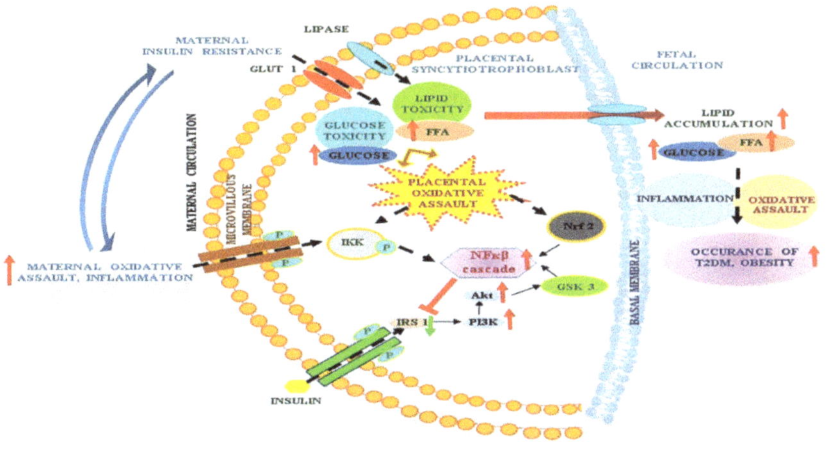

FIGURE 1.3 Relationships between IRS1-mediated pathways, inflammation, and maternal oxidative stress in GDM. In GDM, NFκβ rises due to IKK phosphorylation from maternal oxidative assault, notably in placental syncytiotrophoblasts. Placental oxidative stress worsens with maternal insulin resistance-induced glucose and lipid toxicity, activating NFκβ via Nrf2, heightening fetal inflammation, and risk of GDM and T2DM.

1.2.5 MTNR1B AND GDM

The *MTNR1B* gene is closely linked to regulating glucose levels in the body, affecting essential functions such as the absorption and movement of glucose (Kettunen et al., 2020). The rs10830963 variation in the *MTNR1B* gene has been recognized as a significant factor in glucose metabolism disorders, particularly GDM. Melatonin, by activating *MTNR1B*, enhances the uptake of glucose by promoting the insulin receptor substrate-1/PI3K cascade while simultaneously suppressing the production of insulin by blocking the downstream MAPK signaling cascade (Zhu et al., 2023). The *MTNR1B* gene, which codes for the MT2 melatonin receptor, is present in essential tissues like the human brain, pancreatic islets, and β-cells (Figure 1.4) (Espino et al., 2019). This gene is highly likely to be involved in glycemic and metabolic characteristics. The mutation rs10830963, located inside the 11.5-kb intron of *MTNR1B*, is particularly important in this context (Zhu et al., 2023). In pregnancy, melatonin plays a crucial function in regulating glucose levels. It promotes glucose absorption and increases the production of essential proteins such as GLUT4 and PPARγ in trophoblasts. Curiously, the impact of this phenomenon is diminished when there is a decrease in the expression of MT2 receptors. Within the domain of GDM, three specific SNPs – rs10830962, rs10830963, and rs1387153 – have been detected within the *MTNR1B* gene. The third SNP, rs1387153, has been discovered as a risk factor for GDM in populations of Mexican, Finnish, Danish, and Arab descent (Dias et al., 2018).

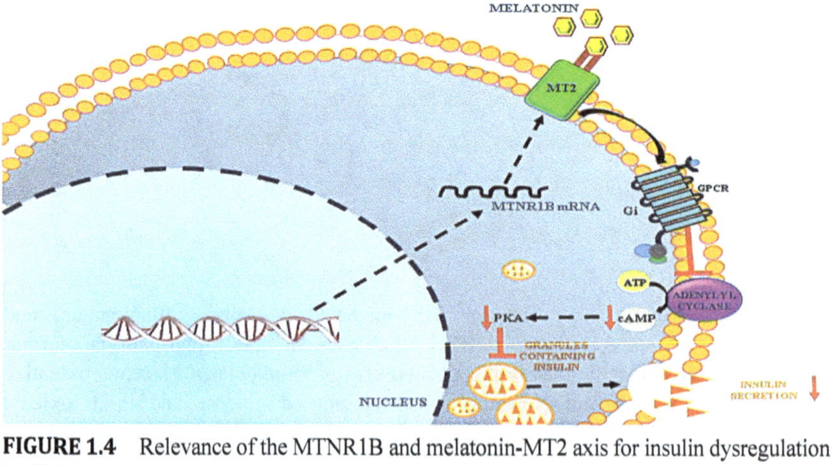

FIGURE 1.4 Relevance of the MTNR1B and melatonin-MT2 axis for insulin dysregulation in GDM.

MTNR1B mRNA encodes MT2. Melatonin binding to MT2 inhibits adenylyl cyclase, decreasing cAMP levels and PKA expression and ultimately reducing insulin secretion in GDM.

1.3 MEMBRANE PROTEINS AND GDM

GDM is characterized by impaired insulin signaling, which prevents the separation of ERp44 from the serotonin transporter (SERT), resulting in a decrease in the absorption of serotonin by the placenta (Perić et al., 2022). In GDM trophoblasts, SERT is trapped by ERp44, which hinders glycosylation and reduces 5-HT uptake. Genetic variables such as TCF7L2 and HHEX can modify insulin production in GDM, promoting its occurrence (Lu et al., 2022). A separate investigation has found the presence of diabetogenic genes *MTNR1B* and *IRS1* in GDM, indicating that membrane proteins and insulin signaling plays a substantial role in the development of GDM (Rosik et al., 2020). Table 1.1 displays instances of membrane proteins and their correlation in GDM.

TABLE 1.1 Membrane Protein Associated with GDM

Membrane Protein	Function in GDM	References
SERT	Insulin signaling defect binds ERp44 to SERT, impacting 5-HT uptake in GDM trophoblasts.	Cooper et al. (2019); Li et al. (2014)
Adipocyte Plasma Membrane-Associated Protein (APMAP)	GDM omental adipose tissue shows impaired insulin signaling and NFκB activation in adipocytes.	Harprecht (2020)
Glucose Transporter Proteins (GLUTs)	Facilitate glucose transport, insert insulin-independent GLUT, and bind vesicles containing insulin-dependent GLUT4.	Feng et al. (2019); Luiken et al. (2020)
GNB3	GNB3 rs5443 polymorphism linked to T2DM and insulin resistance, regulating insulin production.	Нартикоева (2021)
MTNR1B	MTNR1B variations reduce GCK expression cAMP levels, impairing insulin secretion, increasing GDM risk.	Banerjee (2018)

1.4 GENOME-WIDE ASSOCIATION STUDIES AND GLYCEMIC TRAIT ANALYSIS

Genome-wide association studies (GWAS) have significantly transformed our comprehension of the genetic underpinnings of diseases, enabling the detection of genetic variations linked to vulnerability to different circumstances (Uffelmann et al., 2021). Since its establishment in 2005, more than 50,000 connections between illnesses and genetic variations have been documented by GWAS. Nevertheless, only two GWAS have been carried out for GDM, a medical illness that has substantial consequences for the health of both the mother and the fetus. Kwak et al. conducted the initial GWAS specifically targeting GDM. The study was carried out in two stages and focused on Korean women. The first phase involved 468 instances of GDM and 1242 control subjects (Powe et al., 2020). This was followed by a subsequent study in which 931 GDM cases and 783 control subjects were included for replication. Based on these findings, two notable GDM variants have been identified: rs10830962 upstream of MTNR1B and rs7754840 in the intron regions of CDKAL1 (Abu Samra et al., 2022). Around 200 and 81 people, including 115 healthy controls and 103 GDM cases, were the subjects of the second GWAS, which targeted Chinese women (Jääskeläinen et al., 2022). In this investigation, 23 SNPs were shown to be strongly associated with the development of GDM. Four genes—*CTIF, CDH18, PTGIS,* and *SYNPR*—were identified as having a connection to GDM among these SNPs (Wu et al., 2021). The *CDH18, PTGIS,* and *SYNPR* genes are highly abundant in glycometabolism-related cascades, according to additional research in Gene Ontology and the Kyoto Encyclopedia of Genes and Genome (Jääskeläinen et al., 2022).

- **Epigenetic Mechanisms in GDM:** Even though they have the same genetic material, cells have various gene expression patterns. This is due to epigenetic changes. The alterations above, encompassing DNA methylation, histone modifications, and non-coding RNAs (ncRNAs), such as miRNA, actively govern gene activity and expression without modifying the fundamental DNA sequence. Epigenetic alterations can be triggered by environmental and lifestyle variables such as pollution, tobacco smoking, obesity, physical inactivity, and alcohol intake (Mahmoud et al., 2022). It is thought that epigenetic changes significantly influence the onset and progression of GDM, which may influence the health of the offspring. Studies suggest that offspring exposed to GDM have a higher likelihood of experiencing birth abnormalities. Furthermore, scientists like Linares-Pineda et al. (2023) suggest that epigenetic cascades are vital in influencing the development of chronic illnesses, such as T2DM, in adolescent offspring of women with GDM.

1.4.1 DNA METHYLATION DYNAMICS IN GDM

DNA methylation is an essential epigenetic change that involves adding a methyl group to the fifth carbon position of the cytosine nucleotide (Kumar et al., 2018). This modification has regulatory ramifications. The process, facilitated by methyltransferase enzymes (DNMTs), contributes to the regulation of gene expression by either impeding the binding of transcription factors to DNA or employing proteins to suppress gene expression (Lyko et al., 2018). The DNA methylation pattern exhibits variations across different cell types, predominantly occurring at cytosine sites next to guanine (CpG). Cardenas et al. employed bisulphite conversion and the Infinium Methylation EPIC BeadChip to quantify DNA methylation in the fetal placenta of women at 24–30 weeks of gestation following an oral glucose tolerance test. The hypomethylation of four CpG sites in the *PDE4B* gene was linked with glycemia levels two hours after a glucose load in mothers. Furthermore, differential methylation was detected in genes such as BLM, TNFRSF1B, and LDLR, potentially affecting DNA homeostasis, apoptosis, and endocytosis (Cardenas et al., 2018).

A separate investigation employing the Illumina Infinium Human Methylation 450 BeadChip on cord blood identified 4485 distinctively methylated locations, among which 37 CpG sites exhibit potential as clinical indicators for GDM (Dłuski et al., 2021). Examining cascades revealed the importance of the T1DM cascade and the enrichment of cascades related to neuron growth and immunological MHC. Additional research has shown distinct variations in DNA methylation patterns in the adipose tissues of the omentum in patients with GDM. Dias et al. (2022) detected genes exhibiting differential methylation and expression, highlighting the participation of antigen processing and presentation cascades in GDM among Chinese pregnant women. The results of this study highlight the intricate relationship between DNA methylation and the development of GDM, as well as the possible use of DNA methylation as a clinical indicator.

Wang et al. (2021) used Methyl Target sequencing to analyses 337 CpG sites linked to GDM for DNA methylation levels. In addition, eight CpG sites were identified in the qualitative analysis, including RDH 12 and NFATC4, where hypermethylation was linked to an elevated risk of GDM. The study investigated the influence of GDM on leptin levels in newborns, revealing that hypomethylation around the leptin promoter is linked to increased leptin levels in cord blood.

In 2023, there was another study that found that at two different stages of pregnancy, GDM and non-GDM pregnant women had differentially methylated marks. Furthermore, it was discovered that GDM and non-GDM individuals have differing methylation levels at CpG sites within the *DIP2C* and *PTPRN2* genes (Linares-Pineda et al., 2023).

1.4.2 HISTONE MODIFICATIONS IN GESTATIONAL DIABETES MELLITUS

Histones are cationic proteins that are abundant in lysine and arginine residues. Octameric histones receive post-translational modifications (PTM) such as acetylation and methylation, which have an impact on gene expression and the accessibility of chromatin. Studies on GDM have examined histone alterations, specifically emphasizing lysine residues. In case-control research, Hepp et al. examined placental tissues from 40 people with GDM and 40 people without GDM to determine the levels of histone three lysine four trimethylation (H3K4me3) and histone three lysine nine acetylation (H3K9ac) (Hepp et al., 2018). In placentas impacted by GDM, lower levels of H3K9ac were found, although H3K4me3 levels were not significantly different (Dłuski et al., 2021). A study conducted in 2016 examined the histone 3 (H3) dimethylation levels at different time points in 39 people from diverse backgrounds. Those with GDM who developed T2DM after giving birth showed a 50–60% decrease in H3K27 dimethylation compared to those without diabetes at 8–10 and 20 weeks postpartum (Michalczyk et al., 2016). In addition, between 8 and 10 weeks after giving birth, there was a 75% drop in H3K4 dimethylation levels in women with GDM who acquired T2DM after giving birth, as compared to women without T2DM. These findings identify changes in histone modifications linked to GDM (Michalczyk et al., 2016).

1.4.3 MICRORNA-MEDIATED METABOLIC IMPACTS IN OFFSPRING EXPOSED TO GDM

MicroRNA (miRNA) is a short RNA molecule that does not code for proteins (Chen et al., 2020). It has a crucial function in regulating genes by attaching to the untranslated regions (UTRs) of mRNA transcripts. The study investigates the role of particular miRNAs in GDM and their influence on insulin regulation. Feng et al. examined the role of miR-33a-5p in GDM by studying its effects on the rat insulinoma cell line (INS-1 cells). Subjects with GDM showed elevated blood sugar levels and increased expression of miR-33a-5p (Feng et al., 2020). The study identified ATP-binding cassette transporter 1 (ABCA1) as a target of miR-33a-5p in regulating INS-1 cell function. In addition, lnc-DANCR was discovered to be a regulator of miR-33a-5p. Patients with GDM showed increased levels of miR-195-5p, which were positively associated with BMI, fasting glucose, and plasma glucose (Wang et al., 2020). According to functional investigations, Gluconeogenesis was boosted in liver cell lines after suppressing miR-29a. This was due to increased insulin-induced gene 1 (*INSIG1*) expression, which increased phosphoenolpyruvate carboxy kinase 2. Guan et al. (2020) conducted additional experiments targeting miR-21 in patients with GDM and discovered that it was downregulated in GDM cases. A rise in the expression of the gene's target protein, PPARα, which impeded cell growth and invasion, was linked to the gene's diminished activity (Qiu et al., 2020). According to miR-518d, it regulates PPARα expression. The researchers discovered that GDM coincides with increased miR-518d in plasma and placentas. This leads to glucose level abnormalities, which trigger inflammatory responses through the NF-κβ signaling cascade (Qiu et al., 2020). Conversely, overexpression of p21-activated kinase 1 (PAK1) caused cell death and hindered the activity of β-cells. These findings indicate that miR-96 is essential in the development of GDM via controlling the activity of PAK1 and the functioning and survival of β-cells.

1.4.4 FTO-MEDIATED DNA METHYLATION IN GDM

A study by Franzago aims to assess the association between placental DNA methylation and GDM, explicitly focusing on the *FTO* gene (Mehta et al., 2021). While the study did not establish a clear link between FTO

DNA methylation and GDM, it did identify connections between DNA methylation and maternal smoking and lipid profiles in both the GDM and control groups. The study also discovered a link between the FTO rs9939609 gene polymorphism and newborn birthweight. The study investigated the possible effects of maternal smoking and lipid profiles on placental DNA methylation in relation to GDM-related maternal metabolic characteristics. In addition, although the study could not demonstrate a clear correlation between FTO DNA methylation and GDM, it offered a valuable understanding of the complex array of factors that influence the development of obesity and metabolic health issues in children delivered to women with GDM (Franzago et al., 2021). There was no observed link between DNA methylation in the *FTO* gene and GDM in women in the study. At first, relatively low DNA methylation levels were found inside the *FTO* gene promoter, and most CpG dinucleotides were found to be unmethylated (Czogała et al., 2021).

1.5 THE INTERPLAY OF INFLAMMATORY FACTORS AND OXIDATIVE ASSAULT IN DISRUPTED INSULIN CASCADE IN GDM

It is widely recognized that insulin resistance is the primary cause of GDM (Sun et al., 2020). Scientific studies have shown that a modest, systemic inflammation could cause β-cell malfunction before insulin resistance manifests. However, the mother's adipose and skeletal muscle tissues have defective insulin signaling cascades, leading to increased insulin resistance (Figure 1.5) (Szosland et al., 2018). It is normally the binding of insulin to its insulin receptor that initiates the auto-phosphorylation of its tyrosine residues, which in turn starts the glucose regulation process. As a result, insulin receptor substrate 1 (IRS-1) is phosphorylated during this process, triggering additional molecular phosphorylation and activating the PI3K signaling cascade (Zheng et al., 2021). Upon activation, PI3K converts PIP2 to PIP3, phosphatidylinositol (3,4,5)-triphosphate. After that, Akt and its substrate (AS160) are phosphorylated when 3-phosphoinositide-dependent protein kinase 1 (PDK1) is activated (Siess et al., 2019). This mechanism regulates the mobility of glucose transporter 4 (GLUT4) to regulate protein and lipid metabolism and glucose absorption. Evidence shows that key insulin signaling components like IRS1, PIP3, PIK3, and GLUT4 are decreased in GDM pregnancies. Furthermore, individuals afflicted with GDM exhibit an alternative phosphorylation of IRS1 at serine residues. This ailment impedes the PI3K signaling cascade and the efficacy of insulin (Pei et al., 2022).

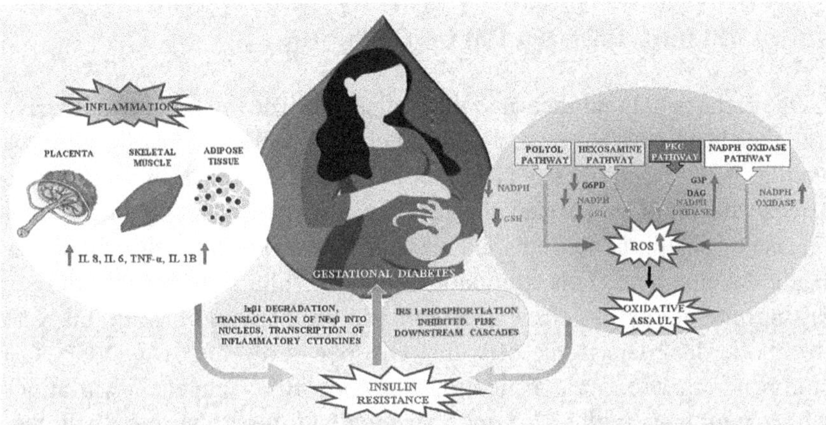

FIGURE 1.5 The interplay of inflammation and oxidative assault in GDM. Elevated levels of inflammatory cytokines (IL-8, IL-6, IL1B, TNFα) indicate heightened inflammation in adipose tissue, skeletal muscle, and placenta during GDM. Metabolic syndrome sees increased ROS due to pathways like polyol, hexosamine, and PKC disruptions. These disturb IRS phosphorylation and NFκβ-mediated cytokine secretion, fostering insulin resistance and GDM development.

In GDM, inflammation is produced by skeletal muscle, adipose tissues, and the placenta. Adipose tissues may interact with the placenta to cause insulin resistance and inflammation (Nguyen-Ngo et al., 2020). Both types of tissues have increased expression of pro-inflammatory markers such as IL-6, IL-8, TNF-α, resistin, and leptin. Leptin levels rise due to an interaction between IL-6 and TNF-α, which amplifies inflammation through a feedback loop. Insulin resistance may be exacerbated when skeletal muscle tissues have elevated TNF-α, which triggers the release of IL-6, IL-8, and monocyte chemotactic protein 1 (MCP-1) (Al-Mansoori et al., 2022). Reduced GLUT4 functioning and disruption of glucose absorption may be caused by increased production of pro-inflammatory cytokines and NF-κβ activation; GDM cases also show elevated levels of the placental pro-inflammatory hormone chorionic gonadotrophin (Olmos-Ortiz et al., 2021). In a high blood sugar milieu, the hexosamine cascade is activated, which inhibits the pentose phosphate cascade. This leads to decreased levels of NADPH and glutathione, worsening oxidative stress. In general, oxidative assault plays a role in developing insulin resistance by activating the JNK and NF-κβ cascades (Siti Hajar., 2018).

1.6 IMPLICATIONS OF GDM ON OFFSPRING

GDM dictates both mothers and their offspring. The offspring tend to have a higher birth weight and are more likely to develop metabolic illnesses such as T2DM and obesity (Kong et al., 2019). Maternal hyperglycemia affects the fetus by passing through the placenta, resulting in a higher release of insulin in the fetus, increased formation of fat cells, and subsequent development. This stimulation causes insulin resistance, leading to lasting alterations in gene expression and an increased susceptibility to metabolic disorders in the offspring (Desoye et al., 2020). The EPOCH study and other recent investigations have identified epigenetic variations between mothers with GDM and those without their offspring. Examination of peripheral and cord blood samples showed notable alterations in DNA methylation in 51 genome regions. The methylation of SH3PXD2A was associated with adipose metabolism, BMI, leptin levels, and subcutaneous adipose tissue in the offspring (Yang et al., 2018). These findings offer essential insights into the enduring consequences of GDM on the metabolic well-being of the offspring.

1.7 CONCLUSION

In conclusion, gestational diabetes mellitus (GDM) poses significant challenges to maternal and child health globally, with potential long-term implications. Exploring miRNAs, genetic variants, and SNPs as biomarkers holds promise for diagnosis and risk assessment. However, their efficacy may vary across populations and environmental contexts, necessitating comprehensive investigations integrating molecular and serum protein biomarkers. Understanding the molecular pathways disrupting glucose homeostasis is critical given the multifactorial nature of GDM, which involves genetic, epigenetic, and environmental factors. Clarifying the link between pregnancy insulin resistance and GDM requires further exploration. Current evidence suggests GDM arises from a combination of factors, each contributing incrementally to risk. Unraveling complex relationships, including potential synergies among polymorphisms, demands further inquiry. A holistic approach considering genetic, epigenetic, and environmental influences is vital. Lifestyle modifications, particularly maintaining a healthy weight, are crucial for GDM prevention, alongside ongoing research to develop tailored treatments. Advancements in personalized medicine and targeted interventions hinge on continued investigation and understanding of these intricate associations.

KEYWORDS

- **endothelial dysfunction**
- **gestational diabetes mellitus**
- **growth factors**
- **insulin resistance**
- **membrane proteins**
- **pro-inflammatory cytokines**
- **single nucleotide polymorphisms**
- **transcription factors**

REFERENCES

Abu Samra, N., Jelinek, H. F., Alsafar, H., Asghar, F., Seoud, M., Hussein, S. M., Mubarak, H. M., Anwar, S., Memon, M., Afify, N., Manzoor, R., Al-Homedi, Z., & Osman, W. (2022). Genomics and epigenomics of gestational diabetes mellitus: Understanding the molecular pathways of the disease pathogenesis. *International Journal of Molecular Sciences, 23*(7), 3514. https://doi.org/10.3390/ijms23073514 (accessed on 24th June 2025).

Amin, U. S. M., Parvez, N., Rahman, T. A., Hasan, M. R., Das, K. C., Jahan, S., Hasanat, M. A., Seraj, Z. I., & Salimullah, M. (2022). CDKAL1 gene rs7756992 A/G and rs7754840 G/C polymorphisms are associated with gestational diabetes mellitus in a sample of Bangladeshi population: Implication for future T2DM prophylaxis. *Diabetology & Metabolic Syndrome, 14*(1), 18. https://doi.org/10.1186/s13098-021-00782-w (accessed on 24th June 2025).

Ballesteros, M., Gil-Lluís, P., Ejarque, M., Diaz-Perdigones, C., Martinez-Guasch, L., Fernández-Veledo, S., Vendrell, J., & Megía, A. (2022). DNA methylation in gestational diabetes and its predictive value for postpartum glucose disturbances. *The Journal of*

Clinical Endocrinology & Metabolism, 107(10), 2748–2757. https://doi.org/10.1210/clinem/dgac462 (accessed on 24th June 2025).

Banerjee, R. R. (2018). Piecing together the puzzle of pancreatic islet adaptation in pregnancy. *Annals of the New York Academy of Sciences, 1411*(1), 120–139. https://doi.org/10.1111/nyas.13552 (accessed on 24th June 2025).

Benny, P., Ahn, H. J., Burlingame, J., Lee, M. J., Miller, C., Chen, J., & Urschitz, J. (2021). Genetic risk factors associated with gestational diabetes in a multi-ethnic population. *PLoS ONE, 16*(12), e0261137. https://doi.org/10.1371/journal.pone.0261137 (accessed on 24th June 2025).

Bernea, E. G., Uyy, E., Mihai, D. A., Ceausu, I., Ionescu-Tirgoviste, C., Suica, V. I., Ivan, L., & Antohe, F. (2022). New born macrosomia in gestational diabetes mellitus. *Experimental and Therapeutic Medicine, 24*(6), 710. https://doi.org/10.3892/etm.2022.11646 (accessed on 24th June 2025).

Blaslov, K., Naranđa, F. S., Kruljac, I., & Renar, I. P. (2018). Treatment approach to type 2 diabetes: Past, present and future. *World Journal of Diabetes, 9*(12), 209–219. https://doi.org/10.4239/wjd.v9.i12.209 (accessed on 24th June 2025).

Cao, M., Zhang, L., Chen, T., Shi, A., Xie, K., Li, Z., Xu, J., Chen, Z., Ji, C., & Wen, J. (2020). Genetic susceptibility to gestational diabetes mellitus in a Chinese population. *Frontiers in Endocrinology, 11*, 247. https://doi.org/10.3389/fendo.2020.00247 (accessed on 24th June 2025).

Capurso, A., Crepaldi, G., & Capurso, C. (2018). Extra-virgin olive oil and type 2 diabetes mellitus. In *Benefits of the Mediterranean Diet in the Elderly Patient* (pp. 57–79). Springer, Cham. https://doi.org/10.1007/978-3-319-78084-9_4 (accessed on 24th June 2025).

Cardenas, A., Gagné-Ouellet, V., Allard, C., Brisson, D., Perron, P., Bouchard, L., & Hivert, M. F. (2018). Placental DNA methylation adaptation to maternal glycemic response in pregnancy. *Diabetes, 67*(8), 1673–1683. https://doi.org/10.2337/db18-0123 (accessed on 24th June 2025).

Chen, L., Wang, C. T., Forsyth, N. R., & Wu, P. (2020). Transcriptional profiling reveals altered biological characteristics of chorionic stem cells from women with gestational diabetes. *Stem Cell Research & Therapy, 11*(1), 319. https://doi.org/10.1186/s13287-020-01828-y (accessed on 24th June 2025).

Chen, X., Guan, N. N., Sun, Y. Z., Li, J. Q., & Qu, J. (2020). MicroRNA-small molecule association identification: From experimental results to computational models. *Briefings in Bioinformatics, 21*(1), 47–61. https://doi.org/10.1093/bib/bby098 (accessed on 24th June 2025).

Choudhury, A. A., & Devi Rajeswari, V. (2021). Gestational diabetes mellitus – A metabolic and reproductive disorder. *Biomedicine & Pharmacotherapy, 143*, 112183. https://doi.org/10.1016/j.biopha.2021.112183 (accessed on 24th June 2025).

Cooper, A., Woulfe, D., & Kilic, F. (2019). Post-translational modifications of serotonin transporter. *Pharmacological Research, 140*, 7–13. https://doi.org/10.1016/j.phrs.2018.10.018 (accessed on 24th June 2025).

Del Bosque-Plata, L., Martínez-Martínez, E., Espinoza-Camacho, M. Á., & Gragnoli, C. (2021). The role of TCF7L2 in type 2 diabetes. *Diabetes, 70*(6), 1220–1228. https://doi.org/10.2337/db20-0573 (accessed on 24th June 2025).

Desoye, G., & Cervar-Zivkovic, M. (2020). Diabetes mellitus, obesity, and the placenta. *Obstetrics and Gynecology Clinics of North America, 47*(1), 65–79. https://doi.org/10.1016/j.ogc.2019.11.001 (accessed on 24th June 2025).

Dias, S., Pheiffer, C., Abrahams, Y., Rheeder, P., & Adam, S. (2018). Molecular biomarkers for gestational diabetes mellitus. *International Journal of Molecular Sciences, 19*(10), 2926. https://doi.org/10.3390/ijms19102926 (accessed on 24th June 2025).

Dias, S., Willmer, T., Adam, S., & Pheiffer, C. (2022). The role of maternal DNA methylation in pregnancies complicated by gestational diabetes. *Frontiers in Clinical Diabetes and Healthcare, 3*, 982665. https://doi.org/10.3389/fcdhc.2022.982665 (accessed on 24th June 2025).

Dłuski, D. F., Wolińska, E., & Skrzypczak, M. (2021). Epigenetic changes in gestational diabetes mellitus. *International Journal of Molecular Sciences, 22*(14), 7649. https://doi.org/10.3390/ijms22147649 (accessed on 24th June 2025).

Ekta, Gupta, M., Kaur, A., Singh, T. G., & Bedi, O. (2020). Pathobiological and molecular connections involved in the high fructose and high fat diet induced diabetes associated nonalcoholic fatty liver disease. *Inflammation Research, 69*(9), 851–867. https://doi.org/10.1007/s00011-020-01373-7 (accessed on 24th June 2025).

Espino, J., Rodríguez, A. B., & Pariente, J. A. (2019). Melatonin and oxidative stress in the diabetic state: Clinical implications and potential therapeutic applications. *Current Medicinal Chemistry, 26*(22), 4178–4190. https://doi.org/10.2174/0929867325666180410094149 (accessed on 24th June 2025).

Feng, Y., Qu, X., Chen, Y., Feng, Q., Zhang, Y., Hu, J., & Li, X. (2020). MicroRNA-33a-5p sponges to inhibit pancreatic β-cell function in gestational diabetes mellitus LncRNA DANCR. *Reproductive Biology and Endocrinology, 18*(1), Article 61. https://doi.org/10.1186/s12958-020-00618-8 (accessed on 24th June 2025).

Franzago, M., Fraticelli, F., Marchioni, M., Di Nicola, M., Di Sebastiano, F., Liberati, M., Stuppia, L., & Vitacolonna, E. (2021). Fat mass and obesity-associated (FTO) gene epigenetic modifications in gestational diabetes: New insights and possible pathophysiological connections. *Acta Diabetologica, 58*(8), 997–1007. https://doi.org/10.1007/s00592-020-01668-5 (accessed on 24th June 2025).

Garg, N., Singh, T. G., Khan, H., Arora, S., Kaur, A., & Mannan, A. (2021). Mechanistic interventions of selected *Ocimum* species in management of diabetes, obesity and liver disorders: Transformative developments from preclinical to clinical approaches. *Biointerface Research in Applied Chemistry, 12*(1), 1304–1323. (accessed on 24th June 2025).

Ghosh, C., Das, N., Saha, S., Kundu, T., Sircar, D., & Roy, P. (2022). Involvement of *Cdkal1* in the etiology of type 2 diabetes mellitus and microvascular diabetic complications: A review. *Journal of Diabetes and Metabolic Disorders, 21*(1), 991–1001. https://doi.org/10.1007/s40200-021-00953-6 (accessed on 24th June 2025).

Guan, C. Y., Tian, S., Cao, J. L., Wang, X. Q., Ma, X., & Xia, H. F. (2020). Down-regulated *miR-21* in gestational diabetes mellitus placenta induces *PPAR-α* to inhibit cell proliferation and infiltration. *Diabetes, Metabolic Syndrome and Obesity: Targets and Therapy, 13*, 3009–3034. https://doi.org/10.2147/DMSO.S253920 (accessed on 24th June 2025).

Harprecht, C. (2020). *Structural analysis of JC polyomavirus inhibitors and receptors* [Doctoral dissertation, Universität Tübingen]. https://doi.org/10.1007/s00894-023-05748-5 (accessed on 24th June 2025).

Hepp, P., Hutter, S., Knabl, J., Hofmann, S., Kuhn, C., Mahner, S., & Jeschke, U. (2018). Histone H3 lysine 9 acetylation is downregulated in GDM placentas and calcitriol supplementation enhanced this effect. *International Journal of Molecular Sciences, 19*(12), 4061. https://doi.org/10.3390/ijms19124061 (accessed on 24th June 2025).

Jääskeläinen, T., & Klemetti, M. M. (2022). Genetic risk factors and gene-lifestyle interactions in gestational diabetes. *Nutrients, 14*(22), 4799. https://doi.org/10.3390/nu14224799 (accessed on 24th June 2025).

Kettunen, J. L. T., & Tuomi, T. (2020). Human physiology of genetic defects causing beta-cell dysfunction. *Journal of Molecular Biology, 432*(5), 1579–1598. https://doi.org/10.1016/j.jmb.2019.12.038 (accessed on 24th June 2025).

Kodama, S., Fujihara, K., Ishiguro, H., Horikawa, C., Ohara, N., Yachi, Y., Tanaka, S., Shimano, H., Kato, K., Hanyu, O., & Sone, H. (2018). Quantitative relationship between cumulative risk alleles based on genome-wide association studies and type 2 diabetes mellitus: A systematic review and meta-analysis. *Journal of Epidemiology, 28*(1), 3–18. https://doi.org/10.2188/jea.JE20160151 (accessed on 24th June 2025).

Kong, L., Nilsson, I. A. K., Gissler, M., & Lavebratt, C. (2019). Associations of maternal diabetes and body mass index with offspring birth weight and prematurity. *JAMA Pediatrics, 173*(4), 371–378. https://doi.org/10.1001/jamapediatrics.2018.5541 (accessed on 24th June 2025).

Kumar, S., Chinnusamy, V., & Mohapatra, T. (2018). Epigenetics of modified DNA bases: 5-methylcytosine and beyond. *Frontiers in Genetics, 9*, 640. https://doi.org/10.3389/fgene.2018.00640 (accessed on 24th June 2025).

Lake, J. A., Dekkers, J. C. M., & Abasht, B. (2021). Genetic basis and identification of candidate genes for wooden breast and white striping in commercial broiler chickens. *Scientific Reports, 11*(1), 6785. https://doi.org/10.1038/s41598-021-86176-4 (accessed on 24th June 2025).

Lenin, M., Ramasamy, R., Kulkarani, S., Ghose, S., & Srinivasan, A. R. S. (2018). Association of *KCNJ11* (rs5219) gene polymorphism with biochemical markers of glycemic status and insulin resistance in gestational diabetes mellitus. *Meta Gene, 16*, 134–138. https://doi.org/10.3390/ijms19102926 (accessed on 24th June 2025).

Li, A., Lin, C., Xie, F., Jin, M., & Lin, F. (2022). Berberine ameliorates insulin resistance by inhibiting IKK/NF-κB, JNK, and IRS-1/AKT signaling pathway in liver of gestational diabetes mellitus rats. *Metabolic Syndrome and Related Disorders, 20*(8), 480–488. https://doi.org/10.1089/met.2022.0017 (accessed on 24th June 2025).

Li, G., Wei, T., Ni, W., Zhang, A., Zhang, J., Xing, Y., & Xing, Q. (2020). Incidence and risk factors of gestational diabetes mellitus: A prospective cohort study in Qingdao, China. *Frontiers in Endocrinology, 11*, 636. https://doi.org/10.3389/fendo.2020.00636 (accessed on 24th June 2025).

Li, M., Rahman, M. L., Wu, J., Ding, M., Chavarro, J. E., Lin, Y., Ley, S. H., Bao, W., Grunnet, L. G., Hinkle, S. N., Thuesen, A. C. B., Yeung, E., Gore-Langton, R. E., Sherman, S., Hjort, L., Kampmann, F. B., Bjerregaard, A. A., Damm, P., Tekola-Ayele, F., … Zhang, C. (2020). Genetic factors and risk of type 2 diabetes among women with a history of gestational diabetes: Findings from two independent populations. *BMJ Open*

Diabetes Research & Care, 8(1), e000850. https://doi.org/10.1136/bmjdrc-2019-000850 (accessed on 24th June 2025).

Li, Y., Cooper, A., Odibo, I. N., Ahmed, A., Murphy, P., Koonce, R., Dajani, N. K., Lowery, C. L., Roberts, D. J., Maroteaux, L., & Kilic, F. (2016). Discrepancy in insulin regulation between gestational diabetes mellitus (GDM) platelets and placenta. *The Journal of Biological Chemistry, 291*(18), 9657–9665. https://doi.org/10.1074/jbc.M116.713693 (accessed on 24th June 2025).

Li, Y., Hadden, C., Singh, P., Mercado, C. P., Murphy, P., Dajani, N. K., Lowery, C. L., Roberts, D. J., Maroteaux, L., & Kilic, F. (2014). GDM-associated insulin deficiency hinders the dissociation of SERT from ERp44 and down-regulates placental 5-HT uptake. *Proceedings of the National Academy of Sciences of the United States of America, 111*(52), E5697–E5705. https://doi.org/10.1073/pnas.1416675112 (accessed on 24th June 2025).

Liao, X., Zhou, Z., & Zhang, X. (2020). Effects of *miR-195-5p* on cell proliferation and apoptosis in gestational diabetes mellitus via targeting *EZH2*. *Molecular Medicine Reports, 22*(2), 803–809. https://doi.org/10.3892/mmr.2020.11142 (accessed on 24th June 2025).

Linares-Pineda, T., Peña-Montero, N., Fragoso-Bargas, N., Gutiérrez-Repiso, C., Lima-Rubio, F., Suarez-Arana, M., Sánchez-Pozo, A., Tinahones, F. J., Molina-Vega, M., Picón-César, M. J., Sommer, C., & Morcillo, S. (2023). Epigenetic marks associated with gestational diabetes mellitus across two time points during pregnancy. *Clinical Epigenetics, 15*(1), 110. https://doi.org/10.1186/s13148-023-01523-8 (accessed on 24th June 2025).

Lu, W., & Hu, C. (2022). Molecular biomarkers for gestational diabetes mellitus and postpartum diabetes. *Chinese Medical Journal, 135*(16), 1940–1951. https://doi.org/10.1097/CM9.0000000000002160 (accessed on 24th June 2025).

Luiken, J. J. F. P., Nabben, M., Neumann, D., & Glatz, J. F. C. (2020). Understanding the distinct subcellular trafficking of CD36 and GLUT4 during the development of myocardial insulin resistance. *Biochimica et Biophysica Acta (BBA) – Molecular Basis of Disease, 1866*(7), 165775. https://doi.org/10.1016/j.bbadis.2020.165775 (accessed on 24th June 2025).

Lyko, F. (2018). The DNA methyltransferase family: A versatile toolkit for epigenetic regulation. *Nature Reviews Genetics, 19*(2), 81–92. https://doi.org/10.1038/nrg.2017.80 (accessed on 24th June 2025).

Mahmoud, A. M. (2022). An overview of epigenetics in obesity: The role of lifestyle and therapeutic interventions. *International Journal of Molecular Sciences, 23*(3), 1341. https://doi.org/10.3390/ijms23031341 (accessed on 24th June 2025).

Mehta, S., Nain, P., Agrawal, B. K., & Singh, R. P. (2022). Vitamin D with calcium supplementation managing glycemic control with HbA1c and improve quality of life in patients with diabetes. *Turkish Journal of Pharmaceutical Sciences, 19*(2), 161–167. https://doi.org/10.4274/tjps.galenos.2021.62357 (accessed on 24th June 2025).

Mehta, S., Nain, P., Agrawal, B. K., Singh, R. P., Kaur, J., Maity, S., Bhattacharjee, A., Peela, J., Nauhria, S., & Nauhria, S. (2021). Effectiveness of empagliflozin with vitamin D supplementation in peripheral neuropathy in type 2 diabetic patients. *Cureus, 13*(12), e20208. https://doi.org/10.7759/cureus.20208 (accessed on 24th June 2025).

Michalczyk, A. A., Dunbar, J. A., Janus, E. D., Best, J. D., Ebeling, P. R., Ackland, M. J., Asproloupos, D., & Ackland, M. L. (2016). Epigenetic markers to predict conversion from gestational diabetes to type 2 diabetes. *The Journal of Clinical Endocrinology and Metabolism, 101*(6), 2396–2404. https://doi.org/10.1210/jc.2015-4206 (accessed on 24th June 2025).

Moini, J., Adams, M., & LoGalbo, A. (2022). *Complications of diabetes mellitus: A global perspective*. CRC Press. (accessed on 24th June 2025).

Nair, S., Ormazabal, V., Lappas, M., McIntyre, H. D., & Salomon, C. (2021). Extracellular vesicles and their potential role inducing changes in maternal insulin sensitivity during gestational diabetes mellitus. *American Journal of Reproductive Immunology, 85*(2), e13361. https://doi.org/10.1111/aji.13361 (accessed on 24th June 2025).

Nguyen-Ngo, C., Jayabalan, N., Haghvirdizadeh, P., Salomon, C., & Lappas, M. (2020). Role of adipose tissue in regulating fetal growth in gestational diabetes mellitus. *Placenta, 102*, 39–48. https://doi.org/10.1016/j.placenta.2020.05.006 (accessed on 24th June 2025).

Nomura, Y., Lambertini, L., Rialdi, A., Lee, M., Mystal, E. Y., Grabie, M., Manaster, I., Huynh, N., Finik, J., Davey, M., Davey, K., Ly, J., Stone, J., Loudon, H., Eglinton, G., Hurd, Y., Newcorn, J. H., & Chen, J. (2014). Global methylation in the placenta and umbilical cord blood from pregnancies with maternal gestational diabetes, preeclampsia, and obesity. *Reproductive Sciences, 21*(1), 131–137. https://doi.org/10.1177/1933719113492206 (accessed on 24th June 2025).

Olmos-Ortiz, A., Flores-Espinosa, P., Díaz, L., Velázquez, P., Ramírez-Isarraraz, C., & Zaga-Clavellina, V. (2021). Immunoendocrine dysregulation during gestational diabetes mellitus: The central role of the placenta. *International Journal of Molecular Sciences, 22*(15), 8087. https://doi.org/10.3390/ijms22158087 (accessed on 24th June 2025).

Omar, G. A., Hegab, W. S., & Ghanem, A. I. (2021). Association among insulin receptor substrate1 genetic polymorphism, sulfonylurea therapeutic efficacy, and insulin resistance in patients with type 2 diabetes mellitus. *Journal of Medicine in Scientific Research, 4*(3), 196. https://doi.org/10.4103/JMISR.JMISR_100_20 (accessed on 24th June 2025).

Panaitescu, A. M., & Peltecu, G. (2016). Gestational diabetes. Obstetrical perspective. *Acta Endocrinologica, 12*(3), 331–334. https://doi.org/10.4183/aeb.2016.331 (accessed on 24th June 2025).

Pei, J., Wang, B., & Wang, D. (2022). Current studies on molecular mechanisms of insulin resistance. *Journal of Diabetes Research, 2022*, 1863429. https://doi.org/10.1155/2022/1863429 (accessed on 24th June 2025).

Perić, M., Bečeheli, I., Čičin-Šain, L., Desoye, G., & Štefulj, J. (2022). Serotonin system in the human placenta – the knowns and unknowns. *Frontiers in Endocrinology, 13*, 1061317. https://doi.org/10.3389/fendo.2022.1061317 (accessed on 24th June 2025).

Pirotta, S., Joham, A., Grieger, J. A., Tay, C. T., Bahri-Khomami, M., Lujan, M., Lim, S. S., & Moran, L. J. (2020). Obesity and the risk of infertility, gestational diabetes, and type 2 diabetes in polycystic ovary syndrome. *Seminars in Reproductive Medicine, 38*(6), 342–351. https://doi.org/10.1055/s-0041-1726866 (accessed on 24th June 2025).

Powe, C. E., & Kwak, S. H. (2020). Genetic studies of gestational diabetes and glucose metabolism in pregnancy. *Current Diabetes Reports, 20*(12), 69. https://doi.org/10.1007/s11892-020-01355-3 (accessed on 24th June 2025).

Powe, C. E., Hivert, M. F., & Udler, M. S. (2020). Defining heterogeneity among women with gestational diabetes mellitus. *Diabetes, 69*(10), 2064–2074. https://doi.org/10.2337/dbi20-0004 (accessed on 24th June 2025).

Qiu, H., Liu, X., Yao, S., Zhou, J., & Zhang, X. (2020). Regulation and mechanism of *miR-518d* through the *PPARα*-mediated *NF-κB* pathway in the development of gestational diabetes mellitus. *Journal of Diabetes Research, 2020*, 7019597. https://doi.org/10.1155/2020/7019597 (accessed on 24th June 2025).

Rasool, S. U. A., Nabi, M., Ashraf, S., & Amin, S. (2022). Insulin receptor substrate 1 *Gly972Arg* (rs1801278) polymorphism is associated with obesity and insulin resistance in Kashmiri women with polycystic ovary syndrome. *Genes, 13*(8), 1463. https://doi.org/10.3390/genes13081463 (accessed on 24th June 2025).

Roep, B. O., Thomaidou, S., van Tienhoven, R., & Zaldumbide, A. (2021). Type 1 diabetes mellitus as a disease of the β-cell (do not blame the immune system?). *Nature Reviews Endocrinology, 17*(3), 150–161. https://doi.org/10.1038/s41574-020-00443-4 (accessed on 24th June 2025).

Sahu, P. K., Sao, R., Mondal, S., Vishwakarma, G., Gupta, S. K., Kumar, V., Singh, S., Sharma, D., & Das, B. K. (2020). Next generation sequencing based forward genetic approaches for identification and mapping of causal mutations in crop plants: A comprehensive review. *Plants, 9*(10), 1355. https://doi.org/10.3390/plants9101355 (accessed on 24th June 2025).

Shankar, A. (2023). A narrative review of pathogenesis of gestational diabetes mellitus. *Student's Journal of Health Research Africa, 4*(12), 12–12. https://doi.org/10.51168/sjhrafrica.v4i12.765 (accessed on 24th June 2025).

Sharma, V. K., & Singh, T. G. (2020). Chronic stress and diabetes mellitus: Interwoven pathologies. *Current Diabetes Reviews, 16*(6), 546–556. https://doi.org/10.2174/1573399815666191111152248 (accessed on 24th June 2025).

Sharma, V. K., Singh, T. G., Dhiman, S., & Garg, N. (2022). Mechanisms of beneficial effects of probiotics in diabetes mellitus. In *Probiotic Research in Therapeutics: Volume 5: Metabolic Diseases and Gut Bacteria* (pp. 97–124). Springer Nature Singapore. (accessed on 24th June 2025).

Siess, K. M., & Leonard, T. A. (2019). Lipid-dependent Akt-ivity: Where, when, and how. *Biochemical Society Transactions, 47*(3), 897–908. https://doi.org/10.1042/BST20190013 (accessed on 24th June 2025).

Singh, R., Rao, H. K., & Singh, T. G. (2020). Advanced glycated end products (AGEs) in diabetes and its complications: An insight. *Plant Archives, 20*(1), 3838–3841. (accessed on 24th June 2025).

Singh, R., Rao, H. K., & Singh, T. G. (2020). Neuropathic pain in diabetes mellitus: Challenges and future trends. *Obesity Medicine, 18*, 100215. (accessed on 24th June 2025).

Singh, S., & Singh, T. G. (2021). Emerging perspectives on mitochondrial dysfunctioning and inflammation in epileptogenesis. *Inflammation Research, 70*(10–12), 1027–1042. https://doi.org/10.1007/s00011-021-01511-9 (accessed on 24th June 2025).

Singh, S., Singh, T. G., Singh, M., Najda, A., Nurzyńska-Wierdak, R., Almeer, R., Kamel, M., & Abdel-Daim, M. M. (2021). Anticonvulsive effects of chondroitin sulfate on pilocarpine an [incomplete entry].

Siti Hajar, A. (2018). *In vitro and in vivo anti-diabetic effects of Marantodes pumilum and Rhinacanthus nasutus and their active compounds* [Doctoral dissertation, University of Malaya]. https://doi.org/10.3390/ph16121692 (accessed on 24th June 2025).

Stern, C., Schwarz, S., Moser, G., Cvitic, S., Jantscher-Krenn, E., Gauster, M., & Hiden, U. (2021). Placental endocrine activity: Adaptation and disruption of maternal glucose metabolism in pregnancy and the influence of fetal sex. *International Journal of Molecular Sciences, 22*(23), 12722. https://doi.org/10.3390/ijms222312722 (accessed on 24th June 2025).

Sun, Y. Y., Juan, J., Xu, Q. Q., Su, R. N., Hirst, J. E., & Yang, H. X. (2020). Increasing insulin resistance predicts adverse pregnancy outcomes in women with gestational diabetes mellitus. *Journal of Diabetes, 12*(6), 438–446. https://doi.org/10.1111/1753-0407.13013 (accessed on 24th June 2025).

Szosland, K., & Lewinski, A. (2018). Insulin resistance–"the good or the bad and ugly." *Neuroendocrinology Letters, 39*(5), 355–362. https://www.termedia.pl/Insulin-resistance-and-prediabetes-diagnosis-and-management,98,45711,1,1.html (accessed on 24th June 2025).

Uffelmann, E., Huang, Q. Q., Munung, N. S., De Vries, J., Okada, Y., Martin, A. R., Martin, H. C., Lappalainen, T., & Posthuma, D. (2021). Genome-wide association studies. *Nature Reviews Methods Primers, 1*(1), 59. https://doi.org/10.3390/ijms23063341 (accessed on 24th June 2025).

Unnikrishnan, B., Singh, A., Rathi, P., Bhat, S. K., Ravishankar, N., Nayak, P. H., & Praveen, O. (2020). Risk factors of gestational diabetes mellitus: A hospital-based pair-matched case-control study in coastal South India. *South African Journal of Obstetrics and Gynaecology, 26*(1), 13–17. https://doi.org/10.7196/sajog.1625 (accessed on 24th June 2025).

Venyo, A. K. G. (2023). Diabetes mellitus: A review and update. *Journal of Ophthalmology Research Reviews & Reports, SRC/JORRR-155.* https://doi.org/10.12998/wjcc.v11.i16.3736 (accessed on 24th June 2025).

Vishwakarma, S., Singh, S., & Singh, T. G. (2022). Pharmacological modulation of cytokines correlating neuroinflammatory cascades in epileptogenesis. *Molecular Biology Reports, 49*(2), 1437–1452. https://doi.org/10.1007/s11033-021-06896-8 (accessed on 24th June 2025).

Wang, J., Pan, Y., Dai, F., Wang, F., Qiu, H., & Huang, X. (2020). Serum *miR-195-5p* is upregulated in gestational diabetes mellitus. *Journal of Clinical Laboratory Analysis, 34*(8), e23325. https://doi.org/10.1002/jcla.23325 (accessed on 24th June 2025).

Wang, X., Huang, J., Zheng, Y., Long, S., Lin, H., Zhang, N., Tian, M., Wu, X., An, R., Ma, S., & Tan, H. (2021). Study on the relationship between DNA methylation of target CpG sites in peripheral blood and gestational diabetes during early pregnancy. *Scientific Reports, 11*(1), 20455. https://doi.org/10.1038/s41598-021-99836-2 (accessed on 24th June 2025).

Wu, L., Fang, C., Zhang, J., Ye, Y., & Zhao, H. (2021). The association between maternal/fetal insulin receptor substrate 1 gene polymorphism rs1801278 and gestational diabetes mellitus in a Chinese population. *Gynecologic and Obstetric Investigation, 86*(1–2), 177–184. https://doi.org/10.1159/000514971 (accessed on 24th June 2025).

Wu, N. N., Zhao, D., Ma, W., Lang, J. N., Liu, S. M., Fu, Y., Wang, X., Wang, Z. W., & Li, Q. (2021). A genome-wide association study of gestational diabetes mellitus in Chinese women. *Journal of Maternal-Fetal & Neonatal Medicine, 34*(10), 1557–1564. https://doi.org/10.1080/14767058.2019.1640205 (accessed on 24th June 2025).

Yang, I. V., Zhang, W., Davidson, E. J., Fingerlin, T. E., Kechris, K., & Dabelea, D. (2018). Epigenetic marks of in utero exposure to gestational diabetes and childhood adiposity outcomes: The EPOCH study. *Diabetic Medicine, 35*(5), 612–620. https://doi.org/10.1111/dme.13604 (accessed on 24th June 2025).

Zhang, P., Deng, M., Li, W., Dai, Q., He, H., Zheng, W., She, L., Xiang, B., Zeng, J., Zhou, F., Guo, Y., & Yang, M. (2022). The correlation between transcription factor 7-like 2 gene polymorphisms and susceptibility of gestational diabetes mellitus in the population of central China: A case-control study. *Frontiers in Endocrinology, 13*, 916590. https://doi.org/10.3389/fendo.2022.916590 (accessed on 24th June 2025).

Zhang, Y., Zhang, T., & Chen, Y. (2018). Comprehensive analysis of gene expression profiles and DNA methylome reveals *Oas1*, *Ppie*, *Polr2g* as pathogenic target genes of gestational diabetes mellitus. *Scientific Reports, 8*(1), 16244. https://doi.org/10.1038/s41598-018-34292-z (accessed on 24th June 2025).

Zheng, M., & Wang, P. (2021). Role of insulin receptor substance-1 modulating PI3K/Akt insulin signaling pathway in Alzheimer's disease. *3 Biotech, 11*(4), 179. https://doi.org/10.1007/s13205-021-02738-3 (accessed on 24th June 2025).

Zhu, H., Zhao, Z. J., Liu, H. Y., Cai, J., Lu, Q. K., Ji, L. D., & Xu, J. (2023). The melatonin receptor 1B gene links circadian rhythms and type 2 diabetes mellitus: An evolutionary story. *Annals of Medicine, 55*(1), 1262–1286. https://doi.org/10.1080/07853890.2023.2191218 (accessed on 24th June 2025).

Ziętek, M., Celewicz, Z., & Szczuko, M. (2021). Short-chain fatty acids, maternal microbiota and metabolism in pregnancy. *Nutrients, 13*(4), 1244. https://doi.org/10.3390/nu13041244 (accessed on 24th June 2025).

CHAPTER 2

Pathophysiological and Clinical Aspects of Gestational Diabetes Mellitus

HENAROOP TIWANA,[1,*] NIDHI GARG,[2] TIRATH GARG,[3] K. A. SHAIMA,[4] and RANIYA MALIK[5]

[1]*Discipline of Pharmacy, Graduate School of Health, University of Technology Sydney, Sydney, New South Wales, Australia*

[2]*Department of Health and Family Welfare, Punjab, India*

[3]*Gian Sagar Dental College and Hospital, Punjab, India*

[4]*Shambhunath Institute of Pharmacy, Jhalwa, Prayagraj, Uttar Pradesh, India*

[5]*Faculty of Health, Australian Research Center in Complementary and Integrative Medicine, University of Technology Sydney, Ultimo, New South Wales, Australia*

*Corresponding author

ABSTRACT

Gestational Diabetes Mellitus (GDM) is an endocrine disease characterized by carbohydrate intolerance with first recognition during pregnancy. It is a widespread disease with a universal prevalence between 3% to 25%. The prevalence of GDM was higher in the age group of 35 years or older (2.4%) than in the 15 to 19 years age group (1.0%). It affects both mother and infant differently, and various factors predispose GDM to development. The causative factors for GDM include increased weight gain during gestation, obesity, increased maternal age, family and individual history of GDM, intrauterine environment (low or high birth weight),

Precision Nutrition and Endocrine Health: Synthesis, Characterization, and Applications.
Thakur Gurjeet Singh and Sanjana Mehta (Eds.)

DOI: 10.1201/9781998511877-2

and other diseases of insulin resistance. The consequences of GDM comprise an increased risk of hypertensive states, hyperinsulinemia and lipid abnormalities that may proceed to the incidence of cardiovascular diseases and the occurrence of metabolic diseases. Initial diagnosis is the key to proper treatment since many symptoms overlap with symptoms of a normal pregnancy. Delay in identifying the cause can lead to risks such as abortion, premature birth, preeclampsia, retroplacental hemorrhage, maternal heart failure, miscarriages, low birth weight and PPH. It can not only be life-threatening but can have a substantial psychological impact on the mother as well. Patient education about effective medical nutrition therapy and self-monitoring blood glucose levels is crucial. An in-depth, comprehensive study of the associated physiological factors, pathological mechanisms and genetic associations would further help in the identification, diagnostic screening and thus effective management of the patient by pharmacological and lifestyle modification strategies to achieve euglycemia and, therefore, end this cycle of transmission. While there are various strategies for the management of GDM, like insulin therapy and modification of lifestyle, there is still a lack of a proper cure or an effective therapeutic regimen for the treatment of GDM. One of the common reasons for this is the poorly defined molecular mechanisms underlying GDM. This chapter describes the pathophysiology of GDM, highlighting the recent pharmacotherapeutic approaches to avoid adverse maternal and fetal side effects of GDM that warrant further exploration.

2.1 INTRODUCTION

Gestational Diabetes Mellitus (GDM) is an endocrine disorder characterized by carbohydrate intolerance with first recognition during pregnancy. The worldwide prevalence of GDM is increasing along with type 2 diabetes. Based on Global Statistics, there are 21.3 million diabetes-associated live births, 86.4% caused by GDM, 6.2% caused by a pre-existing condition of type 1 diabetes mellitus or type 2 diabetes mellitus and 7.4% caused by the detection of type 1 diabetes mellitus and type 2 diabetes mellitus during the first pregnancy (Sharma et al., 2020). GDM affects 5–20% of pregnant women and is responsible for approximately 90–95% of all cases (International et al., 2017). It is a widespread disease with a universal prevalence between 3% to 25%. Results of a recent study have demonstrated that women living in urban areas are more prone to GDM than women living in rural areas. The prevalence of gestational diabetes increases with age (Swaminathan et al., 2020).

The high blood sugar level in GDM adversely affects pregnancy and fetal health. Diabetogenic hormones produced during pregnancy can cause insulin resistance due to the changes in beta cell functions. The highest etiological reasons for GDM were genetic history of the family, increased age of mother, overweight before pregnancy, increased maternal weight gain, and previous history of GDM or glucose intolerance (Ciani et al., 2003), and lowest were westernized diet, ethnicity, genetic polymorphisms, high or low birthweight) and polycystic ovarian syndrome (PCOS) (Anghebem et al., 2017; Ben et al., 2004).

If GDM is untreated, it can lead to perinatal and longer-term maternal and offspring complications, such as caesarean delivery, fetal macrosomia and obesity in the offspring (Bhargava et al., 2022; Buchanan et al., 2012).

Symptoms of GDM include dryness of mouth, polydipsia and frequent urination, but these symptoms are not mainly for gestational diabetes because some of these were also present in normal pregnancy. GDM itself does not show any specific symptoms. In some cases, it was only found when a blood sugar level increased during pregnancy. To prevent adverse fetal and maternal outcomes, it is essential to screen for GDM (Seshiah et al., 2016).

Clinical algorithms have been developed to diagnose and manage GDM. The various diagnostic methods used to screen GDM patients were one- or two-step. These are performed during 24 and 28 weeks of gestation (Seshiah et al., 2016). It is essential to treat GDM promptly because, left on its own, it can rapidly worsen and become life-threatening to the mother and fetus. The initial steps in GDM management are monitoring the blood sugar level daily, eating a balanced diet and exercising. If the higher blood sugar level persists, then treatment is required. Medical Nutrition Therapy (MNT) and physical exercise should be recommended for pregnant women who have tested positive for GDM for the very first time. After doing this for two weeks, 2 hrs PPBS (post-meal) should be carried out. After 2 hr PPBS, if the value is <120 mg/dL, then repeat the test according to the high-risk pregnancy protocol. One monthly test is advised during the second and third trimester of pregnancy. If the 2-hour PPBS value is ≥120 mg/dL, then treatment (metformin or insulin therapy) should be initiated immediately as per the recommendations (Li et al., 2015). So, this chapter highlights recent updates on the pathophysiological and therapeutic aspects of diabetes during pregnancy.

2.2 PREVALENCE FOR GESTATIONAL DIABETES MELLITUS

GDM prevalence is increasing globally. In India, the prevalence rate was between 5 and 14% in urban areas and 1.8% to 13.0% in rural areas. The study's assumption regarding the increasing prevalence of GDM by 2025 was from 62 million people to 79.4 million by 2025. The GDM prevalence rate varied in different parts of India, such as Kashmir (3.8%), Mysore (6.2%), Tamil Nadu (17.9%), Western India (9.5%), Punjab (35%), Lucknow (41%) and so forth (Mithal et al., 2015). According to the International Diabetes Federation (IDF), 14% of pregnancies are affected by GDM, representing approximately 20 million births annually (Gyasi-Antwiet et al., 2020). The prevalence of GDM also varies worldwide, as every country uses its diagnostic criteria to determine its prevalence. Age also affects the prevalence of GDM, as with increasing age, prevalence rises. These results indicated substantial variation in GDM prevalence across states and by individual socioeconomic, demographic and clinical factors (Swaminathan et al., 2020).

2.3 ETIOLOGY FOR GDM

GDM is a metabolic disease with multiple etiologies. The different types of risk factors can be classified into unmodifiable and modifiable factors; unmodifiable factors such as age, ethnicity, previous pregnancies, genetic background and short stature have been identified as independent variables recently. Modifiable known risk factors include obesity, dietary fat, lack of exercise and lifestyle habits like smoking and certain drugs. It has been reported that a vitamin D deficiency might be responsible for the development of GDM (Chen et al., 2015; Mehta et al., 2022). GDM is also linked to antenatal depression, as well as stress (Byrn and Penckofer, 2015). Recent studies have demonstrated that hereditary and environmental factors are also responsible for GDM, but the exact reason is unknown (Singh et al., 2020; Zhang et al., 2018). These risk factors lead to the development of GDM and are responsible for cell dysfunction and decreased insulin sensitivity.

Selective screening of GDM in pregnancy is based on the occurrence of any of these causative factors. The American Diabetes Association's definable risk factors are given below in Table 2.1 (American Diabetes Association 2014).

TABLE 2.1 Causative Factors for Gestational Diabetes Mellitus

Sr. No	Risk Factors
1.	BMI > 25 kg/m2
2.	No physical activity
3.	1st degree relation with diabetes
4.	Ethnic backgrounds
5.	Previous macrosomic child > 9 lb
6.	History of GDM
7.	Increased Blood Pressure
8.	HDL-C < 0.90 mmol/L and/or triglyceride concentration> 2.82 mmol/L
9.	Polycystic ovary syndrome (PCOS)
10.	HbA1c ≥ 5.7% and previous IGT or IFG
11.	Insulin resistance
12.	History of cardiovascular diseases

BMI: Body mass index; HDL: High density lipoprotein; and HbA1c; Glycated haemoglobin.

2.4 SCREENING FOR GDM

Screening is usually carried out at 24–48 weeks of pregnancy. During the initial stages, pregnant women should be diagnosed with T2DM (American College of Obstetricians and Gynecologists, 2013). The recently published guidelines recommended universal screening of GDM, and susceptible women should also undergo regular checkups for early disease management. A few routine tests may be carried out to rule out the presence of GDM through the assessment of associated risk factors in maternal patients, which are as follows:

i. Monitoring of heart rate, blood pressure and weight regularly;
ii. Measurement of the height of uterine fundus;
iii. Pelvic examination to evaluate risks associated with premature birth;
iv. Blood examinations for the measurement of blood sugar, HbA1cand lipid profile;
v. Antibodies testing like anti-insulin antibody, islet cell antibody testing and anti-GAD antibody;
vi. Urine analysis for the estimation of uric acid, protein, glucose, protein, albumin, ketone bodies, N-Acetylgucosaminidase (NAG) and creatinine;

vii. Fetal ultrasound estimates the amount of amniotic fluid, examines fetal development, and evaluates fetal well-being.

One-step and Two-step approaches have been designed for the diagnostic screening of pregnant women for GDM. In the former approach, OGTT is performed without any prior glucose screening, which is also cost-effective. In the two-step approach, GCT is performed as an initial screening process, which measures glucose concentration 1 hour after a load of 50 gm oral glucose. The diagnostic OGTT is performed only in women whose glucose levels exceed acceptable levels.

2.5 DIAGNOSTIC CRITERIA

The primary used two types of criteria for screening of GDM designed for the 3-hour 100-gm OGTT test:

i. Carpenter-Coustan criteria;
ii. The National Diabetes Data Group (NDDG) criteria.

The NDDG criteria were observed as less sensitive for diagnosis of GDM (Cheng et al., 2009). The American Diabetes Association (ADA) criteria for GDM diagnosis consists of initially screening the fasting glucose level and then an OGTT with a 75-gm glucose load with a 1-hour and 2-hour glucose concentration (American Diabetes Association, 2003). The World Health Organization recommends using a 75 gm glucose tolerance test for screening and diagnosis of GDM. Usage of this criteria would double the number of patients diagnosed with GDM. However, there are no additional clinical benefits. This criterion is based upon a single-step method. According to the recommendations of WHO, the guidelines validate a two-h 75-g OGTT test exclusive of last meal timings having a cut-off value of $\geq$140 mg/dL measured by a plasma standardized glucometer (Hasdemir et al., 2014).

Peripheral health workers perform this test for every pregnant woman; the results are noted on the mother-child protection (MCP) card. Based on the OGTT values, a red sticker is pasted onto the cards of GDP-positive patients (Hasdemir et al., 2014).

The screening processes are ideally performed in the third trimester but can be done earlier in highly suspicious cases for undiagnosed T2DM. The procedure involves administering a 50-g oral glucose followed by its serum or plasma measurement after 1 hour. The women who have tested positive (2 hr 75-g OGTT ≥140 mg/dL) for GDM are then registered for subsequent management and follow-up (Hasdemir et al., 2014).

The women who tested negative undergo the OGTT test again at 24–28 weeks to ensure a minimum gap of 4 weeks from the prior test to confirm the diagnosis, as many pregnant women develop glucose intolerance during this phase. In conditions with GDM over 28 weeks, just one test is carried out at the first visit, irrespective of the gestation (Mishra et al., 2018).

The ADA recommendations include a 2-step procedure: Fasting serum glucose concentration > 95mg/dl.

i. 1-hr serum glucose concentration >180 mg/dl, 2-hour serum glucose concentration >155 mg/dl, 3-hour serum glucose concentration >140 mg/dl.

These values are the modifications proposed by Carpenter-Coustan. They are lesser than those values which the Expert Committee recommends on the Diagnosis and Classification of Diabetes Mellitus and the NDDG group (Expert Committee on the Diagnosis and Classification of Diabetes Mellitus, 2003), which used the maximum values of 105, 190, 165, and 145 mg/dL, respectively. Fourth International Workshop recommendation on gestational diabetes also suggests further evaluation of women with random blood glucose values more than 200 mg/dL and fasting glucose values greater than 126mg/dL, as these are strong indicators of diabetes mellitus.

The abnormal rise in serum fasting glucose concentration and HbA1c during 24 to 28 weeks acts as a vital early predictor of infant macrosomia in the obstetrical population (Schrader et al., 1995), which can be reduced from 18% to 7% if serum glucose screening without an oral GTT is done earlier. The data inferred from the result can be used to refer women for dietary or pharmacological treatments and self-blood glucose monitoring to meet the blood glucose targets (Jovanovič et al., 1997).

2.6 PATHOPHYSIOLOGY OF GDM

Gestational diabetes mellitus is a diabetic disease that occurs during pregnancy. It is defined as insufficient glucose utilization in pregnant women's bodies, resulting in high glucose levels in the blood. This condition has implications for both the fetus and mother's health.

The underlying mechanism of GDM involves insulin resistance and malfunctioning of β-cells, which are critical factors in developing the condition. β-cell dysfunction arises when these cells, responsible for storing insulin in response to excessive glucose, malfunction and lose their ability to detect blood glucose levels. This malfunction reduces glucose detection, heightens insulin secretion, and raises blood sugar levels (Weir et al., 2001). Insulin resistance worsens the malfunction of β-cells, resulting in decreased absorption of glucose, high blood sugar levels, and elevated insulin secretion (Ashcroft et al., 2017).

Insulin resistance occurs when β cells become less responsive to insulin release. Insulin resistance at the molecular level usually results from a disruption in insulin signaling, causing inadequate movement of glucose transporter 4 (GLUT4) to the cell's outer layer, which is required for glucose absorption into cells to produce energy. GDM patients demonstrate a 54% decrease in the rate at which glucose is taken up compared to individuals experiencing a normal pregnancy (Catalano et al., 2014). While the number of insulin receptors remains the same, the ability of insulin to send signals is hindered because the receptor is highly phosphorylated at levels of threonine and serine, as compared to tyrosine.

Changes in the expression and phosphorylation of key components in the insulin signaling system, such as phosphatidylinositol 3-kinase (PI3K), insulin receptor substrate (IRS)-1, and GLUT4, have been detected in gestational diabetes mellitus (GDM). Adiponectin and pro-inflammatory cytokines have a function in altering this process. The insulin signaling process entails the insulin binding to the insulin receptor, thereby activating IRS-1. Adiponectin further stimulates IRS-1 via AMP-activated protein kinase (AMPK). IRS-1 furthermore stimulates PI3K, resulting in the conversion of phosphatidylinositol-4, 5-bisphosphate (PIP2) to phosphatidylinositol-3, 4, 5-phosphate (PIP3) by phosphorylation. PIP3 stimulates the activation of Akt2, which then promotes the movement of GLUT4, the protein responsible for transporting glucose into the cells. Conversely, pro-inflammatory cytokines stimulate the activation of protein kinase C (PKC) through IB kinase (IKK), inhibiting IRS-1 as shown in Figure 2.1.

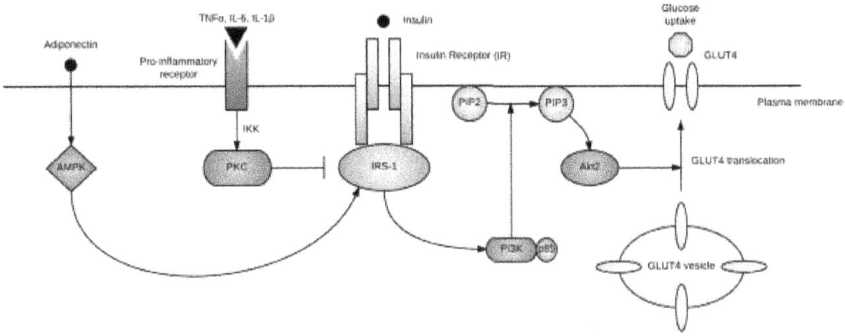

FIGURE 2.1 Mechanism of insulin signalling.

GDM affects multiple organs and systems, including the brain, liver, kidney, adipose tissue, eyes, skin, placenta, and skeletal muscle, as shown in Figure 2.2. During a typical pregnancy, β cells experience an increase in their number (hyperplasia) and an enlargement in size (hypertrophy) to meet the increased metabolic requirements. This leads to elevated blood glucose levels due to reduced insulin sensitivity. After pregnancy, β cells, blood glucose levels, and insulin sensitivity revert to normal. During GDM, the β cells of the pancreas cannot adequately respond to the increased demands of pregnancy. This, along with decreased insulin sensitivity, results in high blood sugar levels, known as hyperglycemia (Goyal et al., 2022).

Neurohormonal dysfunction contributes to the development of GDM by affecting the regulation of cognitive and visual centers, hunger, energy utilization, and basal metabolic rate. This involves both central and peripheral signals. (Mortan et al., 2006; Thorens et al., 2008). Adipokines, such as adiponectin and leptin, which are released by adipose tissue, control this network.

Adiponectin, secreted by adipocytes, controls glucose levels and promotes the breakdown of fatty acids (Williams et al., 2004) state that a reduced adiponectin concentration in GDM hampers insulin signaling. Leptin, released by fat cells, suppresses hunger-inducing substances such as Neuropeptide Y (NPY), leading to decreased appetite and increased energy usage. GDM frequently entails the development of leptin resistance, which leads to elevated levels of leptin in the blood, a condition known as hyperleptinemia. The development of insulin resistance in the placenta during GDM results in elevated leptin levels, promoting amino acid transport across the placenta. This process ultimately leads to the condition known as fetal macrosomia (Perez et al., 2013).

Zonulin (ZO-1), a tight junction protein, controls the gut's permeability. Elevated levels of ZO-1 in the bloodstream are linked to the presence of type 1, type 2, and GDM. Modified intestinal permeability enables inflammatory cytokines to migrate from the intestine into the bloodstream, facilitating systemic insulin resistance development (Backhed et al., 2005).

Homocysteine, produced through the demethylation of Methionine, is associated with GDM due to oxidative stress. Minimal quantities of homocysteine can result in β cell malfunction and hindered insulin production. GDM is linked to micronutrient deficits such as folic acid, B2, B6, and B12 because they maintain homocysteine levels (Debreceni et al., 2014).

The placenta induces insulin resistance during pregnancy through hormone and cytokines secretion. It acts as a barrier between the fetal and maternal surroundings, protecting the fetus from the consequences of hyperglycemia during gestational diabetes mellitus (GDM).

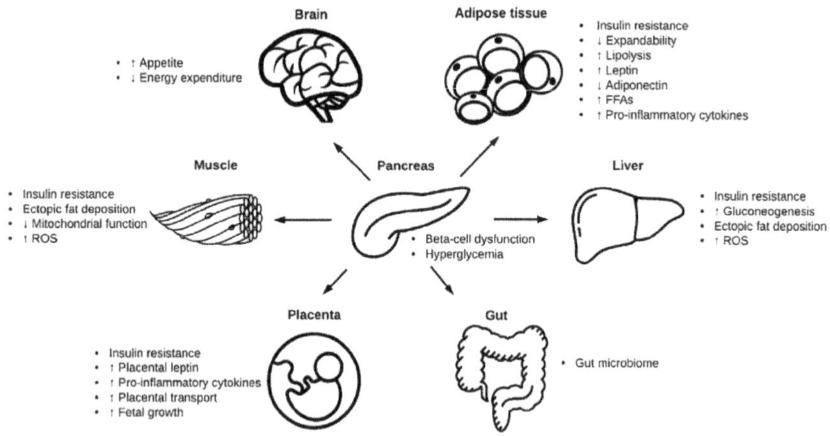

FIGURE 2.2 Organs involved in the pathology of GDM.

Frequently, pancreatic cells cannot react appropriately to an extended excess of energy, which causes resistance to insulin, hyperglycemia, and an increased glucose supply to the growing fetus. Recent evidence has suggested that different variables affect the development of GDM, such as oxidative stress, persistent low-grade inflammation, enhanced gluconeogenesis, and placental effects. Developing effective therapeutic interventions and preventive measures requires a deeper understanding of these complex processes and their function in GDM (Plows et al., 2018).

2.7 COMPLICATIONS OF GDM

GDM has repercussions for both the mother and the fetus, elevating the likelihood of short-term and long-term health complications for both individuals. GDM is associated with prenatal depression during pregnancy (Byrn et al., 2015) and increases the risk of several pregnancy issues, such as more prolonged labor, premature birth, preeclampsia, and, in certain instances, the need for Cesarean section (Tan et al., 2009). According to research conducted by Peters et al. (1996), almost 60% of women diagnosed with GDM ultimately develop T2DM in their later years. Recent research suggests that women who have previously had gestational diabetes mellitus (GDM) experience changes in their blood vessels, making them more susceptible to developing cardiovascular disease (CVD). A study demonstrated that GDM women have a higher risk of CVD, approximately 63%, which can be partially attributed to their BMI (Shostrom et al., 2017).

GDM also affects newborns; during GDM, the fetus produces more insulin and IGF-1 due to an increased transfer of glucose, fatty acids and amino acids across the placenta. This can result in excessive fetal growth, leading to macrosomia at delivery (Schwartz et al., 1994). Increased fetal insulin production is also related to beta cell dysfunction and insulin resistance throughout prenatal development (Fetita et al., 2006). Macrosomia increases the likelihood of shoulder dystocia during childbirth, often requiring the need for cesarean sections. After birth, newborns are more susceptible to experiencing low blood sugar levels after birth, known as hypoglycemia. If not appropriately treated, this condition can lead to brain damage (Gascho et al., 2017; Scifres et al., 2015). There is also evidence indicating a higher likelihood of stillbirth in individuals with GDM (Langer et al., 2005; Rowan et al., 2008).

Long-term neonatal consequences encompass a heightened susceptibility to obesity, neuropsychiatric ailments (such as eating disorders, autism spectrum disorder, obstructive sleep apnea, epilepsy, and infantile spasms), as well as an augmented probability of acquiring T2DM, CVD, and other metabolic illnesses. Children born to moms with GDM have a doubled likelihood of acquiring childhood obesity compared to children born to mothers without diabetes (Tam et al., 2017; Vohr et al., 2008) (Table 2.2).

TABLE 2.2 Complications of Women with Gestational Diabetes Mellitus

Fetal Complications	Maternal Complications
Spontaneous abortion	Obstructed labor
Shoulder dystocia	Polyhydramnios
Intra-uterine death	Prolonged labor
Congenital malformation	Pre-eclampsia
Birth injuries	Uterine atony
Neonatal hypoglycemia	Infection
Respiratory distress syndrome	Cesarean section
Obesity	Postpartum hemorrhage
Fetal Macrosomia	

- **Management of Gestational Diabetes Mellitus:** The screening of GDM women is necessary for the design of a proper therapeutic plan to decrease the associated maternal and fetal comorbidities (Singh et al., 2020; Weir et al., 2001). Patient education plays a vital role and should be carried out for the treatment of women during the gestational period. They should be educated about the disease and effects of GDM along with other measures, including medical nutrition therapies, exercise, management of weight, monitoring of serum blood glucose levels and the usage of pharmacological therapy in the management and treatment of GDM to be followed during labor and post-natal period (Catherine et al., 2010).

2.7.1 PATIENT EDUCATION

The significance of educating women. The disease condition and its management are crucial tasks (Seshiah et al., 2009). They should be aware and follow the drug treatment that is further based on the understanding of the patient about the following points:

i. The implications of GDM
ii. The recommendations related to diet and exercise

iii. Monitoring of blood glucose levels
iv. Insulin administration and dosage adjustment
v. Identification and treatment of consequent hypoglycemia
vi. Measures to reduce the stress
vii. Special attention should also be paid to curtail the anxiety of the women.

The most suitable treatment plan consists of a tailored approach, diet, oral antidiabetic drugs, and insulin therapy according to the response and needs of the individual patients.

2.7.2 MEDICAL NUTRITION THERAPY AND MANAGEMENT OF WEIGHT

Medical nutrition therapy plans designed for managing GDM should be based on the patient's needs (Han et al., 2013; Viana et al., 2014). The food chart should be designed for sufficient calorie intake to promote the mother and fetus's good health, attain the standard glycemic goals, and encourage the maintenance of optimum gestational weight. The suggested daily calorie intake for women with a BMI of 22–25 is 30 kcal/kg and 24 kcal/kg, respectively, and for a BMI of >30 is 12–15 kcal/kg (Gilmartinet al., 2008; Rohilla et al., 2023).

2.4.2.1 GENERAL PRINCIPLES FOR MONITORING THE GLYCEMIC CONTROL

In GDM, successful treatment achievement should be based on maintaining the glycemic control achieved with a dietary or therapeutic regimen. All GDM women should be counselled about nutrition and diet plans to meet pregnancy demands. The predictable increased weight throughout pregnancy is 300 to 400 g/week, whereas overall weight gain weighs up to 10 to 12 kg by each term. Thus, the diet plan aims to supply adequate calories to maintain sufficient nutrition for both mother and fetus and to evade increased weight and related post-prandial hyperglycemia (Mehta et al., 2021; Singh et al., 2020). The second and third trimesters require approximately 300 kcal/day compared to the essential requirement for an ideal body weight of 30 to 40 Kcal/kg (Bühling et al., 2005). The diet plan should be assessed based on Dietary Reference Intakes (DRI). According to DRI, a minimum intake of 175gm of carbohydrates, 71gm of protein, and 28gm of fibers is recommended for GDM women (Management of Diabetes in Pregnancy: Standards of Medical Care in Diabetes, 2019).

2.7.3 EXERCISE

Exercise is one of the vital divisions recommended for treating GDM women because it improves insulin action and reduces the risk of excessive weight gain during pregnancy. Most GDM women respond positively to exercise and diet; pharmacological interventions are unnecessary. Exercise enhances insulin sensitivity, improves fasting and postprandial plasma glucose levels, and decreases insulin need in pregnant women with GDM, as shown in Figure 2.3 (De Barros et al., 2010).

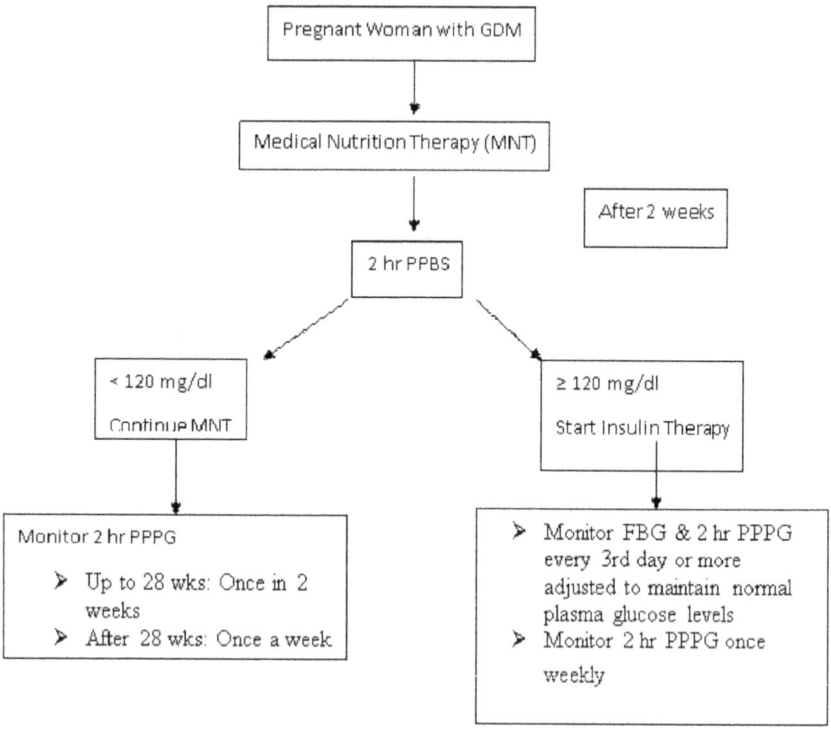

FIGURE 2.3 Management of GDM.

2.8 PHARMACOTHERAPEUTIC INTERVENTIONS

Pharmacotherapeutic interventions are necessary for the management of GDM when non-pharmacological aids such as dietary and medical nutrition therapies and exercise fail to achieve the desired euglycemic state in pregnant mothers.

The pharmacotherapeutic management of the patient is carried out after the proper assessment of the risks and severity associated. The patient is initially managed by the use of non-pharmacological methods to decrease the hyperglycemic levels. If the patient fails to respond, pharmacological therapy is sought for further management. The pharmacological Interventions using antidiabetic medications need to be assessed carefully. Insulin is the mainstay of treatment as it does not cross the placenta; the recommended insulin administration combines short-acting insulin with either long or intermediate-acting agents in divided doses. The insulin doses are adjusted according to the blood sugar levels; a high fasting sugar level is treated by incorporating a night-time intermediate-acting agent, whereas the increased levels of the addition are treated post-meal with a short-acting agent. The usual initiating dose is 0.7–1 unit/kg of body weight. The adjustments of the maintenance doses are then made after proper monitoring of the blood glucose levels (ACOG practice bulletin No. 190: Gestational diabetes mellitus, Committee on Practice Bulletins—Obstetrics 2018).

Insulin Apart and Insulin Lispro are preferred as short-acting agents over regular insulin as they have a faster onset of action that allows their administration at meal timings and not prior as required for the preparations of regular insulin. They do not cross the placenta and permit better control and less hypoglycemic states due to incorrect timings (Anderson et al., 1997). NPH, Glargine and Detemir are the intermediate and long-acting preparations (Herrera et al., 2015; Koren et al., 2015) (Table 2.3).

TABLE 2.3 Commonly Used Preparations of Insulin and Their Properties

Type of Insulin	Generic Name	Onset	Peak	Duration
Rapid-acting	Insulin lispro Insulin Aspart	15 minutes	30–90 minutes	3–5 hrs
Short-acting	Regular insulin	30–60 minutes	2–4 hrs	5–8 hrs
Intermediate-Acting	NPH insulin	1–3 hours	8 hrs	12–16 hrs
Long-acting	Insulin glargine Insulin detemir	1 hour	Peak less	20–26 hrs

Oral antidiabetics are not widely used as they can cross the placenta, which may result in fetal hyperinsulinemia, congenital malformations, neonatal macrosomia, and hypoglycemia.

Metformin is a biguanide that reduces the intestinal absorption of glucose and gluconeogenesis, thereby increasing peripheral glucose uptake. The long-term effects of medication on the fetus are unknown (Eyal et al., 2010), and one study recorded the absence of development till the age of 2 (Wouldes et al., 2015). The drug has limited evidence of its ability to improve pregnancy outcomes (De Leo et al., 2011).

Women with GDM should be adequately counselled about the use of oral antidiabetic medications such as metformin, as it is not superior to insulin and has definitive data about fetal effects. About 24–46% of pregnant women on metformin therapy may need coadministration of insulin for potentiation of glycemic control (Spaulonci et al., 2013). The starting dose of metformin is 500 mg OD for a week, and then the dose is adjusted accordingly. The maximum amount for daily administration in divided doses is 2500–3000 mg. Metformin is contraindicated in patients with improper renal function. The adverse effects associated with metformin treatment occur in 3%-46% of cases (Balsells et al., 2015). The common side effects associated are GIT upset, diarrhea, abdominal pain, higher incidences of preeclampsia, and lactic acidosis; therefore, administration with meals is suitable.

Clinical data do not back up metformin and its effects on long-term pregnancy outcomes, requiring individual experimental analysis. In contrast, the drug is recognized as safe and effectively manages short-term outcomes (Lautatzis et al., 2013).

The sulfonylureas used for GDM include Glyburide, Tolbutamide, and Glibenclamide, which do not cross the placenta. Glyburide is a drug that augments insulin secretion by the pancreas and the extra pancreatic tissues and increases the sensitivity of the peripheral tissues towards insulin. However, it is not used as a first-line agent due to lesser results than the other drugs. The recommended dosage of Glyburide is 2.5–20 mg/day (Langer et al., 2000). However, many patients require the subsequent administration of insulin for adequate glycemic control (Jacobson et al., 2005; Langer et al., 2005; Moore et al., 2010). Sulfa allergy is the contraindication of these drugs. At the same time, different side effects of sulfonylureas included mild GIT effects like nausea, vomiting, diarrhea, and an increased risk of neonatal hypoglycemia and maternal and neonatal weight gain. Specific trials also reported that the women who used Glyburide had increased chances of hypertension and stillbirths than the women who used Insulin medication (Min et al., 2009; Rochon et al., 2006).

Metformin and glyburide are suitable for managing GDM because of their ability to maintain reasonable glycemic control. Due to a lack of proper data on the long-term effects of the medications, pregnant women should be carefully advised about the known and assumed safety and adverse effect profiles of the oral hypoglycemic agents. Antioxidants are used to improve the outcome of pregnancy, as many pieces of evidence relate to the development of diabetes and oxidative stress during pregnancy. Literature evidence also suggests a possible association between the reactive oxygen species and diabetes development during pregnancy (Brownlee et al., 2005; Damasceno et al., 2002).

A recent study demonstrated that using antioxidants significantly decreases the dose of insulin required to manage the sugar level and oxidative markers such as glutathione and superoxide dismutase. The study concluded that the subsequent use of antioxidants in GDM-diagnosed women reverses oxidative stress, which may result in improved neonatal outcomes (Maged et al., 2016).

ACOG recommends the use of insulin as a first-line agent in the treatment of insulin, while oral antidiabetic agents are considered alternative therapies for patients who are unable to adhere to an insulin regimen after a thorough consultation.

2.9 MANAGEMENT DURING THE LABOUR AND POSTNATAL PERIOD

A consensus has not been reached on the most favorable timing and approach for delivering babies to women diagnosed with gestational diabetes mellitus (GDM). Inducing labor is regarded as advantageous in avoiding late neonatal mortality and obstetric difficulties linked to excessive fetal growth (Witkop et al., 2009). As to the guidelines from the American College of Obstetricians and Gynecologists (ACOG), a Caesarean delivery that the mother chooses may be considered if the expected weight of the baby is more than 4.5 kg, to reduce the chances of birth trauma (ACOG Committee on Practice Bulletins, 2005).

Insulin requirements during labor are often diminished due to heightened physical exertion, although certain women may encounter extended periods of fasting. Glucose infusions may be necessary for specific situations to prevent the occurrence of ketosis (Jovanovic et al., 2004). Women who have been treated with pharmacological drugs throughout pregnancy may need insulin during childbirth to control high blood sugar levels, with glucose levels checked every two hours. The Endocrine Society recommends keeping plasma glucose levels between 72–126 mg/dL during childbirth (Blumer et al., 2013). When blood glucose levels are poorly controlled, dextrose should be administered intravenously (IV) or through continuous infusion throughout delivery. Treatment for hyperglycemia should be terminated following the delivery of the fetus.

GDM is commonly recognized as a causative element in the onset of T2DM. Although most of the GDM women have normal blood sugar levels after giving birth, it is essential to closely monitor them after pregnancy to identify any indications of T2DM. It is generally advised to do screenings and monitoring for reduced glucose tolerance for 6–12 weeks following childbirth and then continue monitoring for at least three years afterwards. Aside from engaging in regular physical activity, adopting healthy lifestyles is crucial to minimize the likelihood of getting type 2 diabetes. Mothers who have been diagnosed with GDM should be strongly encouraged to breastfeed sufficiently, starting from delivery and continuing for at least three months after giving birth. This can potentially lower the chances of neonatal hypoglycemia and obesity in the child and also prevent the mother from developing metabolic syndrome and type 2 diabetes. (National Collaborating Centre for Women's and Children's Health 2008, American Association of Diabetes Educators, 2013).

2.10 MANAGEMENT OF PREEXISTING TYPE 1 AND TYPE 2 DIABETES DURING PREGNANCY

Effectively managing preexisting type 1 diabetes and type 2 diabetes during pregnancy necessitates the frequent adjustment of insulin dosage to match the daily needs, with a strong emphasis on the crucial practice of regularly checking blood glucose levels. According to García-Patterson, there is usually an initial rise in insulin requirements during the first trimester of pregnancy, followed by a decline in the following trimesters (García-Patterson et al., 2010; Singh et al., 2022). Women who already have type 1 diabetes may encounter heightened episodes of hypoglycemia. To combat the quick growth in insulin resistance and reach desired blood sugar levels, the insulin dosage is usually raised by 5% starting from the second trimester and then practically doubled by the end of the late third trimester. It is advisable to distribute the total daily insulin dose, allocating a smaller portion for basal administration and a more significant portion for prandial administration. During the final stage of the third trimester, when the body requires less insulin, the management of insulin needs in pregnancy becomes intricate. This sometimes necessitates referring patients to specialized clinics that provide team-based care involving experts from maternal-fetal medicine, endocrinology, and social work.

The current formulations of human insulin that are accessible have been shown in multiple studies (McCance et al., 2008; Pollex et al., 2010; Suffecool et al., 2015) to not pass through the placenta. A comprehensive review by Cochrane found no definitive evidence to suggest that any particular insulin regimen is superior in treating GDM during pregnancy (Neill et al., 2017). GDM during pregnancy is linked to an increased likelihood of having preeclampsia, as stated by Kirsten and Deborah in 2005. Women who are at a high risk of developing preeclampsia after 12 weeks of pregnancy can take low-dose aspirin as a preventive treatment (Henderson et al., 2014; Tiwari et al., 2023). The objective of this method is to decrease the occurrence of illness and the expenses associated with healthcare.

- **Follow Up on GDM:** Frequent follow-up is required in pregnant women with GDM. An OGTT should be performed 6 to 8 weeks post-partum with 75 g oral glucose using the WHO criteria for the non-pregnant population. If the results are expected, GTT is repeated after six and 12 months to establish the progression of glucose tolerance or its average value. Many GDM women may be glucose intolerant (Kale et al., 2004; Singh and Singh 2024). The gestational diabetic women should be advised and counselled regarding the higher risk of developing diabetes mellitus permanently (Damm et al., 2009). The importance of a healthy diet and exercise patterns should be made known to the patients, along with the symptoms of hyperglycemia and hypoglycemia and their management. The preventive measure should begin in the intrauterine period and be maintained throughout early childhood (Jaakko, 2005).

2.11 CONCLUSION

Gestational Diabetes Mellitus, the most common complication of pregnancy, requires proper measures of prevention, treatment and management options to curb adverse pregnancy outcomes and the risk of future metabolic conditions in mothers and their offspring. Timely detection of women with GDM may initiate the implementation of early preventive measures. A proper study of the established and postulated risk factors and universal screening methods need to be carried out for the establishment of suitable prevention strategies, along with proper management of the heart rate, blood pressure, height of uterine fundus and antibody testing. The current diagnostic criteria for OGTT are the Carpenter–Coustan criteria, The National Diabetes Data Group (NDDG) criteria and the ADA procedural recommendations. Complete knowledge about the pathophysiology of GDM and its consequences helps decide effective treatment and prevention strategies to decrease fetal and maternal comorbidities. It is essential to provide patients with information regarding the significance of medical nutrition therapy and self-monitoring glucose levels. The success of treating GDM women is based on preserving the glycemic control obtained by dietary or pharmacological intervention. Thus, all pregnant women diagnosed with GDM should be provided with nutritional counselling. The accepted pharmacological therapy includes the use of insulin or oral antidiabetic drugs. Human insulin is the first-line agent among different insulin analogues, and specific oral anti-diabetic agents like metformin and glyburide have also been used. A treatment program in which diets, oral antidiabetics and insulin medication are recommended according to the needs of the particular patient could be the most viable approach.

KEYWORDS

- **endocrine disorder**
- **GDM**
- **gestational diabetes mellitus**
- **insulin therapy**
- **metformin**
- **pregnancy**

REFERENCES

ACOG Committee on Practice Bulletins. (2005). ACOG Practice Bulletin. Clinical management guidelines for obstetrician-gynecologists. Number 60. Pregestational diabetes mellitus. *Obstetrics and Gynecology, 105*, 675–685. https://doi.org/10.1097/aog.0000000000002960 (accessed on 28th June 2025).

American Association of Diabetes Educators. (2013). Gestational diabetes mellitus AADE practice advisory. https://doi.org/10.1177/2325160314533785 (accessed on 28th June 2025).

American College of Obstetricians and Gynecologists. (2013). Gestational diabetes mellitus. Practice Bulletin No. 137. *Obstetrics and Gynecology, 122*, 406–416. https://doi.org/10.1097/01.aog.0000433006.09219.f1 (accessed on 28th June 2025).

American Diabetes Association. (2003). Gestational diabetes mellitus. *Diabetes Care, 26*(Suppl. 1), S103–S105. https://doi.org/10.2337/diacare.26.2007.S103 (accessed on 28th June 2025).

American Diabetes Association. (2014). Standards of medical care in diabetes. *Diabetes Care, 37*(Suppl. 1), S14–S80. https://doi.org/10.2337/dc14-S014 (accessed on 28th June 2025).

Anderson, J. H., Brunelle, R. L., Koivisto, V. A., Pfutzner, A., Trautmann, M. E., Vignati, L., & DiMarchi, R. (1997). Reduction of postprandial hyperglycemia and frequency of hypoglycemia in IDDM patients on insulin-analog treatment. Multicenter Insulin Lispro Study Group. *Diabetes, 46*(2), 265–270. https://doi.org/10.2337/diab.46.2.265 (accessed on 28th June 2025).

Anghebem-Oliveira, M. I., Martins, B. R., Alberton, D., Ramos, E. A. S., Picheth, G., & Rego, F. G. M. (2017). Type 2 diabetes-associated genetic variants of FTO, LEPR, PPARγ, and TCF7L2 in gestational diabetes in a Brazilian population. *Archives of Endocrinology and Metabolism, 61*(3), 238–248. https://doi.org/10.1590/2359-3997000000258 (accessed on 28th June 2025).

Ashcroft, F. M., Rohm, M., Clark, A., & Brereton, M. F. (2017). Is type 2 diabetes a glycogen storage disease of pancreatic β cells? *Cell Metabolism, 26*, 17–23. https://doi.org/10.1016/j.cmet.2017.05.014 (accessed on 28th June 2025).

Bäckhed, F., Ley, R. E., Sonnenburg, J. L., Peterson, D. A., & Gordon, J. I. (2005). Host-bacterial mutualism in the human intestine. *Science, 307*(5717), 1915–1920. https://doi.org/10.1126/science.1104816 (accessed on 28th June 2025).

Balsells, M., García-Patterson, A., Sola, I., Roqué, M., Gich, I., & Corcoy, R. (2015). Glibenclamide, metformin, and insulin for treating gestational diabetes: A systematic review and meta-analysis. *BMJ, 350*, h102. https://doi.org/10.1136/bmj.h102 (accessed on 28th June 2025).

Ben-Haroush, A., Yogev, Y., & Hod, M. (2004). Epidemiology of gestational diabetes mellitus and its association with type 2 diabetes. *Diabetic Medicine, 21*(2), 103–113. https://doi.org/10.1046/j.1464-5491.2003.00985.x (accessed on 28th June 2025).

Bhargava, S. K., Singh, T. G., Mannan, A., Singh, S., & Gupta, S. (2022). Pharmacological evaluation of *Thuja occidentalis* for the attenuation of nephropathy in streptozotocin-induced diabetes rats. *Obesity Medicine, 31*, 100391. https://doi.org/10.1016/j.obmed.2022.100391 (accessed on 28th June 2025).

Bhargava, S. K., Singh, T. G., Mannan, A., Singh, S., Singh, M., & Gupta, S. (2022). Pharmacological evaluation of *Thuja occidentalis* for the attenuation of neuropathy via AGEs and TNF-α inhibition in diabetic neuropathic rats. *Environmental Science and Pollution Research International, 29*(40), 60542–60557. https://doi.org/10.1007/s11356-022-20106-3 (accessed on 28th June 2025).

Blumer, I., Hadar, E., Hadden, D. R., Jovanović, L., Mestman, J. H., Murad, M. H., & Yogev, Y. (2013). Diabetes and pregnancy: An Endocrine Society clinical practice guideline. *Journal of Clinical Endocrinology and Metabolism, 98*, 4227–4249. https://doi.org/10.1210/jc.2013-2465 (accessed on 28th June 2025).

Brownlee, M. (2005). The pathobiology of diabetic complications: A unifying mechanism. *Diabetes, 54*(6), 1615–1625. http://dx.doi.org/10.2337/diabetes.54.6.1615 (accessed on 28th June 2025).

Buchanan, T. A., Xiang, A. H., & Page, K. A. (2012). Gestational diabetes mellitus: Risks and management during and after pregnancy. *Nature Reviews Endocrinology, 8*(11), 639. https://doi.org/10.1038/nrendo.2012.96 (accessed on 28th June 2025).

Bühling, K. J., Winkel, T., Wolf, C., Kurzidim, B., Mahmoudi, M., Wohlfarth, K., Wäscher, C., Schink, T., & Dudenhausen, W. H. (2005). Optimal timing for postprandial glucose measurement in pregnant women with diabetes and a non-diabetic pregnant population evaluated by the CGMS. *Journal of Perinatal Medicine, 33*(2), 125–131. https://doi.org/10.1515/jpm.2005.024 (accessed on 28th June 2025).

Byrn, M., & Penckofer, S. (2015). The relationship between gestational diabetes and antenatal depression. *Journal of Obstetric, Gynecologic & Neonatal Nursing, 44*(2), 246–255. https://doi.org/10.1111/1552-6909.12554 (accessed on 28th June 2025).

Catalano, P. M. (2014). Trying to understand gestational diabetes. *Diabetic Medicine, 31*, 273–281. https://doi.org/10.1111/dme.12381 (accessed on 28th June 2025).

Catherine, K. (2010). Gestational diabetes: Risks, management, and treatment options. *International Journal of Women's Health, 2*, 339–351. https://doi.org/10.2147/IJWH.S13333 (accessed on 28th June 2025).

Chen, P., Wang, S., Ji, J., Ge, A., Chen, C., Zhu, Y., Xie, N., & Wang, Y. (2015). Risk factors and management of gestational diabetes. *Cell Biochemistry and Biophysics, 71*(2), 689–694. https://doi.org/10.3390/antiox11010129 (accessed on 28th June 2025).

Cheng, Y. W., Block-Kurbisch, I., & Caughey, A. B. (2009). Carpenter-Constant criteria compared with the National Diabetes Data Group thresholds for gestational diabetes mellitus. *Obstetrics and Gynecology, 114*(2 Pt 1), 326–332. https://doi.org/10.1097/aog.0b013e3181ae8d85 (accessed on 28th June 2025).

Cianni, G. D., Miccoli, R., Volpe, L., Lencioni, C., & Di Prato, S. (2003). Intermediate metabolism in normal pregnancy and gestational diabetes. *Diabetes/Metabolism Research and Reviews, 19*, 259–270. http://dx.doi.org/10.1002/dmrr.390 (accessed on 28th June 2025).

Committee on Practice Bulletins—Obstetrics. (2018). ACOG Practice Bulletin No. 190: Gestational diabetes mellitus. *Obstetrics and Gynecology, 131*(2), e49–e64. https://doi.org/10.1097/aog.0000000000002501 (accessed on 28th June 2025).

Damasceno, D. C., Volpato, G. T., de Mattos, P. C. I., & Cunha, R. M. V. (2002). Oxidative stress and diabetes in pregnant rats. *Animal Reproduction Science, 72*(3–4), 235–244. https://doi.org/10.1016/s0378-4320(02)00094-5 (accessed on 28th June 2025).

Damm, P. (2009). Future risk of diabetes in mother and child after gestational diabetes mellitus. *International Journal of Gynecology and Obstetrics, 104*(1), S25–S26. https://doi.org/10.1016/j.ijgo.2008.11.025 (accessed on 28th June 2025).

De Barros, M. C., Lopes, M. A. B., Francisco, R. P. V., Sapienza, A. D., & Zugaib, M. (2010). Resistance exercise and glycemic control in women with gestational diabetes mellitus. *American Journal of Obstetrics and Gynecology, 203*, 556.e1–556.e6. https://doi.org/10.1016/j.ajog.2010.07.015 (accessed on 28th June 2025).

De Leo, V., Musacchio, M. C., Piomboni, P., Di Sabatino, A., & Morgante, G. (2011). The administration of metformin during pregnancy reduces polycystic ovary syndrome-related gestational complications. *European Journal of Obstetrics, Gynecology, and Reproductive Biology, 157*(1), 63–66. https://doi.org/10.1016/j.ejogrb.2011.03.024 (accessed on 28th June 2025).

Debreceni, B., & Debreceni, L. (2014). The role of homocysteine-lowering B vitamins in the primary prevention of cardiovascular disease. *Cardiovascular Therapeutics, 32*(3), 130–138. https://doi.org/10.1111/1755-5922.12064 (accessed on 28th June 2025).

Expert Committee on the Diagnosis and Classification of Diabetes Mellitus. (2003). Report of the expert committee on the diagnosis and classification of diabetes mellitus. *Diabetes Care, 26*(Suppl. 1), S5–S20. https://doi.org/10.2337/diacare.26.2007.S5 (accessed on 28th June 2025).

Eyal, S., Easterling, T. R., Carr, D., Umans, J. G., Miodovnik, M., Hankins, G. D. V., Clark, S. M., Risler, L., Wang, J., Kelly, E. J., Shen, D. D., & Hebert, M. F. (2010). Pharmacokinetics of metformin during pregnancy. *Drug Metabolism and Disposition, 38*(5), 833–840. https://doi.org/10.1155/2014/797681 (accessed on 28th June 2025).

Fetita, L. S., Sobngwi, E., Serradas, P., Calvo, F., & Gautier, J. F. (2006). Consequences of fetal exposure to maternal diabetes in offspring. *The Journal of Clinical Endocrinology & Metabolism, 91*(10), 3718–3724. https://doi.org/10.1210/jc.2006-0624 (accessed on 28th June 2025).

García-Patterson, A., Gich, I., Amini, S. B., Catalano, P. M., de Leiva, A., & Corcoy, R. (2010). Insulin requirements throughout pregnancy in women with type 1 diabetes mellitus: Three direction changes. *Diabetologia, 53*, 446–451. https://doi.org/10.1007/s00125-009-1633-z (accessed on 28th June 2025).

Gascho, C. L. L., Leandro, D. M. K., Silva, T. R., & Silva, J. C. (2017). Predictors of cesarean delivery in pregnant women with gestational diabetes mellitus. *Revista Brasileira de Ginecologia e Obstetrícia, 39*, 60–65. https://doi.org/10.1055/s-0037-1598644 (accessed on 28th June 2025).

Gilmartin, A. B. H., Ural, S. H., & Repke, J. T. (2008). Gestational diabetes mellitus. *Reviews in Obstetrics and Gynecology, 1*, 129–134. http://dx.doi.org/10.3233/NPM-190305 (accessed on 28th June 2025).

Goyal, S., Sood, A., Gautam, I., Pradhan, S., Mondal, P., Singh, G., Jaura, R. S., Singh, T. G., & Sibia, R. S. (2022). Serum protease-activated receptor (PAR-1) levels as a potential biomarker for diagnosis of inflammation in type 2 diabetic patients. *Inflammopharmacology, 30*(5), 1843–1851. https://doi.org/10.1007/s10787-022-01049-0 (accessed on 28th June 2025).

Gyasi-Antwi, P., Walker, L., Moody, C., Okyere, S., Salt, K., Anang, L., … & Adams, G. (2020). Global prevalence of gestational diabetes mellitus: A systematic review and meta-analysis. *New American Journal of Medicine, 1*(3). https://doi.org/10.25159/2520-5293/12158 (accessed on 28th June 2025).

Han, S., Middleton, P., Shepherd, E., van Ryswyk, E., & Crowther, C. A. (2013). Different types of dietary advice for women with gestational diabetes mellitus. *Cochrane Database of Systematic Reviews, 3*, CD009275. https://doi.org/10.3390/nu12103050 (accessed on 28th June 2025).

Hasdemir, P. S., Terzi, H., & Koyuncu, F. M. (2014). Recent advances in the diagnosis and management of gestational diabetes. *Turkish Journal of Obstetrics and Gynecology, 11*(3), 181–185. https://doi.org/10.3390/medsci9040059 (accessed on 28th June 2025).

Henderson, J. T., Whitlock, E. P., O'Conner, E., Senger, C. A., Thompson, J. H., & Rowland, M. G. (2014). Low-dose aspirin for the prevention of morbidity and mortality from preeclampsia: A systematic evidence review for the U.S. Preventive Services Task Force. *Diabetes Care, 42*(Suppl. 1), S171. https://doi.org/10.7326/m13-2844 (accessed on 28th June 2025).

Herrera, K. M., Rosenn, B. M., Foroutan, J., Bimson, B. E., Ibraheemi, Z. A., Moshier, E. L., & Brustman, L. E. (2015). Randomised controlled trial of insulin detemir versus NPH for the treatment of pregnant women with diabetes. *American Journal of Obstetrics and Gynecology, 213*(3), 426.e1–426.e7. http://dx.doi.org/10.1016/j.ajog.2015.06.010 (accessed on 28th June 2025).

Jaakko, T. (2005). A paradigm shift is needed in the primary prevention of type 2 diabetes. In M. Ganz (Ed.), *Prevention of type 2 diabetes* (pp. 153–165). John Wiley & Sons Ltd. https://doi.org/10.2337/dc09-S345 (accessed on 28th June 2025).

Jacobson, G. F., Ramos, G. A., Ching, J. Y., Kirby, R. S., Ferrara, A., & Field, D. R. (2005). Comparison of glyburide and insulin for managing gestational diabetes in a large managed care organisation. *American Journal of Obstetrics and Gynecology, 193*(1), 118–124. https://doi.org/10.1016/j.ajog.2005.11.016 (accessed on 28th June 2025).

Jovanovic, L. (2004). Glucose and insulin requirements during labour and delivery: The case for normoglycemia in pregnancies complicated by diabetes. *Endocrine Practice, 10*(Suppl. 2), 40–45. https://doi.org/10.4158/ep.10.s2.40 (accessed on 28th June 2025).

Jovanović, L., Bevier, W., & Peterson, C. M. (1997). The Santa Barbara County Health Care Services Program: Birth weight change concomitant with screening for and treatment of glucose intolerance of pregnancy: A potential cost-effective intervention? *American Journal of Perinatology, 14*(4), 221–228. https://doi.org/10.2739/kurumemedj.MS65001 (accessed on 28th June 2025).

Kale, S. D., Yajnik, C. S., Kulkarni, S. R., Meenakumari, K., Joglekar, A. A., Khorsand, N., Ladkat, R. S., Ramdas, L. V., & Lubree, H. G. (2004). High risk of diabetes and metabolic syndrome in Indian women with gestational diabetes mellitus. *Diabetic Medicine, 21*, 1257–1259. https://doi.org/10.1111/j.1464-5491.2004.01337.x (accessed on 28th June 2025).

Kirsten, D., & Deborah, H. (2005). Risk factors for preeclampsia at antenatal booking: Systematic review of controlled studies. *BMJ, 330*, 565. https://doi.org/10.1136/bmj.38380.674340.E0 (accessed on 28th June 2025).

Koren, R., Toledano, Y., & Hod, M. (2015). The use of insulin detemir during pregnancy: A safety evaluation. *Expert Opinion on Drug Safety, 14*(4), 593–599. https://doi.org/10.1517/14740338.2015.1013533 (accessed on 28th June 2025).

Langer, O., Conway, D. L., Berkus, M. D., Xenakis, E. M., & Gonzales, O. (2000). A comparison of glyburide and insulin in women with gestational diabetes mellitus. *The New England Journal of Medicine, 343*(16), 1134–1138. https://doi.org/10.1056/nejm200010193431601 (accessed on 28th June 2025).

Langer, O., Yogev, Y., Most, O., & Xenakis, E. M. (2005). Gestational diabetes: The consequences of not treating. *American Journal of Obstetrics and Gynecology, 192*(4), 989–997. https://doi.org/10.1016/j.ajog.2004.11.039 (accessed on 28th June 2025).

Langer, O., Yogev, Y., Xenakis, E. M., & Rosenn, B. (2005). Insulin and glyburide therapy: Dosage, severity level of gestational diabetes, and pregnancy outcome. *American Journal of Obstetrics and Gynecology, 192*(1), 134–139. https://doi.org/10.1016/j.ajog.2004.07.011 (accessed on 28th June 2025).

Lautatzis, M. E., Goulis, D. G., & Vrontakis, M. (2013). Efficacy and safety of metformin during pregnancy in women with gestational diabetes mellitus or polycystic ovary syndrome: A systematic review. *Metabolism, 62*(11), 1522–1534. https://doi.org/10.1016/j.metabol.2013.06.006 (accessed on 28th June 2025).

Li, G., Zhao, S., Cui, S., Li, L., Xu, Y., & Li, Y. (2015). Effect comparison of metformin with insulin treatment for gestational diabetes: A meta-analysis based on RCTs. *Archives of Gynecology and Obstetrics, 292*(1), 111–120. https://doi.org/10.21608/amj.2023.291647 (accessed on 28th June 2025).

Maged, A. M., Torky, H., Fouad, M. A., GadAllah, S. H., Waked, N. M., Gayed, A. S., & Salem, A. K. (2016). Role of antioxidants in gestational diabetes mellitus and relation to fetal outcome: A randomised controlled trial. *Journal of Maternal-Fetal and Neonatal Medicine, 29*(24), 4049–4054. https://doi.org/10.3109/14767058.2016.1154526 (accessed on 28th June 2025).

Management of Diabetes in Pregnancy: Standards of Medical Care in Diabetes 2019. (2019). *Diabetes Care, 42*(Suppl. 1), S165–S172. https://doi.org/10.2337/dc19-s014 (accessed on 28th June 2025).

McCance, D. R., Damm, P., Mathiesen, E. R., Hod, M., Kaaja, R., Dunne, F., Jensen, L. E., & Mersebach, H. (2008). Evaluating insulin antibodies and placental transfer of insulin aspart in pregnant women with type 1 diabetes mellitus. *Diabetologia, 51*, 2141–2143. https://doi.org/10.1007/s00125-008-1120-y (accessed on 28th June 2025).

Mehta, S., Nain, P., Agrawal, B. K., & Singh, R. P. (2022). Vitamin D with calcium supplementation managing glycemic control with HbA1c and improve quality of life in patients with diabetes. *Turkish Journal of Pharmaceutical Sciences, 19*(2), 161–167. https://doi.org/10.4274/tjps.galenos.2021.62357 (accessed on 28th June 2025).

Mehta, S., Nain, P., Agrawal, B. K., Singh, R. P., Kaur, J., Maity, S., Bhattacharjee, A., Peela, J., Nauhria, S., & Nauhria, S. (2021). Effectiveness of empagliflozin with vitamin D supplementation in peripheral neuropathy in type 2 diabetic patients. *Cureus, 13*(12), e20208. https://doi.org/10.7759/cureus.20208 (accessed on 28th June 2025).

Min, J., Park, B., Kim, Y. J., Lee, H., Ha, E., & Park, H. D. (2009). Effect of oxidative stress on birth sizes: Consideration of window from mid-pregnancy to delivery. *Placenta, 30*(5), 418–423. https://doi.org/10.1016/j.placenta.2009.02.007 (accessed on 28th June 2025).

Mishra, S., Bhadoria, A. S., Kishore, S., & Kumar, R. (2018). Gestational diabetes mellitus 2018 guidelines: An update. *PMC US National Library of Medicine*. https://doi.org/10.4103/ijcm.ijcm_298_23 (accessed on 28th June 2025).

Mithal, A., Bansal, B., & Kalra, S. (2015). Gestational diabetes in India: Science and society. *Indian Journal of Endocrinology and Metabolism, 19*(6), 701. https://doi.org/10.4103/2230-8210.164031 (accessed on 28th June 2025).

Moore, L. E., Clokey, D., Rappaport, V. J., & Curet, L. B. (2010). Metformin compared with glyburide in gestational diabetes: A randomised controlled trial. *Obstetrics and Gynecology, 115*(1), 55–59. https://doi.org/10.1097/aog.0b013e3181c52132 (accessed on 28th June 2025).

Morton, G. J., Cummings, D. E., Baskin, D. G., Barsh, G. S., & Schwartz, M. W. (2006). Central nervous system control of food intake and body weight. *Nature, 443*, 289–295. http://dx.doi.org/10.1038/nature05026 (accessed on 28th June 2025).

National Collaborating Centre for Women's and Children's Health. (2008). *Diabetes in pregnancy: Management of diabetes and its complications from preconception to the postnatal period.* London. https://doi.org/10.15277/bjdvd.2015.029 (accessed on 28th June 2025).

Neill, S. M. O., Kenny, L. C., Khashan, A. S., West, H. M., Smyth, R. M., & Kearney, P. M. (2017). Different insulin types and regimens for pregnant women with pre-existing diabetes. *Cochrane Database of Systematic Reviews, 2*, CD011880. http://dx.doi.org/10.1002/14651858.CD011880.pub2 (accessed on 28th June 2025).

Pérez-Pérez, A., Maymó, J. L., Gambino, Y. P., Guadix, P., Dueñas, J. L., Varone, C. L., & Sánchez-Margalet, V. (2013). Activated translation signaling in placenta from pregnant women with gestational diabetes mellitus: Possible role of leptin. *Hormone and Metabolic Research = Hormon- und Stoffwechselforschung = Hormones et Métabolisme, 45*(6), 436–442. https://doi.org/10.1055/s-0032-1333276 (accessed on 28th June 2025).

Peters, R. K., Xiang, A., Kjos, S. L., & Buchanan, T. A. (1996). Long-term diabetogenic effect of single pregnancy in women with previous gestational diabetes mellitus. *The Lancet, 347*(8996), 227–230. https://doi.org/10.1016/s0140-6736(96)90405-5 (accessed on 28th June 2025).

Plows, J. F., Stanley, J. L., Baker, P. N., Reynolds, C. M., & Vickers, M. H. (2018). The pathophysiology of gestational diabetes mellitus. *International Journal of Molecular Sciences, 19*(11), 3342. https://doi.org/10.3390/ijms19113342 (accessed on 28th June 2025).

Plows, J. F., Stanley, J. L., Baker, P. N., Reynolds, C. M., & Vickers, M. H. (2018). The pathophysiology of gestational diabetes mellitus. *International Journal of Molecular Sciences, 19*(11), 3342. https://doi.org/10.3390/ijms19113342 (accessed on 28th June 2025).

Pollex, E. K., Feig, D. S., Lubetsky, A., Yip, P. M., & Koren, G. (2010). Insulin glargine safety in pregnancy: A transplacental transfer study. *Diabetes Care, 33*, 29–33. https://doi.org/10.2337/dc09-1045 (accessed on 28th June 2025).

Putra, I. M. W. A., Fakhrudin, N., Nurrochmad, A., & Wahyuono, S. (2023). A review of medicinal plants with renoprotective activity in diabetic nephropathy animal models. *Life (Basel), 13*(2), 560. https://doi.org/10.3390/life13020560 (accessed on 28th June 2025).

Rochon, M., Rand, L., Roth, L., & Gaddipati, S. (2006). Glyburide for the management of gestational diabetes: Risk factors predictive of failure and associated pregnancy outcomes. *American Journal of Obstetrics and Gynecology, 195*(4), 1090–1094. https://doi.org/10.1016/j.ajog.2006.07.029 (accessed on 28th June 2025).

Rohilla, M., Bansal, R., Garg, A., Dhiman, S., Dhankhar, S., Saini, M., Chauhan, S., Alsubaie, N., Batiha, G. E., Albezrah, N. K. A., & Singh, T. G. (2023). Discussing pathologic mechanisms of diabetic retinopathy & therapeutic potentials of curcumin and β-glucogallin in the management of diabetic retinopathy. *Biomedicine & Pharmacotherapy = Biomedecine & Pharmacotherapie, 169*, 115881. https://doi.org/10.1016/j.biopha.2023.115881 (accessed on 28th June 2025).

Rosenberger, D. C., Blechschmidt, V., Timmerman, H., Wolff, A., & Treede, R. D. (2020). Challenges of neuropathic pain: Focus on diabetic neuropathy. *Journal of Neural Transmission (Vienna), 127*(4), 589–624. https://doi.org/10.1007/s00702-020-02145-7 (accessed on 28th June 2025).

Rowan, J. A., Hague, W. M., Gao, W., Battin, M. R., Moore, M. P., & MiG Trial Investigators. (2008). Metformin versus insulin for the treatment of gestational diabetes. *The New England Journal of Medicine, 358*(19), 2003–2015. https://doi.org/10.1056/NEJMoa0707193 (accessed on 28th June 2025).

Schrader, H. M., Peterson, J. L., Bevier, W. C., & Peterson, C. M. (1995). Fasting plasma glucose and glycosylated protein at 24 to 28 weeks of gestation predict macrosomia in the general obstetric population. *American Journal of Perinatology, 12*(4), 247–251. https://doi.org/10.2337/dc10-1455 (accessed on 28th June 2025).

Schwartz, R., Gruppuso, P. A., Petzold, K., Brambilla, D., Hiilesmaa, V., & Teramo, K. A. (1994). Hyperinsulinemia and macrosomia in the fetus of the diabetic mother. *Diabetes Care, 17*(7), 640–648. https://doi.org/10.2337/diacare.17.7.640 (accessed on 28th June 2025).

Scifres, C. M., Feghali, M., Dumont, T., Althouse, A. D., Speer, P., Caritis, S. N., & Catov, J. M. (2015). Large-for-gestational-age ultrasound diagnosis and risk for cesarean delivery in women with gestational diabetes mellitus. *Obstetrics & Gynecology, 126*(5), 978–986. https://doi.org/10.1097/aog.0000000000001097 (accessed on 28th June 2025).

Seshiah, V., Balaji, V., Balaji, M. S., Paneerselvam, A., & Kapur, A. (2009). Pregnancy and diabetes scenario around the world: India. *International Journal of Gynecology & Obstetrics, 104*, S35–S38. https://doi.org/10.1016/j.ijgo.2008.11.035 (accessed on 28th June 2025).

Seshiah, V., Gupte, S., Datta, M., Kapur, A., & Vijayam, B. (2016). Need for testing glucose tolerance in the early weeks of pregnancy. *Indian Journal of Endocrinology and Metabolism, 20*(1), 43. https://doi.org/10.4103/2230-8210.172238 (accessed on 28th June 2025).

Sharma, V. K., & Singh, T. G. (2020). Chronic stress and diabetes mellitus: Interwoven pathologies. *Current Diabetes Reviews, 16*(6), 546–556. https://doi.org/10.2174/1573399815666191111152248 (accessed on 28th June 2025).

Shostrom, D. C., Sun, Y., Oleson, J. J., Snetselaar, L. G., & Bao, W. (2017). History of gestational diabetes mellitus about cardiovascular disease and cardiovascular risk factors in US women. *Frontiers in Endocrinology, 8*, 144. https://doi.org/10.3389/fendo.2017.00144 (accessed on 28th June 2025).

Singh, R., Farooq, S. A., Mannan, A., Singh, T. G., Najda, A., Ziemann-Gimmel, G., Albadrani, G. M., Sayed, A. A., & Abdel-Daim, M. M. (2022). Animal models of diabetic microvascular complications: Relevance to clinical features. *Biomedicine & Pharmacotherapy = Biomedecine & Pharmacotherapie, 145*, 112305. https://doi.org/10.1016/j.biopha.2021.112305 (accessed on 28th June 2025).

Singh, V. P., Bali, A., Singh, N., & Jaggi, A. S. (2014). Advanced glycation end products and diabetic complications. *Korean Journal of Physiology and Pharmacology, 18*(1), 1–14. https://doi.org/10.4196/kjpp.2014.18.1.1 (accessed on 28th June 2025).

Spaulonci, C. P., Bernardes, L. S., Trindade, T. C., Zugaib, M., & Francisco, R. P. V. (2013). Randomised trial of metformin vs insulin in the management of gestational diabetes. *American Journal of Obstetrics and Gynecology, 209*(1), 34.e1–34.e7. https://doi.org/10.1016/j.ajog.2013.03.022 (accessed on 28th June 2025).

Suffecool, K., Rosenn, B., Niederkofler, E. E., Kiernan, U. A., Foroutan, J., Antwi, K., Ribar, A., Bapat, P., & Koren, G. (2015). Insulin detemir does not cross the human placenta. *Diabetes Care, 38*, e20–e21. http://dx.doi.org/10.2337/dc14-2090 (accessed on 28th June 2025).

Swaminathan, G., Swaminathan, A., & Corsi, D. J. (2020). Prevalence of gestational diabetes in India by individual socioeconomic, demographic, and clinical factors. *JAMA Network Open, 3*(11), e2025074. https://doi.org/10.1001/jamanetworkopen.2020.2507 (accessed on 28th June 2025).

Thorens, B. (2005–2008). Glucose sensing and the pathogenesis of obesity and type 2 diabetes. *International Journal of Obesity, 32*(Suppl. 6), S62–S71. https://doi.org/10.3390/ijms19113342 (accessed on 28th June 2025).

Viana, L. V., Gross, J. L., & Azevedo, M. J. (2014). Dietary intervention in patients with gestational diabetes mellitus: A systematic review and meta-analysis of randomised clinical trials on maternal and newborn outcomes. *Diabetes Care, 37*, 3345–3355. https://doi.org/10.2337/dc14-1530 (accessed on 28th June 2025).

Vohr, B. R., & Boney, C. M. (2008). Gestational diabetes: The forerunner for the development of maternal and childhood obesity and metabolic syndrome. *The Journal of Maternal-Fetal & Neonatal Medicine, 21*(3), 149–157. https://doi.org/10.3390/ijms21145003 (accessed on 28th June 2025).

Wang, D., Li, J., Luo, G., Zhou, J., Wang, N., Wang, S., Zhao, R., Cao, X., Ma, Y., Liu, G., & Hao, L. (2023). Nox4 as a novel therapeutic target for diabetic vascular complications. *Redox Biology, 64*, 102781. https://doi.org/10.1016/j.redox.2023.102781 (accessed on 28th June 2025).

Weir, G. C., Laybutt, D. R., Kaneto, H., Bonner-Weir, S., & Sharma, A. (2001). Beta-cell adaptation and decompensation during the progression of diabetes. *Diabetes, 50*(Suppl. 1), S154–S159. http://dx.doi.org/10.2337/diabetes.50.2007.S154 (accessed on 28th June 2025).

Weir, G. C., Laybutt, D. R., Kaneto, H., Bonner-Weir, S., & Sharma, A. (2001). Beta-cell adaptation and decompensation during the progression of diabetes. *Diabetes, 50*(Suppl. 1), S154. https://doi.org/10.2337/diabetes.50.2007.s154 (accessed on 28th June 2025).

Williams, M. A., Qiu, C., Muy-Rivera, M., Vadachkoria, S., Song, T., & Luthy, D. A. (2004). Plasma adiponectin concentrations in early pregnancy and subsequent risk of gestational diabetes mellitus. *Journal of Clinical Endocrinology and Metabolism, 89*, 2306–2311. https://doi.org/10.1210/jc.2003-031201 (accessed on 28th June 2025).

Witkop, C., Neale, D., Wilson, L. M., Bass, E., & Nicholson, W. (2009). Active compared with expectant delivery management in women with gestational diabetes: A systematic review. *Obstetrics and Gynecology, 113*, 206–217. https://doi.org/10.1097/aog.0b013e31818db36f (accessed on 28th June 2025).

Wouldes, T. A., Battin, M., Coat, S., Rush, E. C., Hague, W. M., & Rowan, J. A. (2015). Neurodevelopmental outcome at two years in offspring of women randomised to metformin or insulin treatment for gestational diabetes. *Archives of Disease in Childhood. Fetal and Neonatal Edition, 101*(6), F488–F493. https://doi.org/10.1136/archdischild-2015-309602 (accessed on 28th June 2025).

Zhang, J., Ma, S., Guo, C., Long, S., Wu, S., & Tan, H. (2018). Research progress on etiology of gestational diabetes mellitus. *Global Health Journal, 2*(4), 19–27. http://dx.doi.org/10.1016/S2414-6447(19)30179-4 (accessed on 28th June 2025).

CHAPTER 3

Endocrine Diseases in Pregnancy and Their Latest Treatment Guidelines

ABRAHAM OLUFEMI ASUKU,[1,2,*] TOHEEB O. OYERINDE,[3]
TOBILOBA SAMUEL OLAJIDE,[3]
GBONJUBOLA OYINLOLA OGUNGBANGBE,[2] and
EBELE JOAN AJAGUN[1]

[1]*Bioresources Development Center, National Biotechnology Development Agency, Ogbomoso, Oyo, Nigeria*

[2]*Department of Physiology, Faculty of Basic Medical Sciences, College of Health Sciences, University of Ilorin, Ilorin, Kwara, Nigeria*

[3]*Laboratory for Experimental and Translational Neurobiology, University of Medical Sciences, Ondo, Nigeria*

*Corresponding author

ABSTRACT

This chapter examines the complex intersection of hormones and pregnancy from a pharmacological approach, with the significant physiological demands that pregnancy places on the endocrine system and the potential consequences for the health of both the mother and the fetus; this chapter will explore the most recent developments in the knowledge and treatment of endocrine disorders during pregnancy, with a focus on the changing field of pharmacological interventions. The first part offers a thorough review of the most prevalent endocrine diseases found in expectant women, including gestational diabetes, thyroid disorders, and adrenal dysfunctions. Each condition is examined in terms of its pathophysiology and effect on the maternal-fetal unit. Special attention

Precision Nutrition and Endocrine Health: Synthesis, Characterization, and Applications.
Thakur Gurjeet Singh and Sanjana Mehta (Eds.)

DOI: 10.1201/9781998511877-3

is given to the dynamic changes in hormone levels, signs and symptoms during pregnancy, and their possible impact on disease progression. The subsequent section will focus on the pharmacological methods to control endocrine disorders during pregnancy. These include drugs, therapy, and so on. Furthermore, the chapter provides a concise view of the difficulties in pharmacological management, stressing the risks and benefits during pregnancy as well as the effects of interactions with other pregnancy-related drugs across the three trimesters. It offers a pharmacologically driven study of the challenges posed by endocrine disorders during pregnancy and the cutting-edge therapeutic methods available to healthcare workers. The chapter ends by reviewing various essential points and stressing the importance of quick and appropriate pharmacological action. It would be a valuable resource for clinicians, researchers, and students wishing to gain a thorough grasp of the complex interactions between endocrinology and pregnancy, emphasizing the most recent developments in pharmaceutical therapies.

3.1 INTRODUCTION

Pregnancy itself induces substantial changes in regular physiological functions and endocrine states due to various influencing factors (Molitch, 2019; Morton and Teasdale, 2022). During pregnancy, there is an augmentation in plasma and red blood cell volume alongside an elevation in the glomerular filtration rate, leading to shifts in the typical hormone levels (Cheung and Lafayette, 2013; Molitch, 2019). Placental hormone production profoundly alters hormone balances and directly impacts the pituitary gland, which is the master gland of the endocrine system (Glezer and Bronstein, 2022; Mehta et al., 2022; Rihal et al., 2023). This, therefore, affects the growth of the developing fetus (Ashique et al., 2022; Johnson et al., 2018). An endocrine disorder in pregnancy pertains to a situation characterized by an irregularity or malfunction within the hormonal system during pregnancy.

In the past, pregnant women were predominantly left out of clinical drug research and the development of new drugs, primarily due to legal and ethical apprehensions (Ren et al., 2021). This omission resulted in the administration of drugs in clinical settings without thorough assessments of their suitability during pregnancy. Regrettably, this situation resulted in women using drugs such as Diethylstilbestrol and thalidomide that thalidomide, which have long been seen to have teratogenic effects (Gao et al., 2020; Hoover et al., 2011). As a result of the possible teratogenic effects over the past 20 years, extensive research has been conducted on this long-standing unresolved medication issue, and guidelines addressing the appropriate use and effectiveness of pharmacotherapy during pregnancy have been developed (Tsakiridis et al., 2022). The changes in the physiological and anatomical condition during pregnancy alter the PD and PK of medications, which can result in either excessive therapy with unforeseen adverse effects or insufficient intervention with poor therapeutic outcomes (Kazma et al., 2020).

3.2 COMMON ENDOCRINE DISORDERS IN PREGNANCY

Common endocrine disorders in pregnancy include various diseases, as shown in Figure 3.1.

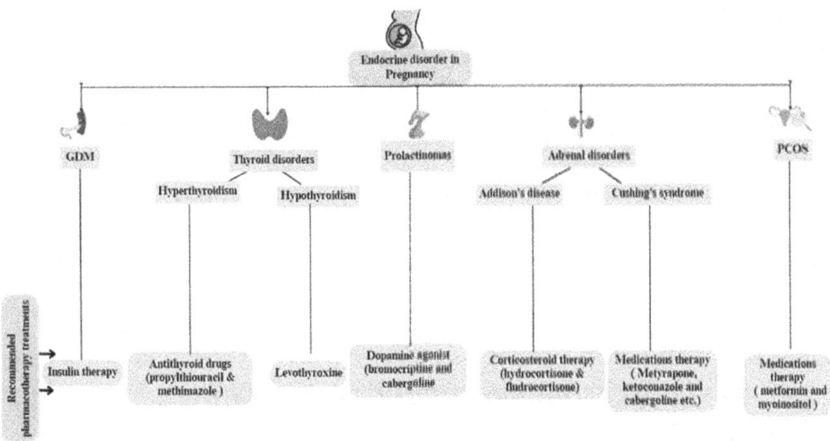

FIGURE 3.1 Endocrine disorders in pregnancy with recommended pharmacotherapy treatments. GDM: gestational diabetes mellitus; PCOS: polycystic ovarian syndrome.

3.2.1 GESTATIONAL DIABETES MELLITUS (GDM)

GDM is a prevalent complication during pregnancy defined by variable degrees of intolerance to glucose that either originates or is first identified during pregnancy (Association, 2012; Buchanan and Xiang, 2005).

As per the latest estimates from the Federation, in 2017, GDM impacts about 14% of pregnancies worldwide, accounting for roughly 18 million births per year. GDM stems from maternal pancreatic β-cell dysfunction, leading to insufficient insulin production, causing difficulties in regulating glucose levels during pregnancy (Plows et al., 2018). The risk factors for this maternal condition involve both non-modifiable elements like familial history of type 2 diabetes mellitus, polycystic ovary syndrome, and ethnic background, as well as easily avoidable factors such as maternal age, pre-pregnancy overweight, obesity, and excessive weight gain during pregnancy (Galtier, 2010; Plows et al., 2018). Insulin, a hormone secreted by the β-cells in the pancreas, facilitates the production and storage of glucose, lipids, and proteins while impeding their breakdown and subsequent release into the bloodstream (Aggarwal et al., 2023; Saltiel, 2016). Insulin resistance is when a normal average or increased insulin level elicits a weakened biological reaction, commonly indicating reduced sensitivity to insulin's role in facilitating the disposal of glucose (Reaven, 2004). According to Zhang et al. (2021), women who are diagnosed with gestational diabetes mellitus (GDM) may have outcomes such as gestational hypertension, preeclampsia, a higher risk of cesarean delivery, and cardiovascular diseases, including an increased likelihood of developing type 2 diabetes mellitus in the future (Metzger et al., 2019; Retnakaran et al., 2010). Moreover, babies given to moms with GDM are also at a larger possibility of suffering significant difficulties, with macrosomia being the most negative effect (Mitanchez, 2010). Considering the extensive ramifications of GDM on both mother and fetal well-being, it necessitates rapid and thorough care.

3.2.2 THYROID DISORDERS DURING PREGNANCY

In pregnancy, thyroid-binding globulin increases, and the thyroid gland undergoes hyperplasia and heightened vascularity. Maternal thyroid function undergoes various alterations during pregnancy, and insufficient adaptation to these changes can result in thyroid dysfunction (Sreelatha et al., 2017). This review focuses mainly on their treatment guidelines, notably the usage of antithyroid medication.

3.2.2.1 HYPOTHYROIDISM IN PREGNANCY

Around 2% to 3% of women are predicted to suffer hypothyroidism when pregnant (Teng et al., 2013). According to Stagnaro-Green, primary maternal hypothyroidism can be described as high Thyroid-Stimulating Hormone (TSH) concentration throughout pregnancy, save for exceptionally uncommon occurrences. During pregnancy, hypothyroidism is classed as either overt hypothyroidism (OH) or subclinical classifications (SCH), depending on the level of thyroid function impairment. Autoimmune thyroiditis, often known as Hashimoto's thyroiditis, is the leading cause of hypothyroidism during pregnancy in regions with appropriate iodine levels (De Groot et al., 2012; Singh et al., 2020). Evidence shows that both low iodine consumption and high iodine levels might potentially contribute to maternal and or fetal hypothyroidism (Connelly et al., 2012; Sang et al., 2012).

3.2.2.2 HYPERTHYROIDISM IN PREGNANCY

Hyperthyroidism develops in 1 or 2 out of every 1000 pregnancies, and it is acknowledged for its link to adverse outcomes for both the fetus and the mother (Cooper and Laurberg, 2013). Graves' disease, an autoimmune disorder triggered by antibodies that activate the stimulating thyroid-stimulating hormone receptor (TSHR), is the most common cause of hyperthyroidism in young women (Alexander et al., 2017; Cooper and Laurberg, 2013). Additional causes, including toxic multinodular goiter, hyperemesis gravidarum, subacute thyroiditis, and toxic adenoma goiter, hyperemesis gravidarum, subacute thyroiditis, and toxic adenoma, might also manifest (Lazarus, 2005). Less common causes comprise disorders including struma ovaria, hydatidiform mole, and documented occurrences involving a TSHR mutation. This mutation was mainly triggered during pregnancy in a family of recurrent gestational thyrotoxicosis due to hypersensitivity to HCG (human chorionic gonadotropin) from the mutant TSHR (Rodien et al., 2004). Maternal hyperthyroidism has been linked to advanced maternal age, multiple previous pregnancies, smoking habits, prior miscarriages, and being overweight or obese. Mothers found to have hyperthyroidism during pregnancy also showed to have higher chances of surgical delivery via cesarean section, placental separation, early deliveries, birthing smaller-than-expected infants for their gestational age, and the necessity for neonatal intensive care unit support (Turunen et al., 2020).

3.2.3 ADRENAL DISORDERS

Adrenal disorders that occur in the course of pregnancy constitute an uncommon and rare complication (Calina et al., 2019). The presentations of these ailments firmly match the signs and symptoms commonly usually associated with pregnancy (Gardella et al., 2022) creating a substantial obstacle in appropriately identifying such disorders.

3.2.3.1 ADDISON'S DISEASE

Addison's disease, also known as primary adrenal insufficiency, is a rare and chronic illness that affects 4 to 11 people out of every 100,000 (Oliveira et al., 2018). It occurs when approximately 90% of the adrenal gland is destroyed and is characterized by deficiencies in both glucocorticoids and mineralocorticoids, stemming from lesions in the adrenal glands caused by various mechanisms. In developed nations, the predominant etiology is autoimmune adrenalitis, constituting more than 70% of all instances of primary hypoadrenalism (Kronenberg et al., 2007). A decrease in weight, anorexia, extreme weariness, postural hypotension, stomach and muscular discomfort, and a low sodium level are the clinical characteristics (Husebye et al., 2021). A pregnant Addison patient is a highly unusual case in clinical practice because women with Addison tend to have lower conception rates and are typically detected even before pregnancy (Ahmed et al., 2021). The low fertility rate is due to the high presence of androgens. When low cortisol levels increase, androgens, particularly dehydroepiandrosterone (DHEA), may increase. Fortunately, with the introduction of glucocorticoid therapy, pregnancy has become less risky for Addison's disease Patients.

3.2.3.2 CUSHING'S SYNDROME

Similar to Addison's disease occurrence, Cushing's syndrome (CS), also referred to as hypercortisolemia, is an uncommon condition that seldom occurs during pregnancy (Pourali et al., 2017). Fewer than 250 cases have been documented, of which less than 100 have undergone active therapy (Sridharan et al., 2021). This relates to the reduced fertility it provides to women owing to abnormalities in the menstrual cycles induced by excessive elevation of cortisol (Bednarek-Tupikowska et al., 2011). In the general population without pregnancy, the projected yearly incidence is 1.2–3.2 cases per million (Hakami et al., 2021). CS can be caused by prolonged abnormal exposure to excess glucocorticoids or increased production of endogenous corticosteroids due to adrenal crisis, thereby leading to unique and significant signs (e.g., fatigue, weight gain, hypertension, edema, and hyperglycemia) and symptoms that are typically synonymous with pregnancy (Pourali et al., 2017). For this reason, CS during pregnancy is typically not identified until mid-gestation (Lindsay and Nieman, 2005). Thus, a detailed grasp of the various signs of CS throughout gestation is critical for efficient therapeutic care.

3.3 TREATMENT GUIDELINES FOR ENDOCRINE DISORDERS IN PREGNANCY

3.3.1 INSULIN THERAPY FOR GDM

Gestational diabetes mellitus contributes to various detrimental implications for both the mother and the developing fetus. These include maternal issues like gestational hypertension, preeclampsia, a higher chance of cesarean delivery, cardiovascular diseases, and a higher chance of developing type 2 diabetes in later life (Metzger et al., 2019; Retnakaran et al., 2010). Prenatal problems, including macrosomia, are also connected with GDM (Olmos et al., 2009; Rihal et al., 2022). Given these implications, addressing GDM requires immediate and focused attention. Among the diverse approaches to managing GDM, pharmacological methods stand out, with insulin therapy as a prime example. Nutrition therapy serves as the primary treatment for GDM. However, in cases where it proves ineffective, insulin therapy (IT) is commonly introduced. Due to its inability to cross the placenta, insulin is the preferred treatment for managing GDM (Association, 2020). As maternal hyperglycemia influences fetal glucose levels, insulin therapy emerges as an efficient method for attaining normal D-glucose levels in the fetus (Sobrevia et al., 2015). Insulin therapy has been linked to beneficial effects, including a reduced incidence of macrosomia (Saez et al., 2018) and a lower rate of cesarean sections, alongside a decrease in cranial-thoracic circumference ratios compared to insulin analogs (You et al., 2016).

3.3.2 ANTITHYROID MEDICATIONS FOR THYROID DISORDERS

Antithyroid drugs, utilized for over half a century, continue to be fundamental in managing thyroid disorders, most especially hyperthyroidism (Cooper, 2005). Antithyroid drugs (e.g., propylthiouracil, methimazole, and carbimazole) are the primary treatment for thyroid disorder in pregnancy (Delitala et al., 2019), although these medications are not devoid of side effects. Antithyroid drugs, classified as thioamides, are relatively uncomplicated molecules of a sulfhydryl group and a thiourea component incorporated into a heterocyclic structure. These thioamides hinder the synthesis of thyroid hormones by impeding the iodination and coupling of tyrosine residues linked to thyroglobulin catalyzed by thyroid peroxidase (Cooper, 2005; Burch and Cooper, 2018). These medications exert other significant effects. Propylthiouracil differs from methimazole or carbimazole in its ability to impede the conversion of thyroxine to triiodothyronine within the thyroid and peripheral tissues. However, this impact is typically insignificant (Cooper, 2005). Nevertheless, earlier studies have indicated a continued elevated risk of perinatal complications despite the treatment of hyperthyroidism with antithyroid drugs (Andersen et al., 2014; Sheehan et al., 2015). Both medications, propylthiouracil and methimazole, cross the placenta and have been connected to fetal abnormalities (Andersen et al., 2016; Nguyen et al., 2018). On the other hand, for the treatment of hypothyroidism, the use of levothyroxine has been used in pregnant women. However, use remains controversial because existing studies have not provided conclusive evidence regarding the positive effects of the treatment on maternal obstetric outcomes or the child's neurodevelopment (Lee and Pearce, 2022).

3.3.5 CORTICOSTEROID THERAPY FOR ADDISON'S DISEASE

Patients with Addison can be adequately treated during pregnancy if carefully monitored, as some case studies have been successfully reported (Lebbe and Arlt, 2013; Margulies et al., 2020). However, in instances of inadequately treated Addison's disease, the growing fetus may not face detriment due to the inherent steroidogenic capabilities of the fetoplacental system (Khakha et al., 2023; Lekarev and New, 2011). However, a study in 2017 indicated that, overall, individuals with Addison's disease face an elevated likelihood of adverse outcomes, encompassing preterm premature rupture of membranes, preterm delivery, and fetal growth restriction (Schneiderman et al., 2017). To have a successful pregnancy outcome for both the mother and the fetus, the use of corticosteroid therapy has been suggested to be the most commonly used treatment (Oliveira et al., 2018). Observing pregnant individuals undergoing steroid replacement poses challenges as symptoms of both over-prescription, such as gestational diabetes, excessive weight gain, and arterial hypertension, and under-prescription, such as low birth weight, the adrenal crisis in the mother and electrolyte imbalance of the medication, often mimic typical manifestations observed in a regular pregnancy (Kumar et al., 2023; Margulies et al., 2020). Therefore, this corticosteroid therapy should be carefully monitored and regulated. The approved FDA drugs for Addison patients are hydrocortisone and fludrocortisone; both drugs have been considered safe during pregnancy when usage and dosage are regulated. In addition, hydrocortisone is also safe for breastfeeding women as its overall excretion into breast milk is considerably low (Lekarev and New, 2011).

3.3.6 TREATMENT FOR CUSHING'S SYNDROME

The therapeutic approach for a patient with CS is highly personalized, with the choice between surgery, medical control of hypercortisolism, or opting for a conservative approach contingent upon factors such as the timing of diagnosis about the stage of gestation, the capability to pinpoint the tumor, the severity of the disease, pre-existing maternal comorbidities, and, ultimately, patient choice (Graillon et al., 2020; Hamblin et al., 2022). Collaboration and synergistic teamwork among diverse disciplines is imperative for optimal treatment (Fountas et al., 2021; Garg et al., 2022). During a normal pregnancy, there is an elevation in ACTH, CRH, cortisol, and urinary-free cortisol levels. Therefore, the administration of dexamethasone does not act as a negative feedback to inhibit cortisol in average pregnant women devoid of CS. Transsphenoidal pituitary surgery is the first-line therapy for patients with CS (Bronstein et al., 2015), while adrenalectomy for adrenal causes of CS, like adenomas and carcinomas, can be performed in both the second and third semesters (Vilar et al., 2007). However, in cases of unsuccessful surgery or in patients who are not surgical candidates, medical therapy like Metyrapone, ketoconazole, cabergoline, cyproheptadine, and aminoglutethimide have been used to control symptoms (Hamblin et al., 2022).

3.4 PHARMACOLOGICAL CONSIDERATION

3.4.1 DRUG SAFETY DURING PREGNANCY

Complete avoidance of pharmacological interventions during pregnancy is not feasible and, in some cases, can pose a detrimental effect on the mother and developing fetus. This is because certain women enter pregnancy with pre-existing medical conditions or known endocrine disorders related to pregnancy, as mentioned in this review. All these disorders necessitate continuous or occasional treatment. The use of inappropriate medication during pregnancy is linked to unfavorable pregnancy outcomes, thus underscoring the importance of establishing a pregnancy drug registry to oversee and ensure the safety of drugs during pregnancy (Choudhary et al., 2021).

In most developing countries, pregnant women frequently resort to over-the-counter medications (Devi et al., 2023; Edet et al., 2023; Rahmani et al., 2019), as four out of five pregnant women receive at least one prescription (Daw et al., 2011). While many over-the-counter drugs are generally safe, certain ones lack proven safety data or are recognized to have adverse effects on the developing fetus because most of these drugs can cross the placenta (Gedeon and Koren, 2006). The safety assessment of specific medications may vary depending on the gestational stage, especially during the first trimester, when the development of the embryo and fetus occurs (Schaefer et al., 2014). Most antacids, kaolin and pectin preparations, acetaminophen, and chlorpheniramine are over-the-counter medications with a good safety record for pregnant women. However, due to possible fetal risks, other OTC medications like atropine/diphenoxylate, pseudoephedrine, and histamine H2-receptor blockers should be used with caution (Black and Hill, 2003; Singh et al., 2020), including many other psychostimulants described by Ross et al. (2015) and numerous drugs listed by Dathe and Schaefer (2019) should be avoided given that some of the congenital disabilities are attributed to maternal drug exposure. It is necessary to look into the risks and benefits of medications and monitor their adjustment during pregnancy.

3.4.2 MONITORING AND ADJUSTING MEDICATIONS

Monitoring and modifying medication during pregnancy is essential to maternal and fetal healthcare throughout the trimester. Physiological and pharmacokinetic changes during pregnancy significantly alter the disposition and reaction to drugs, demanding careful monitoring and modification of prescription regimens (Eke et al., 2023). A comprehensive assessment for monitoring and modifying various pharmaceuticals used throughout all trimesters is essential to minimize the possible hazards of medications on both the mother and fetus (Mehta et al., 2021). The first trimester is the most sensitive stage of embryonic development, as exposure to teratogenic drugs during this stage can have a significant effect on the normal development of the embryo, possibly leading to congenital abnormalities. Therefore, medicines that are teratogenic should be avoided during this time. In addition, maternal health, nausea, and vomiting are prominent throughout the first trimester. Hence, drug-induced emesis should also be avoided if feasible.

3.5 CONCLUSION AND RECOMMENDATION

Pregnancy induces extensive modifications in normal physiological functioning and endocrine states, mediated by many influencing elements. These complicated endocrine variables largely influence fetal development. Among these elements, placental hormones have a substantial effect, generating a hormonal cascade that directly influences the master gland of the body, the pituitary gland. However, the numerous hormones the placenta generates improve nutrition absorption to assist Embryonic Development. The combination of endocrine changes during pregnancy underlines the vital need to maintain hormonal homeostasis. While endocrine problems during pregnancy can lead to unfavorable fetal outcomes and heightened mother morbidity, competent therapy can reduce their effects on both the mother's and child's health. Notably, well-controlled conditions with appropriate treatments demonstrate a minimal impact on the general health of the mother and the growing baby. In some conditions, including adrenal disorders, hyperparathyroidism, or polycystic ovarian syndrome (PCOS), the manifestations closely match the frequent signs and symptoms associated with pregnancy, such as nausea, emesis, increased maternal weight, and exhaustion. This overlap of signs and symptoms provides some substantial issues in identifying between persons with typical pregnancy symptoms and those indicative of underlying endocrine abnormalities. Therefore, the precise identification of these illnesses during pregnancy provides a great difficulty, stressing the necessity for a sophisticated and proactive approach to promote optimal mother and fetal health. In managing different endocrine disorders during pregnancy, if surgery is not an option, the best advice is to use any medication and gather a thorough medical history through a multidisciplinary approach with good communication between the endocrinologist, obstetrician, and pediatrician.

KEYWORDS

- **endocrine disorder**
- **insulin therapy**
- **medication**
- **pharmacological**
- **pregnancy**
- **treatment**

REFERENCES

Adams Waldorf, K. M., & Nelson, J. L. (2008). Autoimmune disease during pregnancy and the microchimerism legacy of pregnancy. *Immunological Investigations, 37*(5–6), 631–644. https://doi.org/10.1080/08820130802205886 (accessed on 28th June 2025).

Ahmed, M., Bashir, M., Okunoye, G. O., & Konje, J. C. (2021). Adrenal disease and pregnancy: An overview. *The Obstetrician & Gynaecologist, 23*(4), 265–277. http://dx.doi.org/10.1111/tog.12761 (accessed on 28th June 2025).

Alexander, E. K., Pearce, E. N., Brent, G. A., Brown, R. S., Chen, H., Dosiou, C., Grobman, W. A., Laurberg, P., Lazarus, J. H., & Mandel, S. J. (2017). 2017 guidelines of the American Thyroid Association for diagnosing and managing thyroid disease during pregnancy and postpartum. *Thyroid, 27*(3), 315–389. https://doi.org/10.1089/thy.2016.0457 (accessed on 28th June 2025).

Amaya García, M., Acosta Feria, M., Soto Moreno, A., Dios Fuentes, E., Navarro González, E., Quijada Thong, D., Del Valle, A., Acosta Delgado, D., & Astorga Jiménez,

R. (2004). Primary hyperparathyroidism in pregnancy. *Gynecological Endocrinology, 19*(2), 111–114. https://doi.org/10.1080/09513590400002334 (accessed on 28th June 2025).

Andersen, S. L., Olsen, J., & Laurberg, P. (2016). Antithyroid drug side effects in the population and pregnancy. *The Journal of Clinical Endocrinology & Metabolism, 101*(4), 1606–1614. https://doi.org/10.1210/jc.2015-4274 (accessed on 28th June 2025).

Andersen, S. L., Olsen, J., Wu, C. S., & Laurberg, P. (2014). Spontaneous abortion, stillbirth and hyperthyroidism: A Danish population-based study. *European Thyroid Journal, 3*(3), 164–172. https://doi.org/10.1159/000365101 (accessed on 28th June 2025).

Anderson, G. M., Kieser, D. C., Steyn, F. J., & Grattan, D. R. (2008). Hypothalamic prolactin receptor messenger ribonucleic acid levels, prolactin signalling, and hyperprolactinemic inhibition of pulsatile luteinising hormone secretion depend on estradiol. *Endocrinology, 149*(4), 1562–1570. https://doi.org/10.1210/en.2007-0867 (accessed on 28th June 2025).

Armanini, D., Boscaro, M., Bordin, L., & Sabbadin, C. (2022). Controversies in the pathogenesis, diagnosis and treatment of PCOS: Focus on insulin resistance, inflammation, and hyperandrogenism. *International Journal of Molecular Sciences, 23*(8), 4110. https://doi.org/10.3390/ijms23084110 (accessed on 28th June 2025).

Artini, P. G., Obino, M. E. R., Sergiampietri, C., Pinelli, S., Papini, F., Casarosa, E., & Cela, V. (2018). PCOS and pregnancy: A review of available therapies to improve the outcome of pregnancy in women with polycystic ovary syndrome. *Expert Review of Endocrinology & Metabolism, 13*(2), 87–98. https://doi.org/10.1080/17446651.2018.1431122 (accessed on 28th June 2025).

Ashique, S., De Rubis, G., Sirohi, E., Mishra, N., Rihan, M., Garg, A., Reyes, R. J., Manandhar, B., Bhatt, S., Jha, N. K., Singh, T. G., Gupta, G., Singh, S. K., Chellappan, D. K., Paudel, K. R., Hansbro, P. M., Oliver, B. G., & Dua, K. (2022). Short chain fatty acids: Fundamental mediators of the gut–lung axis and their involvement in pulmonary diseases. *Chemico-Biological Interactions, 368*, 110231. https://doi.org/10.1016/j.cbi.2022.110231 (accessed on 28th June 2025).

Association, A. D. (2012). Diagnosis and classification of diabetes mellitus. *Diabetes Care, 36*(Supplement_1), S67–S74. https://doi.org/10.2337/dc13-S067 (accessed on 28th June 2025).

Association, A. D. (2015). 12. Management of diabetes in pregnancy. *Diabetes Care, 38*(Supplement_1), S77–S79. https://doi.org/10.2337/dc15-S015 (accessed on 28th June 2025).

Association, A. D. (2020). 14. Management of diabetes in pregnancy: Standards of medical care in diabetes—2020. *Diabetes Care, 43*(Supplement_1), S183–S192. https://doi.org/10.2337/dc20-s014 (accessed on 28th June 2025).

Bahri Khomami, M., Moran, L. J., Kenny, L., Grieger, J. A., Myers, J., Poston, L., McCowan, L., Walker, J., Dekker, G., & Norman, R. (2019). Lifestyle and pregnancy complications in polycystic ovary syndrome: The SCOPE cohort study. *Clinical Endocrinology, 90*(6), 814–821. https://doi.org/10.1111/cen.13954 (accessed on 28th June 2025).

Bednarek-Tupikowska, G., Kubicka, E., Sicińska-Werner, T., Kazimierczak, A., Winowski, J., Tupikowska, M., Janczyszyn, M., & Bolanowski, M. (2011). A case of Cushing's syndrome in pregnancy. *Endokrynologia Polska, 62*(2), 181–185. https://doi.org/10.1007/s11102-014-0627-0 (accessed on 28th June 2025).

Black, R. A., & Hill, D. A. (2003). Over-the-counter medications in pregnancy. *American Family Physician, 67*(12), 2517–2524. https://doi.org/10.1097/nmc.0000000000000537 (accessed on 28th June 2025).

Bronstein, M., Machado, M., & Fragoso, M. (2015). Management of endocrine disease: Management of pregnant patients with Cushing's syndrome. *European Journal of Endocrinology, 173*(2), R85–R91. https://doi.org/10.1530/eje-14-1130 (accessed on 28th June 2025).

Buchanan, T. A., & Xiang, A. H. (2005). Gestational diabetes mellitus. *The Journal of Clinical Investigation, 115*(3), 485–491. https://doi.org/10.1172/jci24531 (accessed on 28th June 2025).

Burch, H. B., & Cooper, D. S. (2018). Antithyroid drug therapy: 70 years later. *European Journal of Endocrinology, 179*(5), R261–R274. https://doi.org/10.1530/eje-18-0678 (accessed on 28th June 2025).

Calina, D., Docea, A. O., Golokhvast, K. S., Sifakis, S., Tsatsakis, A., & Makrigiannakis, A. (2019). Management of endocrinopathies in pregnancy: A review of current evidence. *International Journal of Environmental Research and Public Health, 16*(5), 781. https://doi.org/10.3390/ijerph16050781 (accessed on 28th June 2025).

Cheung, K. L., & Lafayette, R. A. (2013). Renal physiology of pregnancy. *Advances in Chronic Kidney Disease, 20*(3), 209–214. https://doi.org/10.1053/j.ackd.2013.01.012 (accessed on 28th June 2025).

Choudhary, C., Bandyopadhyay, A., Bahadur, A., Chaturvedi, J., Handu, S., & Dhamija, P. (2021). Drug-related adverse pregnancy outcomes at a tertiary care hospital from the foothills of the Himalayas: A prospective observational study. *Journal of Family Medicine and Primary Care, 10*(11), 4176. https://doi.org/10.4103/jfmpc.jfmpc_211_21 (accessed on 28th June 2025).

Cleary, B. J., Butt, H., Strawbridge, J. D., Gallagher, P. J., Fahey, T., & Murphy, D. J. (2010). Medication use in early pregnancy: Prevalence and determinants of use in a prospective cohort of women. *Pharmacoepidemiology and Drug Safety, 19*(4), 408–417. http://dx.doi.org/10.1002/pds.1906 (accessed on 28th June 2025).

Connelly, K. J., Boston, B. A., Pearce, E. N., Sesser, D., Snyder, D., Braverman, L. E., Pino, S., & LaFranchi, S. H. (2012). Congenital hypothyroidism is caused by excess prenatal maternal iodine ingestion. *The Journal of Pediatrics, 161*(4), 760–762. https://doi.org/10.1016/j.jpeds.2012.05.057 (accessed on 28th June 2025).

Cooper, D. S., & Laurberg, P. (2013). Hyperthyroidism in pregnancy. *The Lancet Diabetes & Endocrinology, 1*(3), 238–249. https://doi.org/10.1016/s2213-8587(13)70086 (accessed on 28th June 2025).

Cosimo, C., & Franco, C. (2009). Addison's disease and pregnancy: Case report. *Journal of Prenatal Medicine, 3*(4), 53. https://doi.org/10.3233/npm-190231 (accessed on 28th June 2025).

Cunningham, F. G., Leveno, K. J., Bloom, S. L., Spong, C. Y., Dashe, J. S., Hoffman, B. L., Casey, B. M., & Sheffield, J. S. (2014). *Williams obstetrics* (Vol. 7). McGraw-Hill Medical New York. https://doi.org/10.4236/ahs.2015.44023 (accessed on 28th June 2025).

Dathe, K., & Schaefer, C. (2019). The use of medication in pregnancy. *Deutsches Ärzteblatt International, 116*(46), 783. https://doi.org/10.3238/arztebl.2019.0783 (accessed on 28th June 2025).

Daw, J. R., Hanley, G. E., Greyson, D. L., & Morgan, S. G. (2011). Prescription drug use during pregnancy in developed countries: A systematic review. *Pharmacoepidemiology and Drug Safety, 20*(9), 895–902. https://doi.org/10.1002/pds.2184 (accessed on 28th June 2025).

de Escobar, G. M., Obregón, M. A. J., & del Rey, F. E. (2004). Maternal thyroid hormones early in pregnancy and fetal brain development. *Best Practice & Research Clinical Endocrinology & Metabolism, 18*(2), 225–248. https://doi.org/10.1016/j.beem.2004.03.012 (accessed on 28th June 2025).

De Groot, L., Abalovich, M., Alexander, E. K., Amino, N., Barbour, L., Cobin, R. H., Eastman, C. J., Lazarus, J. H., Luton, D., & Mandel, S. J. (2012). Management of thyroid dysfunction during pregnancy and postpartum: An Endocrine Society clinical practice guideline. *The Journal of Clinical Endocrinology & Metabolism, 97*(8), 2543–2565. https://doi.org/10.1210/jc.2011-2803 (accessed on 28th June 2025).

Delgrange, E., Vasiljevic, A., Wierinckx, A., François, P., Jouanneau, E., Raverot, G., & Trouillas, J. (2015). Expression of estrogen receptor alpha is associated with prolactin pituitary tumour prognosis and supports the sex-related difference in tumour growth. *European Journal of Endocrinology, 172*(6), 791–801. https://doi.org/10.1530/eje-14-0990 (accessed on 28th June 2025).

Delitala, A. P., Capobianco, G., Cherchi, P. L., Dessole, S., & Delitala, G. (2019). Thyroid function and thyroid disorders during pregnancy: A review and care pathway. *Archives of Gynecology and Obstetrics, 299*, 327–338. https://doi.org/10.1007/s00404-018-5018-8 (accessed on 28th June 2025).

Della Corte, L., Foreste, V., Barra, F., Gustavino, C., Alessandri, F., Centurioni, M. G., Ferrero, S., Bifulco, G., & Giampaolino, P. (2020). Current and experimental drug therapy for the treatment of polycystic ovarian syndrome. *Expert Opinion on Investigational Drugs, 29*(8), 819–830. https://doi.org/10.1080/13543784.2020.1781815 (accessed on 28th June 2025).

Devi, S., Chauhan, S., Mannan, A., & Singh, T. G. (2024). Targeting cardiovascular risk factors with eugenol: An anti-inflammatory perspective. *Inflammopharmacology, 32*(1), 307–317. https://doi.org/10.1007/s10787-023-01392-w (accessed on 28th June 2025).

Di Cianni, G., Volpe, L., Ghio, A., Lencioni, C., Cuccuru, I., Benzi, L., & Del Prato, S. (2007). Maternal metabolic control and perinatal outcome in women with gestational diabetes mellitus treated with lispro or aspart insulin: Comparison with regular insulin. *Diabetes Care, 30*(4), e11–e11. https://doi.org/10.2337/dc06-2586 (accessed on 28th June 2025).

Djokanovic, N., Klieger-Grossmann, C., & Koren, G. (2008). Does treatment with bisphosphonates endanger the human pregnancy? *Journal of Obstetrics and Gynaecology Canada, 30*(12), 1146–1148. https://doi.org/10.1016/s1701-2163(16)34026-9 (accessed on 28th June 2025).

Edet, C. K., Wegbom, A. I., Samuel, K. G., Sapira-Ordu, L., Jaja, I. D., Ene-Peter, J., Harold, I., Onyema, C., Pepple, B. G., & Fagbamigbe, A. F. (2023). Prevalence and factors influencing self-medication among pregnant women attending antenatal clinics in urban tertiary hospitals in Nigeria. *BioMed, 3*(1), 166–176. https://doi.org/10.3390/biomed3010014 (accessed on 28th June 2025).

Eke, A. C., Gebreyohannes, R. D., Fernandes, M. F. S., & Pillai, V. C. (2023). Physiologic changes during pregnancy and impact on small-molecule drugs, biologic (monoclonal antibody) disposition, and response. *The Journal of Clinical Pharmacology, 63*, S34–S50. https://doi.org/10.1002/jcph.2227 (accessed on 28th June 2025).

Federation, I. (2017). *IDF Diabetes Atlas* (8th ed.). International Diabetes Federation. https://doi.org/10.1016/j.diabres.2018.02.023 (accessed on 28th June 2025).

Feghali, M., Venkataramanan, R., & Caritis, S. (2015). Pharmacokinetics of drugs in pregnancy. *Seminars in Perinatology.* https://doi.org/10.1053/j.semperi.2015.08.003 (accessed on 28th June 2025).

Fernandino, J. I., Hattori, R. S., Acosta, O. D. M., Strüssmann, C. A., & Somoza, G. M. (2013). Environmental stress-induced testis differentiation: Androgen as a by-product of cortisol inactivation. *General and Comparative Endocrinology, 192*, 36–44. https://doi.org/10.1016/j.ygcen.2013.05.024 (accessed on 28th June 2025).

Fountas, A., Hamblin, R., Criseno, S., & Karavitaki, N. (2021). Multidisciplinary team perspective: A model of care for patients with pituitary tumours. In *Pituitary Tumors* (pp. 679–685). Elsevier. http://dx.doi.org/10.1016/B978-0-12-819949-7.00050-0 (accessed on 28th June 2025).

Frise, C. J., & Williamson, C. (2013). Endocrine disease in pregnancy. *Clinical Medicine, 13*(2), 176. https://doi.org/10.7861/clinmedicine.13-2-176 (accessed on 28th June 2025).

Galtier, F. (2010). Definition, epidemiology, risk factors. *Diabetes & Metabolism, 36*(6 Pt 2), 628–651. https://doi.org/10.1016/j.diabet.2010.11.014 (accessed on 28th June 2025).

Gao, S., Wang, S., Fan, R., & Hu, J. (2020). Recent advances in the molecular mechanism of thalidomide teratogenicity. *Biomedicine & Pharmacotherapy, 127*, 110114. https://doi.org/10.1016/j.biopha.2020.110114 (accessed on 28th June 2025).

Gardella, B., Gritti, A., Scatigno, A. L., Gallotti, A. M. C., Perotti, F., & Dominoni, M. (2022). Adrenal crisis during pregnancy: Case report and obstetric perspective. *Frontiers in Medicine, 9*, 891101. https://doi.org/10.3389/fmed.2022.891101 (accessed on 28th June 2025).

Garg, C., Khan, H., Kaur, A., Singh, T. G., Sharma, V. K., & Singh, S. K. (2022). Therapeutic implications of sonic hedgehog pathway in metabolic disorders: Novel target for effective treatment. *Pharmacological Research, 179*, 106194. https://doi.org/10.1016/j.phrs.2022.106194 (accessed on 28th June 2025).

Gedeon, C., & Koren, G. (2006). We are designing pregnancy-centered medications: Drugs that do not cross the human placenta. *Placenta, 27*(8), 861–868. https://doi.org/10.1016/j.placenta.2005.09.001 (accessed on 28th June 2025).

Graillon, T., Cuny, T., Castinetti, F., Courbiere, B., Cousin, M., Albarel, F., Morange, I., Bruder, N., Brue, T., & Dufour, H. (2020). Surgical indications for pituitary tumours during pregnancy: A literature review. *Pituitary, 23*, 189–199. https://doi.org/10.1007/s11102-019-01004-3 (accessed on 28th June 2025).

Hakami, O. A., Ahmed, S., & Karavitaki, N. (2021). Epidemiology and mortality of Cushing's syndrome. *Best Practice & Research Clinical Endocrinology & Metabolism, 35*(1), 101521. https://doi.org/10.1016/j.beem.2021.101521 (accessed on 28th June 2025).

Hamblin, R., Coulden, A., Fountas, A., & Karavitaki, N. (2022). The diagnosis and management of Cushing's syndrome in pregnancy. *Journal of Neuroendocrinology, 34*(8), e13118. https://doi.org/10.1111/jne.13118 (accessed on 28th June 2025).

Hirsch, D., Kopel, V., Nadler, V., Levy, S., Toledano, Y., & Tsvetov, G. (2015). Pregnancy outcomes in women with primary hyperparathyroidism. *The Journal of Clinical*

Endocrinology & Metabolism, 100(5), 2115–2122. https://doi.org/10.1210/jc.2015-1110 (accessed on 28th June 2025).

Hoover, R. N., Hyer, M., Pfeiffer, R. M., Adam, E., Bond, B., Cheville, A. L., Colton, T., Hartge, P., Hatch, E. E., & Herbst, A. L. (2011). Adverse health outcomes in women exposed in utero to diethylstilbestrol. *New England Journal of Medicine, 365*(14), 1304–1314. https://doi.org/10.1056/nejmoa1013961 (accessed on 28th June 2025).

Husebye, E. S., Pearce, S. H., Krone, N. P., & Kämpe, O. (2021). Adrenal insufficiency. *The Lancet, 397*(10274), 613–629. https://doi.org/10.1016/s0140-6736(21)00136-7 (accessed on 28th June 2025).

Johnson, M. S., Jackson, D. L., & Schust, D. J. (2018). Endocrinology of pregnancy. https://doi.org/10.1002/jcph.2126 (accessed on 28th June 2025).

Kazma, J. M., van den Anker, J., Allegaert, K., Dallmann, A., & Ahmadzia, H. K. (2020). Anatomical and physiological alterations of pregnancy. *Journal of Pharmacokinetics and Pharmacodynamics, 47*(4), 271–285. https://doi.org/10.1007/s10928-020-09677-1 (accessed on 28th June 2025).

Keller-Wood, M., Von Reitzenstein, M., & McCartney, J. (2008). Is the fetal lung a mineralocorticoid receptor target organ? Induction of cortisol-regulated genes in the ovine fetal lung, kidney and small intestine. *Neonatology, 95*(1), 47–60. https://doi.org/10.1159/000151755 (accessed on 28th June 2025).

Khakha, N., Khan, H., Kaur, A., & Singh, T. G. (2023). Therapeutic implications of phosphorylation- and dephosphorylation-dependent factors of cAMP-response element-binding protein (CREB) in neurodegeneration. *Pharmacological Reports: PR, 75*(5), 1152–1165. https://doi.org/10.1007/s43440-023-00526-9 (accessed on 28th June 2025).

Kronenberg, G., Melmed, S., Polonski, K., & Larsen, P. (2007). *Williams endocrinology. Diabetes mellitus and disorders of carbohydrate metabolism*. https://doi.org/10.4183/aeb.2016.113 (accessed on 28th June 2025).

Kumar, M., Nguyen, T. P. N., Kaur, J., Singh, T. G., Soni, D., Singh, R., & Kumar, P. (2023). Opportunities and challenges in application of artificial intelligence in pharmacology. *Pharmacological Reports: PR, 75*(1), 3–18. https://doi.org/10.1007/s43440-022-00445-1 (accessed on 28th June 2025).

Laloi-Michelin, M., Ciraru-Vigneron, N., & Meas, T. (2007). Cabergoline treatment of pregnant women with macroprolactinomas. *International Journal of Gynaecology and Obstetrics, 99*(1), 61–62. https://doi.org/10.1016/j.ijgo.2007.04.027 (accessed on 28th June 2025).

Lazarus, J. H. (2005). Hyperthyroidism during pregnancy: Etiology, diagnosis and management. *Women's Health, 1*(1), 97–104. https://doi.org/10.1517/17455057.1.1.097 (accessed on 28th June 2025).

Lazarus, J., Brown, R. S., Daumerie, C., Hubalewska-Dydejczyk, A., Negro, R., & Vaidya, B. (2014). 2014 European Thyroid Association guidelines for the management of subclinical hypothyroidism in pregnancy and children. *European Thyroid Journal, 3*(2), 76–94. https://doi.org/10.1159/000362597 (accessed on 28th June 2025).

Lebbe, M., & Arlt, W. (2013). What is the best diagnostic and therapeutic management strategy for an Addison patient during pregnancy? *Clinical Endocrinology, 78*(4), 497–502. https://doi.org/10.1111/cen.12097 (accessed on 28th June 2025).

Lee, S. Y., & Pearce, E. N. (2022). Assessment and treatment of thyroid disorders in pregnancy and the postpartum period. *Nature Reviews Endocrinology, 18*(3), 158–171. https://doi.org/10.1038/s41574-021-00604-z (accessed on 28th June 2025).

Lekarev, O., & New, M. I. (2011). Adrenal disease in pregnancy. *Best Practice & Research Clinical Endocrinology & Metabolism, 25*(6), 959–973. https://doi.org/10.1016/j.beem.2011.08.004 (accessed on 28th June 2025).

Li, S., Yang, C., Fan, J., Yao, Y., Lv, X., Guo, Y., & Zhang, S. (2020). Pregnancy-induced Cushing's syndrome with an adrenocortical adenoma overexpressing LH/hCG receptors: A case report. *BMC Endocrine Disorders, 20*(1), 1–6. https://doi.org/10.1186/s12902-020-0539-0 (accessed on 28th June 2025).

Lin, W., Huang, H.-B., Wen, J.-P., Wang, N.-Y., Wang, S.-Y., Wang, C., & Chen, G. (2019). Approach to Cushing's syndrome in pregnancy: Two cases of Cushing's syndrome in pregnancy and a literature review. *Annals of Translational Medicine, 7*(18). https://doi.org/10.21037/atm.2019.07.94 (accessed on 28th June 2025).

Lindsay, J. R., & Nieman, L. K. (2005). The hypothalamic-pituitary-adrenal axis in pregnancy: Challenges in disease detection and treatment. *Endocrine Reviews, 26*(6), 775–799. https://doi.org/10.1210/er.2004-0025 (accessed on 28th June 2025).

Lindsay, J. R., Jonklaas, J., Oldfield, E. H., & Nieman, L. K. (2005). Cushing's syndrome during pregnancy: Personal experience and review of the literature. *The Journal of Clinical Endocrinology & Metabolism, 90*(5), 3077–3083. https://doi.org/10.1210/jc.2004-2361 (accessed on 28th June 2025).

Maiter, D. (2019). Management of dopamine agonist-resistant prolactinoma. *Neuroendocrinology, 109*(1), 42–50. https://doi.org/10.1159/000495775 (accessed on 28th June 2025).

Margulies, S. L., Corrigan, K., Bathgate, S., & Macri, C. (2020). Addison's disease in pregnancy: Case report, management, and literature review. *Journal of Neonatal-Perinatal Medicine, 13*(2), 275–278. https://doi.org/10.3233/npm-190231 (accessed on 28th June 2025).

Mehta, S., Nain, P., Agrawal, B. K., & Singh, R. P. (2022). Vitamin D with calcium supplementation managing glycemic control with HbA1c and improve quality of life in patients with diabetes. *Turkish Journal of Pharmaceutical Sciences, 19*(2), 161–167. https://doi.org/10.4274/tjps.galenos.2021.62357 (accessed on 28th June 2025).

Mehta, S., Nain, P., Agrawal, B. K., Singh, R. P., Kaur, J., Maity, S., Bhattacharjee, A., Peela, J., Nauhria, S., & Nauhria, S. (2021). Effectiveness of empagliflozin with vitamin D supplementation in peripheral neuropathy in type 2 diabetic patients. *Cureus, 13*(12), e20208. https://doi.org/10.7759/cureus.20208 (accessed on 28th June 2025).

Metzger, B. E., Buchanan, T. A., Coustan, D. R., De Leiva, A., Dunger, D. B., Hadden, D. R., Hod, M., Kitzmiller, J. L., Kjos, S. L., & Oats, J. N. (2007). Summary and recommendations of the Fifth International Workshop-Conference on Gestational Diabetes Mellitus. *Diabetes Care, 30*(Supplement_2), S251–S260. https://doi.org/10.2337/dc07-s225 (accessed on 28th June 2025).

Metzger, B. E., Coustan, D. R., & Trimble, E. R. (2019). Hyperglycemia and adverse pregnancy outcomes. *Clinical Chemistry, 65*(7), 937–938. https://doi.org/10.1056/nejmoa0707943 (accessed on 28th June 2025).

Mitanchez, D. (2010). Foetal and neonatal complications in gestational diabetes: Perinatal mortality, congenital malformations, macrosomia, shoulder dystocia, birth injuries, neonatal complications. *Diabetes & Metabolism, 36*(6 Pt 2), 617–627. https://doi.org/10.1016/j.diabet.2010.11.013 (accessed on 28th June 2025).

Mitchell, A. A., Gilboa, S. M., Werler, M. M., Kelley, K. E., Louik, C., Hernández-Díaz, S., & Study, N. B. D. P. (2011). Medication use during pregnancy, with particular focus on prescription drugs: 1976–2008. *American Journal of Obstetrics and Gynecology, 205*(1), 51.e1–51.e8. https://doi.org/10.1016/j.ajog.2011.02.029 (accessed on 28th June 2025).

Molitch, M. E. (2019). *Pregnancy and endocrine disorders, an issue of Endocrinology and Metabolism Clinics of North America* (Vol. 48). Elsevier Health Sciences. https://doi.org/10.1016/j.ecl.2019.06.001 (accessed on 28th June 2025).

Morton, A., & Teasdale, S. (2022). Physiological changes in pregnancy and their influence on the endocrine investigation. *Clinical Endocrinology, 96*(1), 3–11. https://doi.org/10.1111/cen.14624 (accessed on 28th June 2025).

Nguyen, C. T., Sasso, E. B., Barton, L., & Mestman, J. H. (2018). Graves' hyperthyroidism in pregnancy: A clinical review. *Clinical Diabetes and Endocrinology, 4*(1), 1–9. https://doi.org/10.1186/s40842-018-0054-7 (accessed on 28th June 2025).

Oliveira, D., Lages, A., Paiva, S., & Carrilho, F. (2018). Treatment of Addison's disease during pregnancy. *Endocrinology, Diabetes & Metabolism Case Reports, 2018*(1). https://doi.org/10.1530/EDM-17-0179 (accessed on 28th June 2025).

Olmos, P. R., Araya-Del-Pino, A. P., González-Carvello, C. A., Laso-Ulloa, P., Hodgson, M. I., Irribarra, V., Borzone, G. R., Belmar, C., Poblete, A., & Berríos, C. (2009). Near-optimal glycemic control in Chilean women with pregestational type-2 diabetes: Persistent macrosomia relates to maternal pre-pregnancy overweight. *Diabetes Research and Clinical Practice, 85*(1), 53–60. https://doi.org/10.1016/j.bbadis.2017.07.022 (accessed on 28th June 2025).

Oskovi-Kaplan, Z. A., & Ozgu-Erdinc, A. S. (2021). Management of gestational diabetes mellitus. In *Diabetes: From Research to Clinical Practice: Volume 4* (pp. 257–272). https://doi.org/10.1007/5584_2020_552 (accessed on 28th June 2025).

Patti, A. M., Giglio, R. V., Pafili, K., Rizzo, M., & Papanas, N. (2018). Pharmacotherapy for gestational diabetes. *Expert Opinion on Pharmacotherapy, 19*(13), 1407–1414. https://doi.org/10.1080/14656566.2018.1509955 (accessed on 28th June 2025).

Pettitt, D. J., Ospina, P., Kolaczynski, J. W., & Jovanovic, L. (2003). Comparison of an insulin analog, insulin aspart, and regular human insulin with no insulin in gestational diabetes mellitus. *Diabetes Care, 26*(1), 183–186. https://doi.org/10.2337/diacare.26.1.183 (accessed on 28th June 2025).

Plows, J. F., Stanley, J. L., Baker, P. N., Reynolds, C. M., & Vickers, M. H. (2018). The pathophysiology of gestational diabetes mellitus. *International Journal of Molecular Sciences, 19*(11), 3342. https://doi.org/10.3390/ijms19113342 (accessed on 28th June 2025).

Pourali, L., Vatanchi, A. M., & Hamidi, A. (2017). A case of Cushing's syndrome in pregnancy. *Iranian Journal of Medical Sciences, 42*(6), 607. https://doi.org/10.5603/EP.a2020.0089 (accessed on 28th June 2025).

Rahmani, A., Hamanajm, S. A., Fallahi, A., Gheshlagh, R. G., & Dalvand, S. (2019). Prevalence of self-medication among pregnant women: A systematic review and meta-analysis. *Nursing and Midwifery Studies, 8*(4), 169–175. http://dx.doi.org/10.4103/nms.nms_77_18 (accessed on 28th June 2025).

Ravn, P., Gram, F., Andersen, M. S., & Glintborg, D. (2022). Myoinositol vs. metformin in women with polycystic ovary syndrome: A randomized controlled clinical trial. *Metabolites, 12*(12), 1183. https://doi.org/10.3390/metabo12121183 (accessed on 28th June 2025).

Reaven, G. (2004). The metabolic syndrome or the insulin resistance syndrome? Different names, different concepts, and different goals. *Endocrinology and Metabolism Clinics, 33*(2), 283–303. https://doi.org/10.1016/j.ecl.2004.03.002 (accessed on 28th June 2025).

Ren, Z., Bremer, A. A., & Pawlyk, A. C. (2021). Drug development research in pregnant and lactating women. *American Journal of Obstetrics and Gynecology, 225*(1), 33–42. https://doi.org/10.1016/j.ajog.2021.04.227 (accessed on 28th June 2025).

Retnakaran, R., Qi, Y., Connelly, P. W., Sermer, M., Zinman, B., & Hanley, A. J. (2010). Glucose intolerance in pregnancy and postpartum risk of metabolic syndrome in young women. *The Journal of Clinical Endocrinology & Metabolism, 95*(2), 670–677. https://doi.org/10.1210/jc.2009-1990 (accessed on 28th June 2025).

Rihal, V., Khan, H., Kaur, A., & Singh, T. G. (2023). Vitamin D as therapeutic modulator in cerebrovascular diseases: A mechanistic perspectives. *Critical Reviews in Food Science and Nutrition, 63*(25), 7772–7794. https://doi.org/10.1080/10408398.2022.2050349 (accessed on 28th June 2025).

Rihal, V., Khan, H., Kaur, A., Singh, T. G., & Abdel-Daim, M. M. (2022). Therapeutic and mechanistic intervention of vitamin D in neuropsychiatric disorders. *Psychiatry Research, 317*, 114782. https://doi.org/10.1016/j.psychres.2022.114782 (accessed on 28th June 2025).

Rodien, P., Jordan, N., Lefèvre, A., Royer, J., Vasseur, C., Savagner, F., Bourdelot, A., & Rohmer, V. (2004). Abnormal stimulation of the thyrotrophin receptor during gestation. *Human Reproduction Update, 10*(2), 95–105. https://doi.org/10.1093/humupd/dmh008 (accessed on 28th June 2025).

Ross, E. J., Graham, D. L., Money, K. M., & Stanwood, G. D. (2015). Developmental consequences of fetal exposure to drugs: What we know and what we still must learn. *Neuropsychopharmacology, 40*(1), 61–87. https://doi.org/10.1038/npp.2014.147 (accessed on 28th June 2025).

Rovet, J., & Willoughby, K. A. (2010). Maternal thyroid function during pregnancy: Effects on the developing fetal brain. https://doi.org/10.1016/j.neuroscience.2015.09.070 (accessed on 28th June 2025).

Rutgers-Verhage, A. R., Devries, T. W., & Torringa, M. J. L. (2003). No effects of bisphosphonates on the human fetus. *Birth Defects Research Part A: Clinical and Molecular Teratology, 67*(3), 203–204. https://doi.org/10.1002/bdra.10016 (accessed on 28th June 2025).

Saez, T., De Vos, P., Sobrevia, L., & Faas, M. M. (2018). Is there a role for exosomes in foetal endothelial dysfunction in gestational diabetes mellitus? *Placenta, 61*, 48–54. https://doi.org/10.1016/j.placenta.2017.11.007 (accessed on 28th June 2025).

Saltiel, A. R. (2016). Insulin signalling in the control of glucose and lipid homeostasis. In *Metabolic Control* (pp. 51–71). https://doi.org/10.1007/164_2015_14 (accessed on 28th June 2025).

Sang, Z., Wei, W., Zhao, N., Zhang, G., Chen, W., Liu, H., Shen, J., Liu, J., Yan, Y., & Zhang, W. (2012). Thyroid dysfunction during late gestation is associated with excessive iodine intake in pregnant women. *The Journal of Clinical Endocrinology & Metabolism,*

97(8), E1363–E1369. https://doi.org/10.1210/jc.2011-3438 (accessed on 28th June 2025).

Sarayani, A., Albogami, Y., Thai, T. N., Smolinski, N. E., Patel, P., Wang, Y., Nduaguba, S., Rasmussen, S. A., & Winterstein, A. G. (2022). Prenatal exposure to teratogenic medications in the Risk Evaluation and Mitigation Strategies era. *American Journal of Obstetrics and Gynecology, 227*(2), 263.e1–263.e38. https://doi.org/10.1016/j.ajog.2022.01.004 (accessed on 28th June 2025).

Schaefer, C., Peters, P. W., & Miller, R. K. (2014). *Drugs during pregnancy and lactation: Treatment options and risk assessment.* Academic Press. https://doi.org/10.4103/picr.PICR_22_19 (accessed on 28th June 2025).

Scheithauer, B. W., Sano, T., Kovacs, K. T., Young, W. F., Jr, Ryan, N., & Randall, R. V. (1990). The pituitary gland in pregnancy: A clinicopathologic and immunohistochemical study of 69 cases. *Mayo Clinic Proceedings, 65*(4), 461–474. https://doi.org/10.1016/s0025-6196(12)60946 (accessed on 28th June 2025).

Schneiderman, M., Czuzoj-Shulman, N., Spence, A., & Abenhaim, H. (2017). Maternal and neonatal outcomes of pregnancies in women with Addison's disease: A population-based cohort study on 7.7 million births. *BJOG: An International Journal of Obstetrics & Gynaecology, 124*(11), 1772–1779. https://doi.org/10.1111/1471-0528.14448 (accessed on 28th June 2025).

Sheehan, P. M., Nankervis, A., Araujo Júnior, E., & Da Silva Costa, F. (2015). Maternal thyroid disease and preterm birth: Systematic review and meta-analysis. *The Journal of Clinical Endocrinology & Metabolism, 100*(11), 4325–4331. https://doi.org/10.1210/jc.2015-3074 (accessed on 28th June 2025).

Singh, S., Singh, T. G., Mahajan, K., & Dhiman, S. (2020). Medicinal plants used against various inflammatory biomarkers for the management of rheumatoid arthritis. *The Journal of Pharmacy and Pharmacology, 72*(10), 1306–1327. https://doi.org/10.1111/jphp.13326 (accessed on 28th June 2025).

Singh, V. P., Bali, A., Singh, N., & Jaggi, A. S. (2014). Advanced glycation end products and diabetic complications. *The Korean Journal of Physiology & Pharmacology: Official Journal of the Korean Physiological Society and the Korean Society of Pharmacology, 18*(1), 1–14. https://doi.org/10.4196/kjpp.2014.18.1.1 (accessed on 28th June 2025).

Skinningsrud, B., Lie, B. A., Lavant, E., Carlson, J. A., Erlich, H., Akselsen, H. E., Gervin, K., Wolff, A. B., Erichsen, M. M., & Løvås, K. (2011). Multiple loci in the HLA complex are associated with Addison's disease. *The Journal of Clinical Endocrinology & Metabolism, 96*(10), E1703–E1708. https://doi.org/10.1210/jc.2011-0645 (accessed on 28th June 2025).

Sobrevia, L., Salsoso, R., Sáez, T., Sanhueza, C., Pardo, F., & Leiva, A. (2015). Insulin therapy and fetoplacental vascular function in gestational diabetes mellitus. *Experimental Physiology, 100*(3), 231–238. https://doi.org/10.1113/expphysiol.2014.082743 (accessed on 28th June 2025).

Sorenson, R. L., & Brelje, T. C. (2009). Prolactin receptors are critical to the adaptation of islets to pregnancy. *Endocrinology, 150*(4), 1566–1569. https://doi.org/10.1210/en.2008-1710 (accessed on 28th June 2025).

Sreelatha, S., Nadagoudar, S., & Asha, D. L. (2017). The study of maternal and fetal outcomes in pregnant women with thyroid disorders. *International Journal of*

Reproduction, Contraception, Obstetrics and Gynecology, 6(8), 3507–3514. https://doi.org/10.1186/s12884-020-03448 (accessed on 28th June 2025).

Sridharan, K., Sahoo, J., Palui, R., Patil, M., Kamalanathan, S., Ramesh, A., & Kubera, N. (2021). Diagnosis and treatment outcomes of Cushing's disease during pregnancy. *Pituitary, 24*, 670–680. https://doi.org/10.1007/s11102-021-01142-7 (accessed on 28th June 2025).

St-Jean, M., MacKenzie-Feder, J., Bourdeau, I., & Lacroix, A. (2019). Exacerbation of Cushing's syndrome during pregnancy: Stimulation of a cortisol-secreting adrenocortical adenoma by ACTH originating from the fetoplacental unit. *Endocrinology, Diabetes & Metabolism Case Reports, 2019*(1). https://doi.org/10.1530/edm-18-0115 (accessed on 28th June 2025).

Stagnaro-Green, A., Abalovich, M., Alexander, E., Azizi, F., Mestman, J., Negro, R., Nixon, A., Pearce, E. N., Soldin, O. P., & Sullivan, S. (2011). Guidelines of the American Thyroid Association for diagnosing and managing thyroid disease during pregnancy and postpartum. *Thyroid, 21*(10), 1081–1125. https://doi.org/10.1089/thy.2011.0087 (accessed on 28th June 2025).

Teng, W., Shan, Z., Patil-Sisodia, K., & Cooper, D. S. (2013). Hypothyroidism in pregnancy. *The Lancet Diabetes & Endocrinology, 1*(3), 228–237. https://doi.org/10.1016/s2213-8587(13)70109-8 (accessed on 28th June 2025).

Tsakiridis, I., Giouleka, S., Mamopoulos, A., Athanasiadis, A., & Dagklis, T. (2022). Investigation and management of stillbirth: A descriptive review of significant guidelines. *Journal of Perinatal Medicine, 50*(6), 796–813. https://doi.org/10.1515/jpm-2021-0403 (accessed on 28th June 2025).

Turunen, S., Vääräsmäki, M., Lahesmaa-Korpinen, A. M., Leinonen, M. K., Gissler, M., Männistö, T., & Suvanto, E. (2020). Maternal hyperthyroidism and pregnancy outcomes: A population-based cohort study. *Clinical Endocrinology, 93*(6), 721–728. https://doi.org/10.1111/cen.14282 (accessed on 28th June 2025).

Vilar, L., Naves, L. A., Freitas, M. d. C., Moura, E., Canadas, V., Leal, E., Teixeira, L., Gusmão, A., Santos, V., & Campos, R. (2007). Endogenous Cushing's syndrome: Clinical and laboratory features in 73 cases. *Arquivos Brasileiros de Endocrinologia & Metabologia, 51*, 566–574. https://doi.org/10.1590/s0004-27302007000400010 (accessed on 28th June 2025).

Wermers, R. A., Khosla, S., Atkinson, E. J., Achenbach, S. J., Oberg, A. L., Grant, C. S., & Melton III, L. J. (2006). Incidence of primary hyperparathyroidism in Rochester, Minnesota, 1993–2001: An update on the changing epidemiology of the disease. *Journal of Bone and Mineral Research, 21*(1), 171–177. https://doi.org/10.1359/jbmr.050910 (accessed on 28th June 2025).

You, J. Y., Choi, S. J., Roh, C. R., Kim, J. H., & Oh, S. Y. (2016). Pregnancy and neonatal outcomes in gestational diabetes treated with regular insulin or fast-acting insulin analogues. *Gynecologic and Obstetric Investigation, 81*(3), 232–237. https://doi.org/10.1159/000440616 (accessed on 28th June 2025).

Zhang, Y., Xiao, C.-M., Zhang, Y., Chen, Q., Zhang, X.-Q., Li, X.-F., Shao, R.-Y., & Gao, Y.-M. (2021). Factors associated with gestational diabetes mellitus: A meta-analysis. *Journal of Diabetes Research, 2021*, 1–18. https://doi.org/10.1155/2021/6692695 (accessed on 28th June 2025).

CHAPTER 4

Hormone Replacement Therapy: Biological, Pathophysiological, Pharmacological, and Clinical Aspects

SANCHIT DHANKHAR,[1] HIMANSHU SHARMA,[1] NITIKA GARG,[1] POOJA MITTAL,[1,*] SAMRAT CHAUHAN,[1] MONIKA SAINI,[2] THAKUR GURJEET SINGH,[1] SANJANA MEHTA,[1] DIVYA KANWAR,[1] BHAVESH DHARMANI,[1] VISHNU MITTAL,[3] and DINESH KUMAR CHELLAPPAN[4]

[1]*Chitkara College of Pharmacy, Chitkara University, Punjab, India*

[2]*MM College of Pharmacy, Maharishi Markandeshwar (Deemed to be University), Mullana, Ambala, Haryana, India*

[3]*Guru Gobind Singh College of Pharmacy, Haryana, India*

[4]*School of Pharmacy, International Medical University, Bukit Jalil, Kuala Lumpur, Malaysia*

*Corresponding author

ABSTRACT

Hormone replacement treatment (HRT) is a multimodal therapeutic method that addresses the various phases of hormonal imbalance. Outlining the function of hormones in preserving homeostasis and how they affect general health, this chapter explores the complex web of hormone replacement therapy (HRT) and looks at the scientific foundations around it. The pathophysiological analysis of hormone replacement therapy showed the

Precision Nutrition and Endocrine Health: Synthesis, Characterization, and Applications.
Thakur Gurjeet Singh and Sanjana Mehta (Eds.)

DOI: 10.1201/9781998511877-4

complex processes behind the hormone imbalance in a range of clinical conditions. This grasp dictates the pharmacological interventions that examine medication-drug interactions, their transport systems, and dosage forms. It will also highlight the broad range of applications of HRT in patient care as its clinical reputation grows. Thus, in this chapter, we shall discuss the clinical landscape of HRT in different categories. Clinical outcomes, pharmacological concerns, pathophysiological nuances, and biological subtleties contribute to a comprehensive understanding of hormone replacement therapy. In the pursuit of the most excellent possible patient health, this permits informed decision-making.

4.1 INTRODUCTION

The last several decades have seen a progressive increase in the public health issue of menopause, the permanent end of menstruation due to decreasing ovarian function (Bravo et al., 2024). By 2050, there will be 1.6 billion women in the world who are 50 or older. They have an average life expectancy of more than 80 years and can live more than 30 years beyond menopause (Cui et al., 2024). Menopause hormone replacement treatment (HRT) was first developed to treat estrogen deficiency symptoms (Faubion et al., 2022; Martin and Redfern, 2024). In addition, the development of symptoms after stopping HRT and routine assessment of the benefit-risk balance impact the choice to continue medication (Vigneswaran and Hamoda, 2022). A woman should undergo routine medical examinations customized to her unique clinical requirements, considering her cardio-vascular and gynecological risk factors, once she finishes taking hormone replacement therapy (HRT) (Newton et al., 1997).

Finding methods to improve physical function and mobility for the growing elderly population is a top priority in medicine today (Modave et al., 2015). The capacity to perform at our peak level of exercise is among the many vital physical capacities that deteriorate with age. This puts older men at higher risk for frailty and impairment. Additionally, it promotes insulin resistance and the growth of fat tissue (Suominen et al., 2011). This puts older men at higher risk for frailty and impairment (Stout et al., 2017). Anabolism-promoting hormones and locally autocrine/paracrine growth factors that are load-sensitive play a significant role in how muscles react to exercise (Giannoulis et al., 2012). Hormone growth hormone (GH), insulin-like growth factor (IGF-I), and testosterone (T) are intimately linked to muscle protein synthesis and exercise adaptation (Gharahdaghi et al., 2021). Furthermore, T and locally produced IGF-I can stimulate muscle stem cells (Hill and Goldspink et al., 2003). Even while exercise programs improve physical function over time, most senior men do not follow through on them (Stuck et al., 1993). Aging causes both T levels and the GF-I axis to drop sharply. However, more and more research indicates that these changes are necessary to maintain the integrity of bodily function.

According to several research, consuming T increases lean body mass and maximal voluntary strength in elderly, healthy males (Storer et al., 2008). However, the majority of studies revealed that taking GH alone did not affect muscular strength, even while it assisted with some of the undesirable physical changes related to aging (Woodhouse et al., 2006). Growth hormone (GH) and testosterone (T) together have been shown to have a more significant anabolic impact on muscle hypertrophy and protein synthesis than those of either hormone alone (Fink et al., 2018). However, these studies only looked at T and GH's combined effects. A variety of somatic, psychological, and vasomotor symptoms are part of the menopausal syndrome (Muka et al., 2016). is the primary rationale behind the prescription of (HRT), which usually consists of progestin (P) and estrogen (E). hypoestrogenism brought on by early ovarian failure, castration, and hypogonadism (Kwatra and Mukhopadhyay, 2018) or genitourinary problems, preventing bone loss, causing painful vasomotor symptoms (VMS); at the moment, the FDA has granted a license for HRT for these four indications (Paciuc et al., 2020; Patsner, 2008).

Though most women report that their hot flashes are light and sporadic, others report that they are so awful that they interfere with sleep or cause so much anxiety that they interfere with social and professional life. Hot flashes in surgically menopausal women may be more severe and frequent than in naturally menopausal women, particularly within the initial six months following surgery (Mali and Manna et al., 2009). Another factor affecting women's vaginal pH is a decline in the proportion of Lactobacillus-dominated vaginal flora. You may anticipate feeling uncomfortable during sexual activity, have a general lack of enthusiasm for sexual activity, have a higher risk of infection, and have a dry vagina. Low estrogen levels can cause atrophy of the muscles of the urethra, trigone, and pubococcygeal, changing the structure of the urinary system and raising the risk of stress and urge incontinence, urethritis, and cystitis (Bhattacharya et al., 2022). Randomized controlled trials have shown that HRT can effectively cure GSM symptoms and repair the structure of the genitourinary tract as well as lower vaginal pH, thicken vaginal mucosa, and lessen symptoms. Oral ospemifene, low-dose vaginal estrogens, and vaginal DHEA inserts are everyday regimen staples (Pinkerton et al., 2024). Transdermal and oral hormone replacement therapy These are two viable options for women with simultaneous VMS and moderate to severe dyspareunia. Continuous therapy is usually necessary for symptom alleviation, which might take one to three months, as symptoms usually return after therapy is stopped (Ai et al., 2020; Lambalk et al., 2009).

Additionally, 2.5 mg of medroxyprogesterone acetate (MDPA) and 0.625 mg of conjugated equine oestrogens (CEE) were taken daily by 16,000 postmenopausal women with an average age of 64 who were enrolled in the Women's Health Initiative (WHI) trial. Menopausal women's risk of fracture was decreased with HRT. Despite the lack of consensus brought about by research producing inconsistent outcomes over time, the FDA no longer permits HRT for the prevention of cardiovascular disease. HRT was found to increase the risk of cardiovascular events in the WHI study, which involved 16,000 postmenopausal women (mean age 64) who were given 0.625 mg of CEE and 2.5 mg of MDPA daily (Mehedintu et al., 2021).

4.2 AGE-ASSOCIATED ILLNESSES AND HORMONE MISREGULATION

4.2.1 PATHOPHYSIOLOGICAL IMPLICATIONS OF MENOPAUSE

Significant variations in sex hormone levels before and after menopause are the cause of the long-term impacts, which are critical to women's healthy aging. For the brain, heart, and bones to grow and function properly, among other organs, sex hormones are crucial to physiological processes. Because oestrogen exposure causes musculoskeletal and cardiovascular disorders, postmenopausal symptoms are frequently observed (Monteleone et al., 2018). Deterioration of cognition is also linked to hypoestrogenism during menopause. Based on several lines of evidence, menopausal vasomotor symptoms and scorching flashes impair quality of life and are linked to an increased risk of chronic illnesses that require preventive interventions, such as hormone treatment for menopause (Comparetto and Borruto et al., 2023).

Ladies can significantly slow aging by altering their diet, exercising regularly, and taking the appropriate hormone therapies during the "window" of opportunity if they suffer symptoms. In the meantime, customized menopausal hormone treatment can provide postmenopausal women—including those with Genitourinary Menopause Syndrome with symptom alleviation (Johnston et al., 2021).

Women in contemporary industrialized countries may face a range of illnesses associated with decreased oestrogen production, and they might anticipate living for more than 30 years after menopause that occurs on its own. Because of the complex interactions between genetic and epigenetic factors, hormonal alterations during menopause are detrimental to health. Biological aging is accelerated by menopause, mainly when it happens early. Menopause symptoms impact several biological systems. These transient consequences of long-term illnesses that arise during menopause and MT, such as vaginal dryness, mood swings, hot flashes, and altered sleep patterns, are distinct from the long-time consequences of hypoestrogenism and lowered androgen levels, as well as the typical symptoms associated with LMP. Managing VMS and scorching flashes can improve quality of life and reduce the risk of osteoporosis, cardiovascular disease, and cognitive decline. Outside of osteoporosis, an elevated risk of cardiovascular disease and cognitive loss are the other long-term impacts of aging (Ferrucci et al., 2018; Singh et al., 2020). Through several processes, the changes brought about by menopause represent a person's pattern of improving health. The occurrence, persistence, and intensity of symptoms during menopause are "red flags" for healthcare as they need women who are symptomatic to receive extra care (Nappi and Cucinella, 2020). If there are etiopathogenic processes active in VMS that affect long-term effects, or if these symptoms arise concurrently as a sign of a systemic response to sex hormone variations. A higher risk of cardiovascular and cognitive problems might be associated with menopausal symptoms such as mood and sleep disorders.

4.2.2 BONE HEALTH

The rate of bone loss rises with age in fertile women, leading to a significant shift in bone health and a higher risk of fractures and osteoporosis (Lizneva et al., 2018; Thapa et al., 2023). White women's bone mass decreases by 1.8% annually in the femoral neck and 2.5% in the lumbar spine due to variations in Estradiol and Follicle-stimulating hormone

(FSH) levels during MT for ladies aged 50 to 79. Throughout a more than eight-year follow-up period, women with moderate to severe VMS showed lower bone mineral density and more significant risks of hip fractures than women without VMS. Estrogen insufficiency results in altered bone microarchitecture and a reduction in bone mineral density (BMD) (Dhiman et al., 2011; Shen et al., 1995). Estrogens bind to isoforms of the oestrogen receptor alpha, ER-α, and ER-β, stimulating osteoblast development and proliferation in addition to the cessation and mineralization of the bone matrix. However, estrogens also force osteoclasts to undergo apoptosis. There is a link between estrogen and hot flashes because in the absence of estrogens, pro-inflammatory cytokines and increased oxidative stress cause bone resorption (Indran et al., 2016). The rate of cortical bone loss in vertebrae and long bones decreases after menopause. The gradual, visible age-related bone loss begins after 10 years and lasts for life. Several additional risk variables are significant because women who have gone through menopause and have average or slightly lower BMD have a high fracture incidence, with lifetime risks of 15% for hip fractures and 25% for vertebral abnormalities at age 50. People who use specific medications (such as psychiatric meds, ACE inhibitors, thyroid replacement, etc.), smoke, are obese, Hispanic, diabetic, black, or do not get enough vitamin D are more likely to fracture (Mehta et al., 2022; Moen et al., 2017).

4.2.3 THE METABOLIC DISORDER

Following menopause, the prevalence of metabolic syndrome (MS) varied according to the diagnostic criteria: it ranged from 37.17% to 13.60–46.00%. Pregnancy, MT, and polycystic ovarian disease (PCOS) diminish the likelihood of MS in men compared to women. Postmenopausal women had higher odds of high systemic blood pressure, poor HDL cholesterol, high triglyceride levels, high waist circumference, and fasting blood glucose when compared to premenopausal women. Postmenopausal women exhibited a higher overall pooled odds ratio (POR) for MS of 3.54 (OR 2.74), depending on the classification criteria. At least three of these outcomes should be seen if you have MS. When comparing women with VMS to women without symptoms, there is a greater prevalence of Multiple sclerosis (MS) is linked to low levels of HDL-C in plasma, obesity, high blood pressure, hyperglycemia, and hypertriglyceridemia (Batista et al., 2016; Sharma et al., 2022).

4.2.4 CARDIOVASCULAR RISK

Heart disease is the most significant cause of death for women after menopause, and multiple sclerosis is known to cause blood clots often (Padro et al., 2021). When comparing the clinical manifestation of CVD to males, there is a ten-year lag due to the robust defense that estrogens provide up to LMP. Records show that beyond 75 years of age, women have cardiovascular disease (CVD) at a greater frequency than men. After an acute myocardial infarction, conventional risk variables had longer-term and more noticeable impacts on women than on men. Women are more likely than men to suffer cardiovascular disease (CVD), even though type 2 diabetes affects both sexes more frequently (Ai et al., 2019). Increased CVD morbidity and death are linked to DM2 in both sexes (Mehta et al., 2021). There is inconclusive evidence that estrogen levels impact the glucose balance during MT. Women who have previous experience with gestational diabetes and hypertensive problems during pregnancy, a prolonged menstrual cycle, or other common female-specific comorbidities are more likely to develop cardiovascular disease due to hormonal imbalance. Cardiovascular disease risk factors include menopause itself, and evidence from women who go through early menopause supports this theory (Furman et al., 1997).

Likewise, a unilateral salpingo-oophorectomy alone has a 4.55 relative risk of cardiovascular disease and a 1.25 relative risk of early menopause (Mannan et al., 2023; Santen et al., 2010). Women with poorer stroke-free survival in the past and Significant coronary disease history increased the likelihood of early menopause-related cardiovascular disease and stroke in the future. After menopause, a woman's lowered estradiol levels and increased visceral fat deposition particularly her heart fat increase her risk of cardiovascular disease (CVD). FSH hormone controls insulin resistance, atherosclerosis, dyslipidemia, fat accumulation, and type 2 diabetes. For women of whatever age, weight, or ethnicity, the first year after, a significant increase in antiatherogenic impact marks LMP and decreases in menopause after. However, it is still a powerful predictor of women's cardiovascular mortality. Women are more likely to die from coronary heart disease when they have high triglycerides and low HDL cholesterol. Decreased synthesis of the cardioprotective nitric oxide, activation of the renin system, and formation and proliferation of vascular smooth muscle cells are all impacted by the loss in endothelial cell function brought on by hypoestrogenism during menopause. A surge in the powerful vasoconstrictor endothelin, angiotensin, and an overall increase in salt sensitivity are the reasons why postmenopausal women have systemic hypertension more than twice as frequently as premenopausal women do (Pillow et al., 2019; Sharma et al., 2021).

4.2.5 ANDROGEN DEFICIENCY IN MEN

Determining androgen insufficiency is difficult because of the term's complex historical background and constantly evolving biochemical, pathologic, and physiological implications. The "androgen deficiency" refers to a condition in which the hypothalamic-pituitary axis (I) is malfunctioning, (II) the testes are malfunctioning, resulting in insufficient production of testosterone (T). Male hypogonadism, a collection of symptoms, is medically considered to be inextricably tied to androgen insufficiency, brought on by either a lack of androgens or the incapacity of sex hormones to activate in the body's effector organs fully.

Male hypogonadism symptoms might vary in severity according to when androgen insufficiency occurs. Regarding the MetS specifically, this is a reference to LOH. Mature male anatomy and secondary sex characteristics are unaffected by low androgen levels (LOH), which begin after puberty (Corona et al., 2013). LOH symptoms might be difficult to identify since they often appear part of the average age. These symptoms are low libido, impotence, and other sexual problems; depression; exhaustion; hot flashes; and a decline in bone density and muscle mass (Table 4.1). Because it might be difficult to pinpoint these symptoms in some instances (30–59%), questionnaires may have limited specificity symptom evaluation plays a critical role in deciding who should have laboratory T testing; generally speaking, healthy, asymptomatic males do not fulfil the requirements (Thakur et al., 2020; Thapa et al., 2021).

Before discussing specific thresholds for insufficient androgen, it is imperative to highlight the intricacy of the T-test. The bioavailability of T is made up of several elements. The following are the four types of testosterone that are present in the blood: (i) firmly bound to SHBG, making up about 44% of the total; (ii) loosely bound to albumin, making up about 50%; (iii) weakly attached to CBG, making up about four percent; and, lastly, unrestricted or free testosterone, making up around two to three percent. The free and the T bound to CBG and albumin comprise T's active or bioavailable form. To develop a normal T reference range, no sample of guys of reproductive age with typical libido and fertility has been employed. More than three orders of magnitude can separate T within the population. Furthermore, in younger guys, T can vary by up to 50% across the day and season. Standard T tests lose some sensitivity when T levels drop below normal. Like MetS, several organizations have developed guidelines detailing androgen's specific characteristics and deficiencies. There are some points regarding standards that appear to be universally accepted. There is no established threshold for low testosterone (TT), although generally speaking, when evaluating FT in males with a borderline result, one of two methods should be utilized: equilibrium dialysis or measuring SHBG and computing FT level. Alternative FT evaluation techniques are thought to be unreliable. More recent research has concentrated on broadening the definition of androgen deficiencies/hypogonadism to include molecular-cell processes Apart from the customary evaluation of the hormones in circulation. Examples of these proteins are the androgen receptor (AR) and its action-modifying variants since heat-shock protein 70, which suppresses regulated androgen transcription. This research has given us a biological foundation for understanding why some people might have symptoms of androgen insufficiency even when their lab tests show normal findings.

While there is irrefutable evidence that links androgen deficiency to MetS, which is probably complex and multifaceted, what specific mechanism causes low T levels in boys with MetS (Table 4.1).

TABLE 4.1 Male Hypogonadism's Metabolic Syndrome-Related Mechanism

System	Remark
The hormone Leptin	Reduced T synthesis due to direct influence on Leydig cells
Inflammation	Testing the disruption of testicular steroid production
Elevated activity of the aromatase	The hypothalamus and pituitary glands' negative feedback on hypogonadotropic hypogonadism is enhanced by elevated T estradiol conversion.
Diminished SHBG	Diminished TT Independent risk factor for DM with low SHBG
Apnea during sleep	Pituitary and hypothalamic suppression to hypogonadism hypogonadotropic
Internalized opioid	Reduced secretion of LH
Testicular surroundings	elevated fever in the testicles

TT: total testosterone; LH: Luteinizing hormone, or. SHBG; and T: testosterone.

The efficacy of several treatments for androgen deficiency linked to MetS is not well supported by randomly controlled studies (Liu et al., 2004). Comparing past studies could be difficult due to differences in language, patient demographics, and treatment aims. There are two primary methods for categorizing treatments: (i) the use of non-surgical or surgical therapy and (ii) the identification of androgen deficiency or MetS as the primary cause of the condition.

4.3 TREATMENT

4.3.1 BEHAVIORAL MODIFICATION

Many randomized controlled experiments have looked into how weight reduction affects androgen levels. There is conflicting evidence; although some studies reveal no relationship between T and diet, others indicate that T rises with a low-calorie diet. In the current meta-analysis, TT of obese males improved with weight loss ($P < 0.0001$). An examination of the included publications using meta-regression revealed that testosterone levels were more significant in older men and males without diabetes ($P < 0.0001$). According to the previously mentioned mechanisms, weight loss was linked to a low estradiol level and a high level of gonadotropin. The study conducted by Niskanen et al. showed a direct relation between the improvement in testosterone and the quantity of weight lost.

4.3.2 GONADOTROPIN-RELEASING HORMONE (GNRH) AND GONADOTROPIN

The administration of pulsatile GnRH injections and gonadotropins has proven beneficial for fertile males with low sperm counts. Due to their high cost and complex administration, these medications are rarely advised as the first line of therapy unless fertility is an issue. Information about the use of this male agent with MetS is scarce.

4.3.3 TESTOSTERONE REPLACEMENT THERAPY (TRT)

Until now, six random control trials have examined TRT quality in guys with diabetes or MetS. During 57 weeks, 483 individuals were monitored in these randomized controlled trials (RCTs). In males with MetS, A mean decrease of 4.1 cm in waist circumference ($P = 0.03$), an average increase of 0.48 mmol/L ($P < 0.001$) in fasting blood glucose levels, and a mean decrease of 0.4 nmol/L in triglyceride levels were all seen with TRT, according to a recent meta-analysis. Because TRT lowers cytokine production from a pathophysiologic standpoint, it is thought to have an anti-inflammatory impact and benefit men with MetS.

4.3.4 ANTIESTROGENS

Selective oestrogen receptor modulators (SERMs) antagonistically influence the oestrogen receptors in the pituitary gland and the brain to regulate the release of gonadotropins in males. Your body reacts to SERM by increasing the production of FSH, LH, and testosterone. Clomiphene citrate therapy is used in guys with erectile dysfunction and secondary hypogonadism, markedly raising LH, FSH, TT, and FT. Given that males with MetS experience estrogen-mediated hypogonadism, this medication may be beneficial for them.

4.3.5 BARIATRIC SURGERY

Following bariatric surgery, both sex-related quality of life and erectile dysfunction significantly improve, and a positive impact on the levels of TT appears to surpass the benefits of weight reduction without surgery. For instance, TT improved following bariatric surgery, according to a recent meta-analysis. TT growth was more closely associated with bariatric surgery than a low-calorie diet. There have been just two randomized controlled trials on hypogonadism with bariatric surgery. Around 20 males comprised the control group; after the 20-month follow-up, Reis et al. discovered that the gastric bypass group had higher TT, FT, and FSH levels. Mingrone and colleagues randomly allocated 27 male subjects to receive either dietary modification or malabsorptive surgery throughout their one-year trial. Compared with males randomly allocated to a low-calorie diet, the SHBG level rose considerably in those who received malabsorptive surgery.

4.3.6 PROCEDURE: VARICOCELECTOMY

Although varicocele has traditionally been linked to male infertility, recent studies suggest that low T levels may also be at risk due to this condition

(Pastuzak and Wang et al., 2016; Rihal et al., 2022). The particular processes via which varicocele inhibits testicular function are still unknown, and the majority of the empirical data that is now available comes from infertile people. Recent research has demonstrated that infertile males with varicocele who undergo microsurgical varicocelectomy had higher T levels.

Ozturk et al. sought to determine the impact of MetS on varicocele repair success rates. Around 48 men with MetS and 56 without had varicocele repair. Upon two years of follow-up, the rate of spontaneous pregnancies in the non-MetS group was 45%, but the rate in the MetS group was 34%. T levels may rise in hypogonadism patients after varicocelectomy who are fertile, despite the lack of scientific evidence at this time.

4.4 OTHER HEALTH CONDITIONS IMPROVED BY HRT

4.4.1 THE THYROID CONDITIONS

Thyroid hormone replacement medication has been used for treating hypothyroidism for over one century, and its general effectiveness is undeniable. Palpitations occur during the absorption phase, when serum triiodothyronine (T3) levels rise to supranormal levels, and desiccated thyroid also contains thyroxine (T4). Liothyronine (T3) has the same issue and needs to be taken twice daily due to its short half-life. Levothyroxine (L-T4) synthesized has several advantages: Completely functional and potentially protective against disease, extrathyroidal conversion of T4 to T3 yields around 80% of the daily rate of T3 synthesis. One pill a day is plenty because of its lengthy half-life; thus, it is okay to forget to take a tablet periodically. It is the preferred treatment now that L-T4 does not result in any additional deaths after Prolonged usage. Normalizing serum thyroid stimulating hormone (TSH) levels can be achieved by administering 1.6 μg/kg of T4 on average daily. Due to this, serum-free T4 (fT4) concentrations are either modestly raised or fall within the upper half of the reference range for normative values (Faheema et al., 2016). The thyroid gland would typically provide 20% of the daily rate of T3 synthesis, which has to be replaced to generate T4, probably the reason for the elevated fT4 levels. The 75 to 250 μg range is relatively wide for the daily maintenance dosage of T4. Precise dosage estimation is possible by measuring TSH and fT4 in a blood sample obtained shortly before ingesting the subsequent T4 pill. It is best to avoid taking drugs that interfere with the metabolism or absorption of T4 when pregnant, and patients on certain medicines may need to have their dosages changed. Laboratory testing should not be performed earlier because a new equilibrium is formed after around six weeks. Once the maintenance dosage is steady, an annual check-up is usually sufficient. Based on the total amount of L-T4 replacement experience, several locations have been determined to be of concern. First, there is not always a bioequivalence between brand names and generics. For instance, people on T4 replacement frequently have a subnormal TSH. Approximately 0.1 mU/l of TSH is linked to not an increased fracture rate but rather a risk of atrial fibrillation and bone loss. Thus, maintaining TSH over the artificial cutoff of 0.2 mU/l is ideal.

Numerous medical professionals have observed that a small proportion of hypothyroid individuals nevertheless experience symptoms like sadness, tiredness, and cognitive deficits, even when biochemical testing indicates that the thyroid is operating adequately. Various organs get various amounts of T3; therefore, there may be a physiological foundation for these symptoms. For example, local deiodinase type II activity mainly determines the brain's T3 concentration. That being said, it is interesting that several psychometric scores in patients with hypothyroidism showed a significant improvement with conversion from 50μg of T4 to 12.5μg of T3. Further investigation is urgently needed to validate this. Some hypothyroid individuals may have more quality-of-life improvement from a slow-release formulation that combines T4 and T3 than from T4 therapy alone.

T4 and T3 replacement treatment can thus be considered an experimental strategy. Notwithstanding the results, it is clear that scientists are once again focused on developing the most effective thyroid hormone replacement treatment (Okosieme et al., 2011; Saklani et al., 2022). nevertheless, minor changes could be required because of the varying absorption rates: You may use 10 μg of T3 and 100 vg of T4 as an estimate. Lastly, slow-release formulations are needed to avoid the adverse cardiac consequences of high blood T3 levels during absorption.

4.4.2 ADRENAL INSUFFICIENCY

Replacement treatment includes mineralocorticoids, glucocorticoids, and adrenal androgen precursors (Hahner et al., 2021). In cases when hormone replacement treatment is initiated for recently diagnosed adrenal insufficiency, results are rapid and impressive. Regretfully, even with tried-and-true replacement methods, individuals with adrenal insufficiency may not always fully recover and may have a shorter life expectancy. This has caused an evaluation of the current replacement strategies. Dehydroepiandrosterone (DHEA) has been demonstrated in several studies to improve sexual function and general health, suggesting that it may be an added advantage of therapy. However, DHEA alone cannot normalize subjective health state, and no long-term studies with the substance have been conducted. When patients with freshly diagnosed adrenal insufficiency begin hormone replacement therapy, the results are striking and manifest quickly. Novel formulations of delayed-release glucocorticoids that may help to restore the circadian rhythm are being studied in ongoing clinical studies (Johannsson et al., 2014; Kaur et al., 2023). However, whether or not this method genuinely enhances patients' health is still up for discussion. Considerable steps must be taken to prevent adrenal crises in those with AI diagnoses. Patient education is a critical component of an efficient preventive strategy. We have discovered that people with knowledge of adrenal crisis avoidance often assist clinicians who do not.

4.5 FUTURE DIRECTIONS

It makes sense to suggest hormone replacement treatment (HRT) to both sexes in order to prevent the health issues brought on by hormone deficiencies. Many persons with VMS and GSM have found relief from their symptoms by using HRT, which also prevents bone loss and the associated fractures. Each woman should carefully consider the dangers and advantages of an HRT regimen, as these considerations vary according to the particular regimen, dose, mode of administration, length of therapy, initial dosage, and necessity of a preventative. Regularly reassessing the advantages and disadvantages of hormone replacement therapy is crucial. While treating menopausal symptoms with medications and cognitive-behavioral therapy can help affected women live better in the short term, long-term strategies to lower the dangers associated with menopause are still required. A typical medical condition that often remains undiagnosed and untreated is hypogonadism, especially in guys above a specific age. It can cause a variety of symptoms. There is strong evidence that problems with body composition and sexual function can be resolved with testosterone replacement therapy (TRT). While research on bone mineral density is consistent, there is little conflicting information regarding insulin sensitivity, mood, glycemic control, lipid profiles, and cognitive function. Years of studies have shown that the concern expressed by certain doctors over the possibility that testosterone replacement therapy may lead to prostate cancer is unjustified. Longer trials—say, 10 years or more—would provide even more convincing results. The subject also touches on other issues that need more research. Physicians who serve most patients in primary care must make extra effort to recognize and treat hypogonadism in those who show symptoms. As per the most recent guidelines, men should undergo testing for testosterone if they exhibit signs of hypogonadism, and it should be a routine component of screenings for men's health starting between the ages of 40 and 50. Transdermal testosterone replacement treatment may be beneficial for a patient whose total testosterone level in blood is below 300 ng/dL and who exhibits symptoms. A physician should discuss these benefits with the patient. After beginning TRT, patients should have evaluations of their response and side effects every three to six months, and therapy modifications should be made as necessary.

KEYWORDS

- **bariatric surgery**
- **bone disorders**
- **hormone replacement therapy**
- **hypogonadism**
- **oestrogen**
- **testosterone**

REFERENCES

Al Saedi, A., Stupka, N., & Duque, G. (2020). Pathogenesis of osteoporosis. *Bone Regulators and Osteoporosis Therapy, 353–367.* https://doi.org/10.1007/164_2020_358 (accessed on 28th June 2025).

Al-Salameh, A., Chanson, P., Bucher, S., Ringa, V., & Becquemont, L. (2019, February). Cardiovascular disease in type 2 diabetes: A review of sex-related differences in predisposition and prevention. In *Mayo Clinic Proceedings, 94*(2), 287–308. https://doi.org/10.1016/j.mayocp.2018.08.007 (accessed on 28th June 2025).

Batista, A. P., Ambrosim, T. V., Nascimento Neto, R. M. D., Pimenta, F. A. P., Freitas, S. N. D., Lauria, M. W., & Coelho, G. L. L. M. (2016). Hypovitaminosis D is associated with visceral adiposity and high low-density lipoprotein and triglyceride levels in alternating shift workers. https://doi.org/10.14740/jem340w (accessed on 28th June 2025).

Bhattacharya, T., Soares, G. A. B. E., Chopra, H., Rahman, M. M., Hasan, Z., Swain, S. S., & Cavalu, S. (2022). Applications of phyto-nanotechnology for the treatment of neurodegenerative disorders. *Materials, 15*(3), 804. https://doi.org/10.3390/chemosensors11100528 (accessed on 28th June 2025).

Bravo, B., Penedo, L., Carvalho, R., Dal Vesco, C., Calomeni, M., Gapanowicz, D., … & Renke, G. (2024). Dermatological changes during menopause and HRT: What to expect? *Cosmetics, 11*(1), 9. https://doi.org/10.3390/cosmetics11010009 (accessed on 28th June 2025).

Comparetto, C., & Borruto, F. (2023). Treatments and management of menopausal symptoms: Current status and future challenges. *OBM Geriatrics, 7*(3), 1–47. https://doi.org/10.21926/obm.geriatr.2303248 (accessed on 28th June 2025).

Corona, G., Rastrelli, G., & Maggi, M. (2013). Diagnosis and treatment of late-onset hypogonadism: Systematic review and meta-analysis of TRT outcomes. *Best Practice & Research Clinical Endocrinology & Metabolism, 27*(4), 557–579. https://doi.org/10.1007/s40618-022-01859-7 (accessed on 28th June 2025).

Cui, J., Ding, R., Liu, H., Ma, M., Zuo, R., & Liu, X. (2024). Trends in the incidence and survival of cancer in individuals aged 55 years and older in the United States, 1975–2019. *BMC Public Health, 24*(1), 72. https://doi.org/10.1186/s12889-023-17571-x (accessed on 28th June 2025).

Faheema Farvin, N. (2016). A study on the prevalence of subclinical hypothyroidism among pregnant women (Doctoral dissertation, Madras Medical College, Chennai). https://doi.org/10.1155/2021/5515831 (accessed on 28th June 2025).

Faubion, S. S., Crandall, C. J., Davis, L., El Khoudary, S. R., Hodis, H. N., Lobo, R. A., … & Wolfman, W. (2022). The 2022 hormone therapy position statement of the North American Menopause Society. *Menopause, 29*(7), 767–794. https://doi.org/10.1097/gme.0000000000002028 (accessed on 28th June 2025).

Ferrucci, L., & Fabbri, E. (2018). Inflammageing: Chronic inflammation in ageing, cardiovascular disease, and frailty. *Nature Reviews Cardiology, 15*(9), 505–522. https://doi.org/10.1038/s41569-018-0064-2 (accessed on 28th June 2025).

Fink, J., Schoenfeld, B. J., & Nakazato, K. (2018). The role of hormones in muscle hypertrophy. *The Physician and Sports Medicine, 46*(1), 129–134. https://doi.org/10.1080/00913847.2018.1406778 (accessed on 28th June 2025).

Furman, C. S. (1997). *Turning point: The myths and realities of menopause.* Oxford University Press. https://doi.org/10.1016/S0749-3797(18)30226-5 (accessed on 28th June 2025).

Gharahdaghi, N., Phillips, B. E., Szewczyk, N. J., Smith, K., Wilkinson, D. J., & Atherton, P. J. (2021). Links between testosterone, oestrogen, and the growth hormone/insulin-like growth factor axis and resistance exercise muscle adaptations. *Frontiers in Physiology, 11*, 621226. https://doi.org/10.3389/fphys.2020.621226 (accessed on 28th June 2025).

Giannoulis, M. G., Martin, F. C., Nair, K. S., Umpleby, A. M., & Sonksen, P. (2012). Hormone replacement therapy and physical function in healthy older men: Time to talk hormones? *Endocrine Reviews, 33*(3), 314–377. https://doi.org/10.1210/er.2012-1002 (accessed on 28th June 2025).

Hahner, S., Ross, R. J., Arlt, W., Bancos, I., Burger-Stritt, S., Torpy, D. J., & Quinkler, M. (2021). Adrenal insufficiency. *Nature Reviews Disease Primers, 7*(1), 19. https://doi.org/10.1038/s41572-021-00252-7 (accessed on 28th June 2025).

Hill, M., & Goldspink, G. (2003). Expression and splicing of the insulin-like growth factor gene in rodent muscle is associated with muscle satellite (stem) cell activation following local tissue damage. *The Journal of Physiology, 549*(2), 409–418. https://doi.org/10.1113/jphysiol.2002.035832 (accessed on 28th June 2025).

Indran, I. R., Liang, R. L. Z., Min, T. E., & Yong, E. L. (2016). Preclinical studies and clinical evaluation of compounds from the genus *Epimedium* for osteoporosis and bone health. *Pharmacology & Therapeutics, 162*, 188–205. https://doi.org/10.1016/j.pharmthera.2016.01.015 (accessed on 28th June 2025).

Johannsson, G., Skrtic, S., Lennernäs, H., Quinkler, M., & Stewart, P. M. (2014). Improving outcomes in patients with adrenal insufficiency: A review of current and future treatments. *Current Medical Research and Opinion, 30*(9), 1833–1847. https://doi.org/10.1185/03007995.2014.925865 (accessed on 28th June 2025).

Johnston, S., Bouchard, C., Fortier, M., & Wolfman, W. (2021). Guideline no. 422b: Menopause and genitourinary health. *Journal of Obstetrics and Gynaecology Canada, 43*(11), 1301–1307. https://doi.org/10.1016/j.jogc.2021.09.001 (accessed on 28th June 2025).

Kaur, M., Nagpal, M., Grewal, A. K., Chauhan, S., Dora, C. P., & Singh, T. G. (2023). Molecular complex of HSIM-loaded polymeric nanoparticles: Potential carriers in osteoporosis. *Current Drug Targets, 24*(13), 1066–1078. https://doi.org/10.2174/1389450124666230915092910 (accessed on 28th June 2025).

Kwatra, G., & Mukhopadhyay, S. (2018). Topical corticosteroids: Pharmacology. In *A Treatise on Topical Corticosteroids in Dermatology: Use, Misuse and Abuse* (pp. 11–22). https://doi.org/10.1007/978-981-10-4609-4_2 (accessed on 28th June 2025).

Lambalk, C. B., Van Disseldorp, J., De Koning, C. H., & Broekmans, F. J. (2009). Testing ovarian reserve to predict age at menopause. *Maturitas, 63*(4), 280–291. https://doi.org/10.1016/j.maturitas.2009.06.007 (accessed on 28th June 2025).

Liu, P. Y., Swerdloff, R. S., & Veldhuis, J. D. (2004). The rationale, efficacy and safety of androgen therapy in older men: Future research and current practice recommendations. *The Journal of Clinical Endocrinology & Metabolism, 89*(10), 4789–4796. https://doi.org/10.1210/jc.2004-0807 (accessed on 28th June 2025).

Lizneva, D., Yuen, T., Sun, L., Kim, S. M., Atabiekov, I., Munshi, L. B., … & Zaidi, M. (2018). Emerging concepts in the epidemiology, pathophysiology, and clinical care of osteoporosis across the menopausal transition. *Matrix Biology, 71*, 70–81. https://doi.org/10.1016/j.matbio.2018.05.001 (accessed on 28th June 2025).

Mali, H. S., & Manna, A. (2009). Current status and application of abrasive flow finishing processes: A review. *Proceedings of the Institution of Mechanical*

Engineers, Part B: Journal of Engineering Manufacture, 223(7), 809–820. https://doi.org/10.1243/09544054JEM1311 (accessed on 28th June 2025).

Mannan, A., Kakkar, C., Dhiman, S., & Singh, T. G. (2023). Advancing the frontiers of adaptive cell therapy: A transformative mechanistic journey from preclinical to clinical settings. *International Immunopharmacology, 125*, 111095. https://doi.org/10.1016/j.intimp.2023.111095 (accessed on 28th June 2025).

Martin, H., & Redfern, A. (2024). Bone mineral density fall during aromatase inhibitor treatment may predict lower breast cancer recurrence. *Cancer Medicine.* https://doi.org/10.1002/cam4.6846 (accessed on 28th June 2025).

Mehedintu, C., Carp-Veliscu, A., Plotogea, M., Edu, A., Petca, A., Dumitrascu, M., … & Antonovici, M. R. (2021). Benefits and risks of hormonal replacement therapy. *Romanian Journal of Medical Practice, 16*(6), 82. https://doi.org/10.3389/fendo.2021.564781 (accessed on 28th June 2025).

Mehta, S., Nain, P., Agrawal, B. K., & Singh, R. P. (2022). Vitamin D with calcium supplementation managing glycemic control with HbA1c and improve quality of life in patients with diabetes. *Turkish Journal of Pharmaceutical Sciences, 19*(2), 161–167. https://doi.org/10.4274/tjps.galenos.2021.62357 (accessed on 28th June 2025).

Mehta, S., Nain, P., Agrawal, B. K., Singh, R. P., Kaur, J., Maity, S., Bhattacharjee, A., Peela, J., Nauhria, S., & Nauhria, S. (2021). Effectiveness of empagliflozin with vitamin D supplementation in peripheral neuropathy in type 2 diabetic patients. *Cureus, 13*(12), e20208. https://doi.org/10.7759/cureus.20208 (accessed on 28th June 2025).

Modave, F., Bian, J., Leavitt, T., Bromwell, J., Harris III, C., & Vincent, H. (2015). Low quality of free coaching apps with respect to the American College of Sports Medicine Guidelines: A review of current mobile apps. *JMIR mHealth and uHealth, 3*(3), e4669. https://doi.org/10.2196/mhealth.4669 (accessed on 28th June 2025).

Moen, J. (2017). *Basic health care series: Obesity.* Vij Books India Pvt Ltd. https://doi.org/10.1016/B978-0-323-90446-9.00008-3 (accessed on 28th June 2025).

Monteleone, P., Mascagni, G., Giannini, A., Genazzani, A. R., & Simoncini, T. (2018). Symptoms of menopause—Global prevalence, physiology and implications. *Nature Reviews Endocrinology, 14*(4), 199–215. https://doi.org/10.1038/nrendo.2017.180 (accessed on 28th June 2025).

Muka, T., Oliver-Williams, C., Colpani, V., Kunutsor, S., Chowdhury, S., Chowdhury, R., … & Franco, O. H. (2016). Association of vasomotor and other menopausal symptoms with risk of cardiovascular disease: A systematic review and meta-analysis. *PLOS ONE, 11*(6), e0157417. https://doi.org/10.1371/journal.pone.0157417 (accessed on 28th June 2025).

Nappi, R. E., & Cucinella, L. (2020). Long-term consequences of menopause. In *Female Reproductive Dysfunction* (pp. 1–13). https://doi.org/10.1007/978-3-030-03594-5_17-1 (accessed on 28th June 2025).

Newton, K. M., Lacroix, A. Z., Leveille, S. G., Rutter, C., Keenan, N. L., & Anderson, L. A. (1997). Women's beliefs and decisions about hormone replacement therapy. *Journal of Women's Health, 6*(4), 459–465. https://doi.org/10.1089/jwh.1997.6.459 (accessed on 28th June 2025).

Okosieme, O. E. (2011). Thyroid hormone replacement: Current status and challenges. *Expert Opinion on Pharmacotherapy, 12*(15), 2315–2328. https://doi.org/10.1517/14656566.2011.600307 (accessed on 28th June 2025).

Paciuc, J. (2020). Hormone therapy in menopause. In *Hormonal Pathology of the Uterus* (pp. 89–120). https://doi.org/10.1007/978-3-030-38474-6_6 (accessed on 28th June 2025).

Padro, T., Muñoz-Garcia, N., Peña, E., & Badimon, L. (2021). Sex differences and emerging new risk factors for atherosclerosis and its thrombotic complications. *Current Pharmaceutical Design, 27*(29), 3186–3197. https://doi.org/10.3390/ijms24097910 (accessed on 28th June 2025).

Pastuszak, A. W., & Wang, R. (2015). Varicocele and testicular function. *Asian Journal of Andrology, 17*(4), 659. https://doi.org/10.4103/1008-682X.153539 (accessed on 28th June 2025).

Patsner, B. (2008). Pharmacy compounding of bioidentical hormone replacement therapy (BHRT): A proposed new approach to justify FDA regulation of these prescription drugs. *Food and Drug Law Journal, 63*(2), 459–491. https://doi.org/10.4065/mcp.2010.0714 (accessed on 28th June 2025).

Pinkerton, J. V., Vaughan, M. H., & Kaunitz, A. M. (2024). Hormonal medications for genitourinary syndrome of menopause. *Clinical Obstetrics and Gynecology, 67*(1), 68–78. https://doi.org/10.1097/grf.0000000000000835 (accessed on 28th June 2025).

Pollow, D. P., Uhlorn, J., Husband, N., & Brooks, H. L. (2019). Regulation of postmenopausal hypertension. In *Sex Differences in Cardiovascular Physiology and Pathophysiology* (pp. 105–118). https://doi.org/10.2165/11588030-000000000-00000 (accessed on 28th June 2025).

Rihal, V., Khan, H., Kaur, A., Singh, T. G., & Abdel-Daim, M. M. (2022). Therapeutic and mechanistic intervention of vitamin D in neuropsychiatric disorders. *Psychiatry Research, 317*, 114782. https://doi.org/10.1016/j.psychres.2022.114782 (accessed on 28th June 2025).

Saklani, P., Khan, H., Gupta, S., Kaur, A., & Singh, T. G. (2022). Neuropeptides: Potential neuroprotective agents in ischemic injury. *Life Sciences, 288*, 120186. https://doi.org/10.1016/j.lfs.2021.120186 (accessed on 28th June 2025).

Santen, R. J., Allred, D. C., Ardoin, S. P., Archer, D. F., Boyd, N., Braunstein, G. D., … & Utian, W. H. (2010). Postmenopausal hormone therapy: An Endocrine Society scientific statement. *The Journal of Clinical Endocrinology & Metabolism, 95*(7_Supplement_1), S1–S66. https://doi.org/10.1210/jc.2009-2509 (accessed on 28th June 2025).

Sharma, V. K., Singh, T. G., & Mehta, V. (2021). Stressed mitochondria: A target to intrude Alzheimer's disease. *Mitochondrion, 59*, 48–57. https://doi.org/10.1016/j.mito.2021.04.004 (accessed on 28th June 2025).

Sharma, V., Singh, T. G., & Mannan, A. (2022). Therapeutic implications of glucose transporters (GLUT) in cerebral ischemia. *Neurochemical Research, 47*(8), 2173–2186. https://doi.org/10.1007/s11064-022-03620-1 (accessed on 28th June 2025).

Shen, V., Birchman, R., Xu, R., Lindsay, R., & Dempster, D. W. (1995). Short-term changes in histomorphometric and biochemical turnover markers and bone mineral density in estrogen- and/or dietary calcium-deficient rats. *Bone, 16*(1), 149–156. https://doi.org/10.1016/8756-3282(95)80026-M (accessed on 28th June 2025).

Singh, S., Singh, T. G., Mahajan, K., & Dhiman, S. (2020). Medicinal plants used against various inflammatory biomarkers for the management of rheumatoid arthritis. *The Journal of Pharmacy and Pharmacology, 72*(10), 1306–1327. https://doi.org/10.1111/jphp.13326 (accessed on 28th June 2025).

Storer, T. W., Woodhouse, L., Magliano, L., Singh, A. B., Dzekov, C., Dzekov, J., & Bhasin, S. (2008). Changes in muscle mass, muscle strength, and power but not physical function are related to testosterone dose in healthy older men. *Journal of the American Geriatrics Society, 56*(11), 1991–1999. https://doi.org/10.1111/j.1532-5415.2008.01927.x (accessed on 28th June 2025).

Stout, M. B., Justice, J. N., Nicklas, B. J., & Kirkland, J. L. (2017). Physiological aging: Links among adipose tissue dysfunction, diabetes, and frailty. *Physiology, 32*(1), 9–19. https://doi.org/10.1152/physiol.00012.2016 (accessed on 28th June 2025).

Stuck, A. E., Siu, A. L., Wieland, G. D., Rubenstein, L. Z., & Adams, J. (1993). Comprehensive geriatric assessment: A meta-analysis of controlled trials. *The Lancet, 342*(8878), 1032–1036. https://doi.org/10.1016/0140-6736(93)92884-V (accessed on 28th June 2025).

Suominen, H. (2011). Ageing and maximal physical performance. *European Review of Aging and Physical Activity, 8*, 37–42. https://doi.org/10.1007/s10522-016-9641-0 (accessed on 28th June 2025).

Thakur, A. K., Chellappan, D. K., Dua, K., Mehta, M., Satija, S., & Singh, I. (2020). Patented therapeutic drug delivery strategies for targeting pulmonary diseases. *Expert Opinion on Therapeutic Patents, 30*(5), 375–387. https://doi.org/10.1080/13543776.2020.1741547 (accessed on 28th June 2025).

Thapa, K., Khan, H., Kaur, G., Kumar, P., & Singh, T. G. (2023). Therapeutic targeting of angiopoietins in tumor angiogenesis and cancer development. *Biochemical and Biophysical Research Communications, 687*, 149130. https://doi.org/10.1016/j.bbrc.2023.149130 (accessed on 28th June 2025).

Thapa, K., Khan, H., Singh, T. G., & Kaur, A. (2021). Traumatic brain injury: Mechanistic insight on pathophysiology and potential therapeutic targets. *Journal of Molecular Neuroscience: MN, 71*(9), 1725–1742. https://doi.org/10.1007/s12031-021-01841-7 (accessed on 28th June 2025).

Vigneswaran, K., & Hamoda, H. (2022). Hormone replacement therapy – Current recommendations. *Best Practice & Research Clinical Obstetrics & Gynaecology, 81*, 8–21. https://doi.org/10.1016/j.bpobgyn.2021.12.001 (accessed on 28th June 2025).

Wong, W. F., Ang, K. P., Sethi, G., & Looi, C. Y. (2023). Recent advancement of medical patch for transdermal drug delivery. *Medicina (Kaunas, Lithuania), 59*(4), 778. https://doi.org/10.3390/medicina59040778 (accessed on 28th June 2025).

Woodhouse, L. J., Mukherjee, A., Shalet, S. M., & Ezzat, S. (2006). The influence of growth hormone status on physical impairments, functional limitations, and health-related quality of life in adults. *Endocrine Reviews, 27*(3), 287–317. https://doi.org/10.1210/er.2004-0022 (accessed on 28th June 2025).

CHAPTER 5

Understanding Lesch-Nyhan Syndrome: Overview and Pharmacotherapeutic Strategies

SAKSHI MALIK,[1,*] HAROON RIASAT,[2] and DANIA MUGHAL[3]

[1]*Acute and General Medicine, Hull University Teaching Hospitals NHS Trust, Hull, United Kingdom*

[2]*Diabetes and Endocrinology, Hull University Teaching Hospitals NHS Trust, Hull, United Kingdom*

[3]*Pediatric Diabetes, North Lincolnshire and Goole NHS Trust, Grimsby, United Kingdom*

*Corresponding author

ABSTRACT

Lesch-Nyhan Syndrome is a rare genetic disorder related to chromosome X and characterized by a mutation in the *HGPRT1* gene. This mutation leads to a deficiency of the enzyme hypoxanthine-guanine phosphoribosyl transferase (HGPRT). The lack of HGPRT results in the accumulation of uric acid in all body fluids, which in turn causes severe neurological and behavioral symptoms.Self-mutilating behavior, characterized by lip and finger biting, is a hallmark feature of this syndrome. High uric acid levels result in the accumulation of sodium urate crystals in joints, kidneys, the Central Nervous System, and other parts of the body, resulting in swelling of the joints, severe kidney problems, and neurological features. Symptom control is the mainstay of the treatment. Allopurinol can prevent excessive amounts of uric acid accumulation in joints. Kidney stones in Lesch-Nyhan

Precision Nutrition and Endocrine Health: Synthesis, Characterization, and Applications.
Thakur Gurjeet Singh and Sanjana Mehta (Eds.)

DOI: 10.1201/9781998511877-5

Syndrome can be treated with lithotripsy, while physiotherapy is recommended to prevent contractures. However, no standard treatment currently exists to address the neurological symptoms of Lesh-Nyhan Syndrome. A variety of patients can benefit from drugs like diazepam, phenobarbital, haloperidol, levodopa, or carbidopa. Further research into more options, such as targeted gene therapy for the definitive management of the condition, is required to develop a standard treatment.

5.1 INTRODUCTION

Lesch-Nyhan Syndrome is a genetic disorder caused by a deficiency in the enzyme hypoxanthine-guanine phosphoribosyltransferase (HGPRT), leading to an inborn error in purine metabolism which results in overproduction of uric acid manifesting in the form of lithiasis, gout and a spectrum of neurological features. Lesch-Nyhan syndrome is the most severe form of the HGPRT enzymatic deficiency, the neurological manifestations of which include cognitive and attention deficit, severe action dystonia, ballismus, choreoathetosis and self-injurious behavior (Bell et al., 2016). The deficiency of HGPRT enzymatic activity is linked to two OMIM entities. Leshc-Nyhan Syndrome (OMIM 300322), first described by M. Lesch and W. Nyhan in 1964, is associated with complete HGPRT deficiency. In 1967, a partial deficiency of HGPRT activity was described, termed Kelly-Seegmiller syndrome or HGPRT-related gout (OMIM 300323) (Kelley et al., 1967). This form of HGPRT deficiency manifested as gouty features with minimal neurological symptoms. A continuous spectrum of neurological features is found between two syndromes, and the sufferers are called Lesch Nyhan variants presenting with HGPRT-related gout with variable degrees of neurological involvement.

5.2 EPIDEMIOLOGY AND CLINICAL FEATURES

The disease has an estimated prevalence of 1 in 380,000 live births. The HGPRT enzyme is encoded by a single structural gene located on the long arm of the X-chromosome at Xq26. Being an X-linked recessive condition, the affected population is males. Females are usually carriers and thus asymptomatic. Patients with Lesch-Nyhan syndrome appear normal at birth. One of the earliest signs is noticing orange crystals in the diapers, i.e., crystalluria due to urinary tract obstruction.

Psychomotor delay becomes apparent within 3–6 months. Also, delayed achievement of neck holding and sitting with hypotonia and athetoid movements raises suspicion of an abnormality needing further attention.

Obsessive-compulsive self-injurious behavior is the hallmark feature of this syndrome, which typically manifests between the ages of 2 and 16 years (Nyhan et al., 1972).

This behavior becomes apparent in the form of lip biting and finger chewing. Aggressive behavior is episodic; generally, children with Lesch-Nyhan syndrome are cheerful and engaging when restrained. After using specific tests for motor function evaluation, all Lesch-Nyhan variants and patients with Lesch-Nyhan syndrome have variable degrees of mental retardation, along with a variable degree of attention deficit disorders. The neuro-behavioral symptoms can be markedly optimized by environmental factors like familiarization with the environment and, most importantly, education (Jinnah et al., 2006).

Patients can frequently present with hematological abnormalities like megaloblastic anemia, and in some rare cases, microcytic anemia can also be present.

Renal and joint symptoms related to hyperuricemia are present in all Lesch-Nyhan syndrome cases, including urolithiasis or nephrolithiasis, gouty arthritis, and juvenile arthritis. Rarely, in cases of delayed diagnosis, patients can present with renal failure or acidosis.

5.3 DIAGNOSIS

The diagnosis of Lesch-Nyhan syndrome is based on clinical features, biochemical findings, and enzymatic and molecular tests. Children born with the syndrome are normal at birth. The apparent psychomotor delay raises suspicion of an abnormality, requiring further investigations. Other clinical features significantly pointing towards the condition are cognitive and behavioral abnormality, self-mutilating behavior, and gouty features.

5.3.1 BIOCHEMICAL FEATURES

Hyperuricemia and hyperuricosuria are biochemical findings that help diagnose the condition. In cases of psychomotor delay, it is important to consider early evaluation of serum and urine uric acid levels as part of the differential diagnosis. Urine uric acid/creatinine ratio can also be used as a screening test for diagnosing inherited disorders of purine metabolism. However, the values are age-specific and should be interpreted according to the patient's age. Plasma concentration of uric acid and other purine metabolites is markedly raised (Kaufman et al., 1968; Singh et al., 2021; Torres et al., 2007).

5.3.2 ENZYMATIC TESTS

HGPRT activity determination in hemolysate, red cells, and fibroblasts helps diagnose the condition. In HGPRT deficient patients/Lesch-Nyhan variants, 0–10% HGRPT activity is observed in hemolysates, whereas HGPRT activity is undetectable in patients with Lesch-Nyhan syndrome (Rylance et al., 1982).

5.3.3 MOLECULAR TESTS

Molecular tests facilitate prenatal diagnosis of the condition through amniocentesis, which can be performed at 15–18 weeks or chorionic villous sampling at about 10–12 weeks of gestation. While Lesch-Nyhan Syndrome follows an X- linked recessive inheritance pattern, about 30% of the patients' mothers are not carriers, depicting that LNS can result from *de novo* mutations (Hara et al., 1982). HGPRT-deficient individuals show HGPRT mRNA expression, and molecular diagnosis can be made firm by cDNA sequencing. A very high degree of heterogeneity is noted in mutations in HGPRT-deficient individuals in terms of type and location within the gene, ranging from point mutations to deletion, insertion, and duplication. HGPRT variants are noted to result from single-point mutations, while Lesch-Nyhan syndrome results from mutations affecting the size of the resultant protein (Bhargava et al., 2022; De Gregorio et al., 2005; Ogasawara et al., 1989).

5.4 TREATMENT

- **Optimizing the Serum Uric Acid Levels:** Uric acid overproduction can result in crystalluria, acute arthritis, gouty arthritis, nephrolithiasis or urolithiasis. Xanthine oxidase inhibitors (Allopurinol) can block the enzyme xanthine oxidase and prevent the production of uric acid from xanthine and hypoxanthine (Kelley et al., 1969;

Singh et al., 2020). Upon confirmation of the diagnosis, initiating allopurinol therapy is crucial. The recommended starting dose is 5–10 mg/kg/day, adjusting as needed to maintain high normal serum uric acid levels and achieve a urinary uric acid/ creatinine ratio below 1. Treatment with allopurinol is proven to be highly efficacious leading to approximately a 50% reduction in serum uric acid levels and a substantial decrease of about 74% in the urinary uric acid/creatinine ratio. Though allopurinol is generally safe to use for the treatment of overproduction of uric acid, xanthine lithiasis can develop in some cases, which can be prevented by serial measurement of urinary oxypurinol, the level of which should be targeted to corresponding to certain levels of uric acid excretion (Torres et al., 2007).

- **Managing Motor Symptoms:** Since the cause of neurological dysfunction is unknown, the available therapy targets symptom control. No medication has been found to control the extrapyramidal symptoms effectively. Spasticity and dystonia can be effectively managed using benzodiazepines and GABA inhibitors, e.g., baclofen (Jinnah et al., 2006; Sharma et al., 2023). Referral to physical rehabilitation is one of the mainstays of the treatment. Appropriate walking aids, special devices to aid hand control of objects, and posture management are advised to improve quality of life.
- **Managing Behavioral Problems:** A combination of behavioral and pharmacological treatment and physical retainment can manage self-mutilating behavior. Aggressive behavior is sometimes shown against friends or family members, which can be because of stress or anxiety. Stressful situations can be managed using behavioral management strategies like de-escalation. Pharmacological therapy using benzodiazepines and carbamazepine can also be used to improve symptoms related to stress/anxiety. The mainstay for the management of self-harm is physical retainment, for example, using elbow restraints to avoid finger biting and using dental guards to avoid cheek biting.

It was believed that the decreased concentration of purines in the cells of LNS patients is because of the failure of purine recycling. HGPRT deficiency is supposed to have minimal effect on the concentration of purine in these cells as the deficiency can be compensated by increasing the *de novo* purine synthesis (Nyhan et al., 1997). On the contrary, in experimental studies, administration of purine did not improve behavioral or neurological symptoms but helped reduce uric acid excretion and combat megaloblastic anemia in some LNS patients (Mehta et al., 2021; Torres and Puig, 2007). Another study showed some improvement in behavioral symptoms with the administration of purine. However, the resulting renal failure due to the overproduction of insoluble metabolites urged the abandonment of this treatment (Ceccarelli et al., 1974; Kumar et al., 2023).

Some early studies proved that the administration of 5-hydroxytryptophan, carbidopa and imipramine can improve the self-injurious behavior in LNS patients, but the effect tends to be temporary and usually lasts only a few weeks (Nyhan et al., 1980, 2000; Soni et al., 2024).

Most later studies on LNS patients have focused on providing evidence suggesting dopaminergic deficiency in LNS patients. Positron Emission Tomography (PET) studies depicting DOPA decarboxylase activity have evidenced that LNS patients have significantly reduced dopaminergic production and storage compared to controls (Ernst et al., 1996; Khan et al., 2022; Sharma et al., 2021; Wong et al., 1996). Following this evidence, trials have been made to increase the level of dopamine in the brain with a compound called L-dopa, which is converted to dopamine by DOPA decarboxylase. However, the current evidence suggests very minimal to no improvement in self-mutilating behavior and the effect is temporary (Ciaranello et al., 1976; Hunter et al., 1996; Jankovic et al., 1988; Manzke et al., 1986; Mittal et al., 2023; Mizuno and Yugari, 1975; Rebai et al., 2014; Schneider et al., 2006; Serrano et al., 2008; Singh et al., 2021; Visser et al., 2011).

A dramatic and persistent improvement in self-injurious behavior over several years is observed when LNS patients are treated with S-adenyl methionine (SAM) with an intent to decrease transaminase levels, which are usually elevated in LNS patients due to regular fentanyl administration (Dolcetta et al., 2013; Glick et al., 2006; Lauber et al., 2016; Mehta et al., 2022).

Some experimental studies have suggested that gabapentin can improve self-inflicting behavior. Other management options without proven efficacy are botulinum toxin and deep brain stimulation. Further treatment options using molecular testing and gene therapy are yet to be explored.

5.5 CONCLUSION

Since Lesch and Nyhan's first recognition of the syndrome in 1964, the syndrome has attracted the interest of many clinicians and scientists worldwide. Trials have been made to understand the genetic basis of the condition, the effect of HGPRT deficiency, the symptoms caused by the overproduction of uric acid, therapeutics to manage the joint manifestations, neuropathological and behavioral manifestations, yet the effective management of the condition with the available options is questionable.

To develop better management options, the underlying etiology of the disease must be fully understood. Future studies should examine the mechanisms behind the beneficial effects of the available treatment options that have notably shown positive results, such as deep brain stimulation and SAM administration. Conducting more experimental studies in this area to support or reject the available hypotheses is advisable.

Various LNS models have been devised, but the treatments that showed positive results in the LNS models could not replicate the same levels of improvement in the human brain, meaning that the complete biochemical picture of HGPRT deficiency has not yet been successfully created. Understanding the currently known biochemical abnormalities involved in the condition, new strategic models need to be devised in combination with newer and more effective methods of investigation to gain a greater understanding of the etiology and develop more effective interventions.

KEYWORDS

- **allopurinol therapy**
- **experimental therapies**
- **genetic disorder**
- ***HGPRT1 gene***
- **molecular diagnosis**
- **X-linked genetic disorder**

REFERENCES

Anderson, L. T., Herrmann, L., & Dancis, J. (1976). The effect of L-5-hydroxytryptophan on self-mutilation in Lesch-Nyhan disease: A negative report. *Neuropädiatrie, 7*(4), 439–442. https://doi.org/10.1055/s-0028-1091644 (accessed on 28th June 2025).

Bell, S., Kolobova, I., Crapper, L., & Ernst, C. (2016). Lesch-Nyhan syndrome: Models, theories, and therapies. *Molecular Syndromology, 7*(6), 302–311. https://doi.org/10.1159/000449296 (accessed on 28th June 2025).

Bhargava, S. K., Singh, T. G., Mannan, A., Singh, S., Singh, M., & Gupta, S. (2022). Pharmacological evaluation of *Thuja occidentalis* for the attenuation of neuropathy via AGEs and TNF-α inhibition in diabetic neuropathic rats. *Environmental Science and Pollution Research International, 29*(40), 60542–60557. https://doi.org/10.1007/s11356-022-20106-3 (accessed on 28th June 2025).

Ceccarelli, M., Ciompi, M. L., & Pasero, G. (1974). Acute renal failure during adenine therapy in Lesch-Nyhan syndrome. *Advances in Experimental Medicine and Biology, 41*, 671–675. https://doi.org/10.1007/978-1-4757-1433-3_38 (accessed on 28th June 2025).

Ciaranello, R. D., Anders, T. F., Barchas, J. D., Berger, P. A., & Cann, H. M. (1976). The use of 5-hydroxytryptophan in a child with Lesch-Nyhan syndrome. *Child Psychiatry and Human Development, 7*(2), 127–133. https://doi.org/10.1007/BF01464036 (accessed on 28th June 2025).

De Gregorio, L., Jinnah, H. A., Harris, J. C., Nyhan, W. L., Schretlen, D. J., Trombley, L. M., & O'Neill, J. P. (2005). Lesch-Nyhan disease in a female with a clinically normal monozygotic twin. *Molecular Genetics and Metabolism, 85*(1), 70–77. https://doi.org/10.1016/j.ymgme.2004.11.009 (accessed on 28th June 2025).

Dolcetta, D., Parmigiani, P., Salmaso, L., Bernardelle, R., Cesari, U., Andrighetto, G., Baschirotto, G., Nyhan, W. L., & Hladnik, U. (2013). Quantitative evaluation of the clinical effects of S-adenosylmethionine on mood and behavior in Lesch-Nyhan patients. *Nucleosides, Nucleotides & Nucleic Acids, 32*(4), 174–188. https://doi.org/10.1080/15257770.2013.774012 (accessed on 28th June 2025).

Ernst, M., Zametkin, A. J., Matochik, J. A., Pascualvaca, D., Jons, P. H., Hardy, K., Hankerson, J. G., Doudet, D. J., & Cohen, R. M. (1996). Presynaptic dopaminergic deficits in Lesch-Nyhan disease. *The New England Journal of Medicine, 334*(24), 1568–1572. https://doi.org/10.1056/NEJM199606133342403 (accessed on 28th June 2025).

Glick, N. (2006). Dramatic reduction in self-injury in Lesch-Nyhan disease following S-adenosylmethionine administration. *Journal of Inherited Metabolic Disease, 29*(5), 687. https://doi.org/10.1007/s10545-006-0229-8 (accessed on 28th June 2025).

Hunter, T. C., Melancon, S. B., Dallaire, L., Taft, S., Skopek, T. R., Albertini, R. J., & O'Neill, J. P. (1996). Germinal HPRT splice donor site mutation results in multiple RNA splicing products in T-lymphocyte cultures. *Somatic Cell and Molecular Genetics, 22*(2), 145–150. https://doi.org/10.1007/BF02369904 (accessed on 28th June 2025).

Jankovic, J., Caskey, T. C., Stout, J. T., & Butler, I. J. (1988). Lesch-Nyhan syndrome: A study of motor behavior and cerebrospinal fluid neurotransmitters. *Annals of Neurology, 23*(5), 466–469. https://doi.org/10.1002/ana.410230507 (accessed on 28th June 2025).

Jinnah, H. A., Visser, J. E., Harris, J. C., Verdu, A., Larovere, L., Ceballos-Picot, I., Gonzalez-Alegre, P., Neychev, V., Torres, R. J., Dulac, O., Desguerre, I., Schretlen, D. J., Robey, K. L., Barabas, G., Bloem, B. R., Nyhan, W., De Kremer, R., Eddey, G. E., Puig, J. G., & Lesch-Nyhan Disease International Study Group. (2006). Delineation of the motor disorder of Lesch-Nyhan disease. *Brain: A Journal of Neurology, 129*(Pt 5), 1201–1217. https://doi.org/10.1093/brain/awl056 (accessed on 28th June 2025).

Kaufman, J. M., Greene, M. L., & Seegmiller, J. E. (1968). Urine uric acid to creatinine ratio – a screening test for inherited disorders of purine metabolism. *The Journal of Pediatrics, 73*(4), 583–592. https://doi.org/10.1016/s0022-3476(68)80274-4 (accessed on 28th June 2025).

Kelley, W. N., Greene, M. L., Rosenbloom, F. M., Henderson, J. F., & Seegmiller, J. E. (1969). Hypoxanthine-guanine phosphoribosyltransferase deficiency in gout. *Annals of Internal Medicine, 70*(1), 155–206. https://doi.org/10.7326/0003-4819-70-1-155 (accessed on 28th June 2025).

Kelley, W. N., Rosenbloom, F. M., Henderson, J. F., & Seegmiller, J. E. (1967). A specific enzyme defect in gout associated with overproduction of uric acid. *Proceedings of the National Academy of Sciences of the United States of America, 57*(6), 1735–1739. https://doi.org/10.1073/pnas.57.6.1735 (accessed on 28th June 2025).

Khan, H., Tiwari, C., Grewal, A. K., Singh, T. G., Chauhan, S., & Batiha, G. E. (2022). Pharmacological modulation of phosphodiesterase-7 as a novel strategy for neurodegenerative disorders. *Inflammopharmacology, 30*(6), 2051–2061. https://doi.org/10.1007/s10787-022-01072-1 (accessed on 28th June 2025).

Kumar, M., Kaur, K., & Singh, T. G. (2023). Neuroprotective effects of carbonic anhydrase inhibition and cyclic adenosine monophosphate activation in mouse model of transient global cerebral ischemia and reperfusion. *Neuromolecular Medicine, 25*(2), 217–229. https://doi.org/10.1007/s12017-022-08728-9 (accessed on 28th June 2025).

Lama, A., Pirozzi, C., Avagliano, C., Annunziata, C., Mollica, M. P., Calignano, A., Meli, R., & Mattace Raso, G. (2020). Nutraceuticals: An integrative approach to starve Parkinson's disease. *Brain, Behavior, & Immunity – Health, 2*, 100037. https://doi.org/10.1016/j.bbih.2020.100037 (accessed on 28th June 2025).

Lauber, M., Plecko, B., Pfiffner, M., Nuoffer, J. M., & Häberle, J. (2017). The effect of S-adenosylmethionine on self-mutilation in a patient with Lesch-Nyhan disease. *JIMD Reports, 32*, 51–57. https://doi.org/10.1007/8904_2016_571 (accessed on 28th June 2025).

Manzke, H., Gustmann, H., Koke, H. G., & Nyhan, W. L. (1986). Hypoxanthine and tetrahydrobiopterin treatment of a patient with features of the Lesch-Nyhan syndrome. *Advances in Experimental Medicine and Biology, 195* Pt A, 197–203. https://doi.org/10.1007/978-1-4684-5104-7_31 (accessed on 28th June 2025).

Maruta, K., Ohi, T., Yamada, Y., Goto, H., Ogasawara, N., & Matsukura, S. (1997). *No to shinkei = Brain and Nerve, 49*(11), 1009–1013.

Mehta, S., Nain, P., Agrawal, B. K., & Singh, R. P. (2022). Vitamin D with calcium supplementation managing glycemic control with HbA1c and improve quality of life in patients with diabetes. *Turkish Journal of Pharmaceutical Sciences, 19*(2), 161–167. https://doi.org/10.4274/tjps.galenos.2021.62357 (accessed on 28th June 2025).

Mehta, S., Nain, P., Agrawal, B. K., Singh, R. P., Kaur, J., Maity, S., Bhattacharjee, A., Peela, J., Nauhria, S., & Nauhria, S. (2021). Effectiveness of empagliflozin with vitamin

D supplementation in peripheral neuropathy in type 2 diabetic patients. *Cureus, 13*(12), e20208. https://doi.org/10.7759/cureus.20208 (accessed on 28th June 2025).

Mittal, P., Dhankhar, S., Chauhan, S., Garg, N., Bhattacharya, T., Ali, M., Chaudhary, A. A., Rudayni, H. A., Al-Zharani, M., Ahmad, W., Khan, S. U., Singh, T. G., & Mujwar, S. (2023). A review on natural antioxidants for their role in the treatment of Parkinson's disease. *Pharmaceuticals (Basel, Switzerland), 16*(7), 908. https://doi.org/10.3390/ph16070908 (accessed on 28th June 2025).

Nyhan, W. L. (1972). Clinical features of the Lesch-Nyhan syndrome. *Archives of Internal Medicine, 130*(2), 186–192. https://doi.org/10.1001/archinte.1972.03650020016004 (accessed on 28th June 2025).

Nyhan, W. L. (1997). The recognition of Lesch-Nyhan syndrome as an inborn error of purine metabolism. *Journal of Inherited Metabolic Disease, 20*(2), 171–178. https://doi.org/10.1023/a:1005348504512 (accessed on 28th June 2025).

Nyhan, W. L. (2000). Dopamine function in Lesch-Nyhan disease. *Environmental Health Perspectives, 108* Suppl 3, 409–411. https://doi.org/10.1289/ehp.00108s3409 (accessed on 28th June 2025).

Nyhan, W. L., Johnson, H. G., Kaufman, I. A., & Jones, K. L. (1980). Serotonergic approaches to the modification of behavior in the Lesch-Nyhan syndrome. *Applied Research in Mental Retardation, 1*(1–2), 25–40. https://doi.org/10.1016/0270-3092(80)90014-4 (accessed on 28th June 2025).

Ogasawara, N., Stout, J. T., Goto, H., Sonta, S., Matsumoto, A., & Caskey, C. T. (1989). Molecular analysis of a female Lesch-Nyhan patient. *The Journal of Clinical Investigation, 84*(3), 1024–1027. https://doi.org/10.1172/JCI114224 (accessed on 28th June 2025).

Rylance, H. J., Wallace, R. C., & Nuki, G. (1982). Hypoxanthine-guanine phosphoribosyl transferase: Assay using high performance liquid chromatography. *Clinica Chimica Acta, 121*(2), 159–165. https://doi.org/10.1016/0009-8981(82)90054-7 (accessed on 28th June 2025).

Schneider, S. A., Aggarwal, A., Bhatt, M., Dupont, E., Tisch, S., Limousin, P., Lee, P., Quinn, N., & Bhatia, K. P. (2006). Severe tongue protrusion dystonia: Clinical syndromes and possible treatment. *Neurology, 67*(6), 940–943. https://doi.org/10.1212/01.wnl.0000237446.06971.72 (accessed on 28th June 2025).

Serrano, M., Pérez-Dueñas, B., Ormazábal, A., Artuch, R., Campistol, J., Torres, R. J., & García-Cazorla, A. (2008). Levodopa therapy in a Lesch-Nyhan disease patient: Pathological, biochemical, neuroimaging, and therapeutic remarks. *Movement Disorders: Official Journal of the Movement Disorder Society, 23*(9), 1297–1300.

Sharma, T., Kaur, D., Grewal, A. K., & Singh, T. G. (2021). Therapies modulating insulin resistance in Parkinson's disease: A cross talk. *Neuroscience Letters, 749*, 135754. https://doi.org/10.1016/j.neulet.2021.135754 (accessed on 28th June 2025).

Sharma, V. K., Singh, T. G., Mehta, V., & Mannan, A. (2023). Biomarkers: Role and scope in neurological disorders. *Neurochemical Research, 48*(7), 2029–2058. https://doi.org/10.1007/s11064-023-03873-4 (accessed on 28th June 2025).

Singh, H. P., Singh, T. G., & Singh, R. (2020). Sinapic acid attenuates cisplatin-induced nephrotoxicity through peroxisome proliferator-activated receptor gamma agonism in rats. *Journal of Pharmacy & Bioallied Sciences, 12*(2), 146–154. https://doi.org/10.4103/jpbs.JPBS_220_19 (accessed on 28th June 2025).

Singh, S., Singh, T. G., Rehni, A. K., Sharma, V., Singh, M., & Kaur, R. (2021). Reviving mitochondrial bioenergetics: A relevant approach in epilepsy. *Mitochondrion, 58*, 213–226. https://doi.org/10.1016/j.mito.2021.03.009 (accessed on 28th June 2025).

Singh, S., Singh, T. G., Singh, M., Najda, A., Nurzyńska-Wierdak, R., Almeer, R., Kamel, M., & Abdel-Daim, M. M. (2021). Anticonvulsive effects of chondroitin sulfate on pilocarpine and pentylenetetrazole induced epileptogenesis in mice. *Molecules (Basel, Switzerland), 26*(22), 6773. https://doi.org/10.3390/molecules26226773 (accessed on 28th June 2025).

Torres, R. J., & Puig, J. G. (2007). Hypoxanthine-guanine phosphoribosyltransferase (HPRT) deficiency: Lesch-Nyhan syndrome. *Orphanet Journal of Rare Diseases, 2*, 48. https://doi.org/10.1186/1750-1172-2-48 (accessed on 28th June 2025).

Torres, R. J., Prior, C., & Puig, J. G. (2007). Efficacy and safety of allopurinol in patients with hypoxanthine-guanine phosphoribosyltransferase deficiency. *Metabolism: Clinical and Experimental, 56*(9), 1179–1186. https://doi.org/10.1016/j.metabol.2007.04.013 (accessed on 28th June 2025).

Visser, J. E., Schretlen, D. J., Bloem, B. R., & Jinnah, H. A. (2011). Levodopa is not a useful treatment for Lesch-Nyhan disease. *Movement Disorders: Official Journal of the Movement Disorder Society, 26*(4), 746–749. https://doi.org/10.1002/mds.23478 (accessed on 28th June 2025).

Wong, D. F., Harris, J. C., Naidu, S., Yokoi, F., Marenco, S., Dannals, R. F., Ravert, H. T., Yaster, M., Evans, A., Rousset, O., Bryan, R. N., Gjedde, A., Kuhar, M. J., & Breese, G. R. (1996). Dopamine transporters are markedly reduced in Lesch-Nyhan disease in vivo. *Proceedings of the National Academy of Sciences of the United States of America, 93*(11), 5539–5543. https://doi.org/10.1073/pnas.93.11.5539 (accessed on 28th June 2025).

CHAPTER 6

Proteomics in Pediatric Endocrine and Metabolic Disorders: Applications and Implications

NEELPARNA INDU,[1] ANIRBAN HAIT,[1] ATHARVA ANAND MAHAJAN,[2] SAHELI BANERJEE,[3] RANIT MONDAL,[4] ANUVAB DEY,[5] SUBHROJYOTI GHOSH,[6,*] and BRIAN G. OLIVER[7,8]

[1]*Department of Biotechnology, Heritage Institute of Technology, Kolkata, West Bengal, India*

[2]*Tata Memorial Center, Advanced Center for Treatment, Research and Education, Mumbai, Maharashtra, India*

[3]*Department of Chemistry and Chemical Biology, Indian Institute of Technology (Indian School of Mines), Dhanbad, Jharkhand, India*

[4]*Department of Pharmaceutical Technology, Jadavpur University, Kolkata, West Bengal, India*

[5]*Department of Biosciences and Bioengineering, Indian Institute of Technology Guwahati, Assam, India*

[6]*Department of Biotechnology, Indian Institute of Technology Madras, Chennai, Tamil Nadu, India*

[7]*School of Life Sciences, University of Technology Sydney, Sydney, New South Wales, Australia*

[8]*Woolcock Institute of Medical Research, University of Sydney, Sydney, New South Wales, Australia*

*Corresponding author

Precision Nutrition and Endocrine Health: Synthesis, Characterization, and Applications.
Thakur Gurjeet Singh and Sanjana Mehta (Eds.)

DOI: 10.1201/9781998511877-6

ABSTRACT

The objective of proteomics, a cutting-edge field driven by technology, is to understand the pathophysiologic mechanisms of the underlying diseases. The current revolution in proteomics has led to the identification of precise biomarkers for diagnosis, therapy, and prediction that, when combined, will enable successful, patient-specific, tailored approaches by the basic principles of predictive, preventive, and personalized medicine. Mass spectrometry-based proteomics finds a broad range of applications in pediatric endocrinology, including type-1 diabetes, thyroid disease, adrenal disease, metabolic syndrome, and inborn errors of metabolism (IEM). These applications include accurate diagnosis, early detection of specific at-risk populations to prevent potential complications or disease manifestation, and neonatal screening. Urinemic is a rapidly growing field in pediatric proteomics since urine sample collection from a child is more accessible as it is a non-invasive procedure. Analysis of metabolites in urine is suggested for children suspected to bear different inborn errors of metabolism. We now know that urine includes many proteins, contrary to previously believed. The field of proteomics holds many promises for novel biomarkers in pediatric applications. Future efforts are anticipated to contribute to the creation of marker panels and standardization of procedures, ultimately aiding in the early diagnosis of pediatric illnesses, prognostication, and therapeutic follow-up.

6.1 INTRODUCTION

The emerging field of predictive, preventive, personalized medicine (PPPM) aims to revolutionize healthcare by offering individualized risk assessments, preventive strategies, and tailored therapeutic options based on the Unique characteristics of each patient and their disease, considering both genetic and environmental factors (Golubnitschaja et al., 2016). A deeper understanding of disease mechanisms is crucial to achieving this goal, allowing for identifying subtle differences that make each patient unique (Golubnitschaja et al., 2014; Kaur et al., 2023). Reliable biomarkers play a pivotal role in PPPM, serving as objective indicators of normal biological processes, pathogenic developments, or responses to therapeutic interventions (Biomarkers and Surrogate Endpoints: Preferred Definitions and Conceptual Framework, 2001). Proteomics, a technology-driven science focused on studying proteins, their modifications, interactions, and changes resulting from diseases or external factors, plays a crucial role in identifying novel therapeutic and diagnostic biomarkers (Tsangaris, 2009). Proteomic analyses are considered the "gold standard" for measuring various molecules, including steroid hormones, and have significantly advanced analytical specificity and sensitivity (Kosteria et al., 2018a). In endocrinology and metabolism, proteomics research has enhanced our understanding of disease processes and shed light on poorly studied pathways leading to complications. Proteomics has been integral in investigating endocrine diseases throughout childhood, from early fetal stages to newborn screening programs, offering insights into the molecular pathophysiology of rare metabolic disorders (Garg et al., 2022; Sabbagh et al., 2016).

6.2 FUNDAMENTALS OF PROTEOMICS

Proteomics, the large-scale study of proteins, is crucial in unravelling the molecular complexities of pediatric endocrine and metabolic disorders. By examining the complete set of proteins expressed in biological systems, proteomics contributes to a deeper understanding of disease mechanisms, identification of biomarkers, and development of targeted therapeutic strategies. Proteomics is a fundamental tool in understanding pediatric endocrine and metabolic disorders by providing a comprehensive view of the protein landscape. Its applications in biomarker discovery, elucidating protein-protein interactions, and exploring post-translational modifications contribute to advancing both basic research and clinical interventions. As proteomic technologies evolve, they promise to play a pivotal role in improving the diagnosis, treatment, and management of pediatric patients with endocrine and metabolic disorders. Figure 6.1 depicts the fundamentals of proteomics.

6.2.1 OVERVIEW OF PROTEOMICS

Proteomics is a fascinating type of 'omics' that has grown incredibly fast, particularly in the therapeutics industry. Prof. Dr. Marc Wilkins developed the notion of the proteome and coined the term in 1994 to denote the "PROTEin complement of a genOME" (Aslam et al., 2017; Sharma and Singh, 2020; Wilkins et al., 1996). The large-scale study of proteins, their structure, and their physiological role or functions is known as proteomics. In every form of life, proteins are fundamental macromolecules or cellular components. The term "Proteomics" resembled the word "genome" quite a bit. The word "proteome" combines the terms "genome" and "protein."

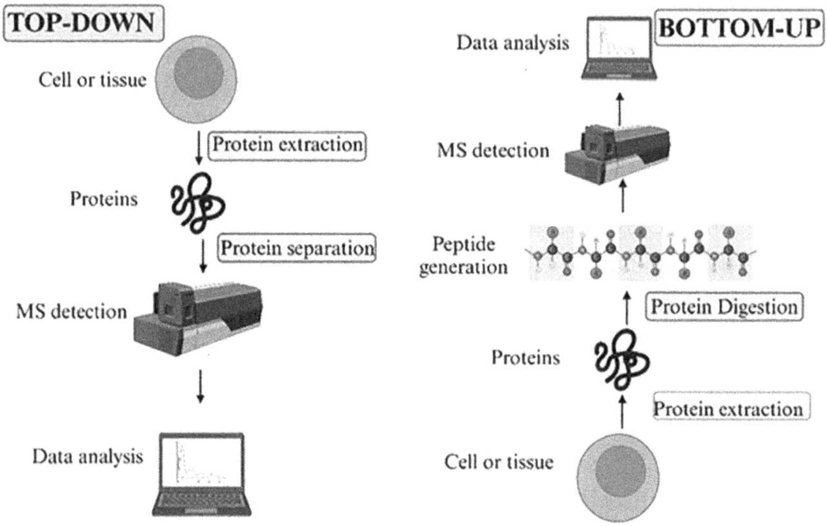

FIGURE 6.1 Fundamentals of proteomics. Proteomics can be used in two ways: top-down and bottom-up. At the top, the whole proteasome is analysed, whereas the proteins are degraded at the bottom, and *de novo* synthesis occurs.

To put it precisely and specifically, the proteome is the whole complement, database, or set of proteins a living being produces. "proteome" refers to a broad range of changes organisms undergo, including modifications or alterations resulting in native protein. These days, postgenomic and systems biology techniques rely heavily on proteomics to uncover important diagnostic and prognostic biomarkers and comprehend the molecular mechanisms behind both healthy and disease phenotypes (Veenstra et al., 2004). Since proteins can be found in samples, proteomics aims to determine their abundance, location, post-translational modifications, isoforms, and molecular interactions, in addition to identifying any proteins that may be present (Holman et al., 2013). Nearly one million human proteins are thought to exist, and many of them have modifications such as post-translational modifications (PTMs) (Holman et al., 2013; Sood et al., 2023). Still, an estimated 26000–31000 proteins are predicted to be encoded by the human genome (Vercauteren et al., 2004). Shotgun proteomics, one-dimensional (1D) and two-dimensional (2D) gel electrophoresis (2-DE), and protein microarrays can be employed in tissues, organelles, and cells. Proteomics has emerged at the convergence of computer science, bioinformatics, physics, and biochemistry (Chandramouli and Qian, 2009).

6.2.2 TECHNIQUES AND METHODOLOGIES

Proteomics favors various techniques for the separation of complicated protein or peptide samples: high-performance liquid chromatography (HPLC), one-dimensional gel electrophoresis (1D-GE), two-dimensional gel electrophoresis (2D-DIGE), and denaturing polyacrylamide gel electrophoresis (PAGE) or sodium dodecyl sulfate-polyacrylamide gel electrophoresis (SDS-PAGE) (Chandramouli and Qian, 2009).

6.2.2.1 GEL ELECTROPHORESIS

The analysis of complicated samples in separation sciences is facilitated by the constant trend toward high-resolution separations. Since biological samples are frequently highly complicated, this is very strong in that field. Proteins are incredibly complex analytes with a solid propensity to precipitate, making protein electrophoretic separations no exception to this rule. Two high-performance protein electrophoretic separation methods were available at the start of the 1970s:

i. SDS, as originally describes by Laemmli and subsequently refined, rapidly gained popularity and remains widely utilized in protein electrophoresis today.
ii. denaturing isoelectric focusing, as previously described, by Gronow and Griffith (Rabilloud and Lelong, 2011).

1-DE can separate proteins ranging in molecular weight from 10 kDa to 300 kDa. It uses sodium dodecyl sulphate (SDS), a detergent that denatures tertiary structures linked by disulphide and combines them with a negative charge corresponding to their volume. This makes it possible to determine molecular weights (Chen et al., 2015). SDS-PAGE can be used to measure protein purification, determine sample purity, and determine the molecular weights of proteins that are not known (Brunelle and Green, 2014).

Protein molecules differ in molecular weight and isoelectric point, which allows 2-DE to distinguish proteins more effectively than 1-DE (Chen et al., 2015). The protein is divided into two distinct dimensions, which results in a higher resolution than 1-DE. Proteins are separated in 1-DE according to net charge, whereas in 2-DE, they are separated according to molecular mass and isoelectric point. PTMs and phosphorylation are examples of the various protein forms this method can identify. Using 2-DE, some proteins resulting from various proteolysis processes and alternative mRNA splicing can be identified (Brunelle and Green, 2014). A crucial stage in the procedure affecting the outcomes' dependability and quality is sample preparation for two-dimensional gel electrophoresis (2DGE). The first step is to take proteins from the biological sample (e.g., cells or tissues). Typically, a procedure known as protein extraction is used to do this. The sample type will determine which extraction buffer is to be used. For the extraction of mammalian cells, for instance, a radioimmunoprecipitation assay (RIPA) buffer is frequently utilized. Protease inhibitors must be added to the extraction solution to stop proteases from breaking down proteins. Proteins in the extraction buffer are distributed uniformly due to homogenization. After extraction, the total protein level should be quantified using suitable tests, such as the Bradford or bicinchoninic acid (BCA) assay (Bradford, 1976). Protein quantification is crucial for loading similar amounts of protein in future phases to compare the samples effectively.

Proteins are typically solubilized in a denaturing buffer. Urea, which aids in protein unfolding, and a polar detergent (such as sodium dodecyl sulphate, or SDS), which aids in protein denaturation, are commonly used as the primary ingredients of this buffer. Reducing agents such as 2-mercaptoethanol and dithiothreitol, or DTT, are administered to proteins to break disulphide bonds and denaturize them (Ashique et al., 2022; Görg et al., 2000).

In the next step, the whole gel material is prepared for the first dimension of 2DGE, isoelectric focusing (IEF). IEF is an electrophoretic technique used for separating amphoteric molecules such as proteins and peptides based on their charge, determined by the pKa values of proton-accepting sites within the molecule. These sites include the side chains of arginine, lysine, histidine, aspartic acid and glutamic acid residues, as well as the free amines and carboxylic acids found at the N- and C- termini of proteins and peptides (Görg et al., 2000). The isoelectric point (pI) of an amphoteric molecule is the pH at which the molecule carries no net charge, owing to its physiochemical properties. To achieve high resolution isoelectric focusing (IEF), it is essential to prevent the formation of protein aggregates and complexes in the sample. This is typically achieved by conditioning the sample with a high concentration of chaotropic agents, zwitterionic detergents, reducing thiols, and carrier ampholytes. Additionally, it is crucial to remove non-protein based ions from the sample to maintain high electrical resistance, enabling the application of a strong electric field (8000–10,000 v) while minimizing current flow (Hoving et al., 2000).

Protein precipitation techniques are frequently employed to reduce the quantity of such pollutants. Molecular sieves of thin polyacrylamide gel with an immobilized pH gradient (IPG) are used in modern IEF techniques for 2D gel electrophoresis. The matrix should not restrict high-molecular-weight proteins, so the gels have a low acrylamide concentration (typically 4–5% total acrylamide). An electric field is then applied after introducing proteins into this medium. In an electric field, positively charges proteins migrate towards the cathode when they are positioned in a pH gradient lower (more acidic) than their isoelectric point (pI). Conversely, proteins move towards the anode when placed in a pH gradient higher (more alkaline) than their pI. The pH at which a protein is electrically neutral is defined as its pI. Proteins positioned at the pH gradient's point equal to their pI experience no net movement in the electric field. This cessation of migration at their pI is termed "focusing." Towards the end of an isoelectric focusing (IEF) run, proteins become highly concentrated at their respective isoelectric points, which enhances detection sensitivity. Narrow gradient intervals and longer separation lengths allow for the differentiation of even minute charge changes and improve resolution. If desired, marker proteins can be used to estimate the isoelectric points of the proteins using a calibration curve (Pergande and Cologna, 2017; Sharma et al., 2021).

In 2D gel electrophoresis, sodium dodecyl sulphate-polyacrylamide gel electrophoresis, or SDS-PAGE, is the second dimension for sorting proteins according to their molecular weight. This procedure denatures proteins and coats them with the negatively charged detergent SDS. Once protein samples are prepared, they are applied onto a polyacrylamide gel and subjected to an electric field. This electric field causes the proteins to migrate through the gel matrix, primarily based on their size. Because the negative charge is proportional to the mass of the protein, SDS ensures that the separation predominantly reflects molecular weight. The proteins are dyed for visibility following electrophoresis, typically with silver or Coomassie Blue stain. SDS-PAGE is frequently used to characterize proteins in diverse biological contexts, determine protein expression levels, and purify proteins (Laemmli, 1970; Nowakowski et al., 2014).

6.2.2.2 MASS SPECTROMETRY (MS)

Mass spectrometry (MS) is a highly effective analytical technique used for both qualitative and quantitative analysis, enabling the identification and precise measurement of a wide range of clinically relevant analytes. MS extends analytical capabilities to clinical applications with gas or liquid chromatography. Moreover, MS is a crucial analytical tool in proteomics because of its capacity to detect and quantify proteins (Király et al., 2016; Matthiesen and Bunkenborg, 2013; Mehta et al., 2022; Rihal et al., 2022; Zhang et al., 2010). Mass spectrometry data are reported in terms of the mass-to-charge ratio, denoted as m/z, where m represents the molecular weight of the ion in Daltons, z indicates the number of charges carried by the ion (Urban, 2016). In small molecules (<1000 Da), where typically only one charge is present, the mass of the molecular ion is equal to its m/z value (Sugai, 2017). However, more giant molecules—like proteins or peptides—usually have more than one ionic charge when measured; as a result, the z value is more than 1. The m/z value in these circumstances will be a portion of the ion's mass (Domon and Aebersold, 2006).

Successful MS requires careful sample preparation, especially when working with complicated matrices like those in clinical chemistry. Usually, this entails taking one or more of the subsequent actions: (i) precipitation of proteins followed by filtration or centrifugation; (ii) extraction in solid phase; (iii) extraction in liquid phase; (iv) enrichment by affinity; or (v) derivatization (Wilschefski and Baxter, 2019). Derivatization chemically changes the Target compounds to perform MS analysis more successfully (Finoulst et al., 2011; Singh et al., 2020). Derivatization typically entails including a distinct functional group (Guerrasio et al., 2013). Depending on the application, derivatization can have a variety of objectives, but the most common ones are (i) higher volatility; (ii) increased thermal stability; (iii) altered chromatographic properties; (iv) increased ionization efficiency; and (v) advantageous fragmentation properties, or a mix of these (Khan et al., 2021; Vilbaste et al., 2020).

A mass spectrometer transforms molecules into ions, subsequently controlled by magnetic and electric fields (Domon and Aebersold, 2006). Three key elements are needed for this, and they are as follows:

i. **Ion Source:** The device ionizes the material after a sample is placed into the mass spectrometer (Olshina and Sharon, 2016).

ii. **Mass Analyzer:** The apparatus sorts the ions according to their mass-to-charge ratio (m/z).

iii. **Detector:** The mass spectrum chart shows the measured and exhibited ions.

The ionization of atoms and molecules is a prerequisite for their acceleration via the mass spectrometer and subsequent detection (Bantscheff et al., 2007). An ionization source will initially provide a positive charge to the sample molecule in the mass spectrometer. By taking out a valence electron, this positive charge is obtained. Protons can also be added to produce a positive electrical charge. The ionized molecule disintegrates into smaller pieces, separated in the mass analyzer based on their mass-to-charge ratio (Király et al., 2016). Interestingly, only the cationic pieces are isolated. Neutral species in a mass spectrometer can go undetected because they can either be absorbed by the device or eliminated by vacuum. Neutral species in a mass spectrometer can go undetected because they can either be absorbed by the device or eliminated by vacuum (Haag, 2016).

The data from the mass spectrometer will be analyzed by making a chart. In mass spectrometry, the mass-to-charge ratio (m/z) is typically plotted on the x-axis, while the relative intensity is plotted on the y-axis (Olshina and Sharon, 2016; Singh et al., 2020). The relative intensity of the ion is normalized to 100% on the y-axis, with all subsequent ion peaks plotted relative to this value. The molecular ion peak is the parent peak because its weight corresponds to the sample's (Buchberger et al., 2018). For example, if the material in the mass spectrometer were hexane, the m/z would be 86 since hexane has a molecular weight of 86 g/mol. Furthermore, as each atom has a different isotope, the peak at m/z = 87 would be categorized as the m+1 peak if it exists (Haag, 2016).

6.2.2.3 PROTEIN MICROARRAY

Protein microarrays are versatile and high-throughput tools that enable the simultaneous analysis of various proteins for various applications, including protein-protein interactions, biomarker discovery, and drug development. The principles of protein microarrays involve immobilizing proteins onto a solid surface, systematic arrangement in an array format, incubation with biological samples, and subsequent detection and analysis of protein interactions (Schena et al., 1995).

The immobilization of proteins is a crucial step, and various methods can be employed. Common approaches include direct spotting, where proteins are physically deposited onto a substrate, and indirect methods, such as chemical coupling or affinity capture, where proteins are attached via specific ligands or antibodies (MacBeath and Schreiber, 2000).

The array format allows for the spatial organization of multiple proteins on a single surface, facilitating the parallel analysis of interactions. This feature is particularly advantageous for studying complex biological processes involving numerous proteins simultaneously (Zhu et al., 2001).

During the assay, the protein microarray is exposed to a biological sample, such as cell lysate, serum, or other protein mixtures. Interactions between immobilized proteins and components in the sample, such as protein-protein interactions or binding events, are detected. Depending on the specific experimental requirements, detection methods include fluorescence, chemiluminescence, or label-free techniques (Paweletz et al., 2001; Zhu et al., 2001).

The utilization of protein microarrays has expanded across diverse research areas due to their ability to provide high-throughput, multiplexed data. They have been applied in cancer research, immunology, and drug discovery.

Protein microarrays aid in the diagnosis and treatment of diseases in several ways:

Protein microarrays enable the identification of potential biomarkers associated with pediatric endocrine and metabolic disorders. By analyzing the protein expression profiles in patient samples, researchers can discover novel markers indicating disease presence, progression, or response to treatment (Kosteria et al., 2018b; Liotta et al., 2003; Rifai et al., 2006).

Endocrine disorders often involve dysregulation of hormone levels. Protein microarrays can profile hormones' expression, post-translational modifications, and their receptors, providing insights into the underlying mechanisms of disorders such as diabetes, growth hormone, and thyroid disorders in pediatric patients (Zhu et al., 2003).

Protein microarrays contribute to the era of personalized medicine by enabling the profiling of individual patient samples. This allows for a more tailored approach to diagnosis and treatment, considering the unique molecular characteristics of each pediatric patient (Paweletz et al., 2001).

Protein microarrays can untangle the intricate molecular pathways underlying pediatric endocrine and metabolic disorders, improving our knowledge of disease etiology.

6.2.3 CHALLENGES AND ADVANCES IN PEDIATRIC APPLICATIONS

Pediatric proteomics applications face many multifaceted challenges as the samples are collected from children. Therefore, several ethical concerns are present in these applications.

Getting enough biological samples from Pediatric patients can be difficult because of restricted blood volume, ethical concerns, and challenges with obtaining tissues. In Pediatric research, micro-sampling methods like dried blood spot (DBS) analysis are emerging to address sample restrictions (Weiss and Kim, 2012).

The proteomic analysis must consider the variability of pediatric disorders to provide precise diagnoses and individualized treatment plans. Integrating multi-omics methods brings together proteomics, genomes, and metabolomics, offering a more thorough understanding of pediatric disorders (Weiss and Kim, 2012).

Proteomics data standardization is essential for cross-platform and cross-study comparisons. Furthermore, analyzing large-scale proteomic datasets can be challenging. The development of standardized procedures and bioinformatic instruments facilitates the interpretation of proteomic results and improves data repeatability (Barsnes and Vaudel, 2018).

Proteomic research with children presents ethical questions about agreement, consent, and the use of private health data. Updated guidelines and ethical frameworks emphasize the protection of pediatric research subjects, concession, and informed permission (Knoppers and Chadwick, 2005).

Validating proteomic biomarkers for therapeutic application in pediatric illnesses involves overcoming repeatability, sensitivity, and specificity issues. Collaborative efforts and longitudinal research facilitate the rigorous validation of identified biomarkers and help translate them into therapeutic applications (Rifai et al., 2006).

Due to the rapid improvements in proteomics technology, it can be difficult for researchers to acquire and integrate new technologies. Proteomic analyses in pediatric research are becoming more sensitive, accurate, and accessible thanks to ongoing breakthroughs like mass spectrometry and high-throughput approaches (Domon and Aebersold, 2006).

6.3 PEDIATRIC ENDOCRINE DISORDERS

6.3.1 DIABETES MELLITUS IN CHILDREN

Diabetes mellitus encompasses a group of metabolic disorders marked by chronic hyperglycemia due to deficiencies in insulin secretion, insulin action, or both. Individuals, particularly children with absolute insulin deficiency and significant hyperglycemia, may experience symptoms sucg as polyuria, polydipsia, polyphagia, weight loss and blurred vision (Yau et al., 2000).

- **Proteomic Insights into Type 1 Diabetes:** The autoimmune destruction of insulin-secreting β-cells and other congenital (genetic abnormalities in the creation or function of the endocrine pancreas) or acquired (relapsing pancreatitis and pancreatectomy) disorders can result in absolute insulin deficiency (Yau et al., 2000).
- **Type 2 Diabetes in Paediatric Patients:** Type 2 diabetes mellitus (T2DM) is the most common prevalent form of diabetes, characterized by insulin resistance in peripheral tissues (muscle, fat, and liver) and increasing β cell failure. It is particularly evident when insulin secretion is impaired in response to glucose stimulation, the liver produces more glucose than usual, and there are no signs of pancreatic autoimmunity. The epidemic of obesity and T2DM continues to affect more younger adults and children than in the past (Yau et al., 2000).

6.3.2 GROWTH HORMONE DEFICIENCY

Growth hormone (GH) deficiency (GHD) in children is defined as impaired. The pituitary gland produces GH, resulting in growth failure. With an estimated rate of 1 patient per 4000–10,000 live births, isolated GHD might have a variety of causes, some of which are yet unknown. When treating children with low stature with recombinant human growth hormone, the correct diagnosis is still crucial in enabling them to reach their genetically determined adult height (Ranke, 2021).

6.3.3 THYROID DISORDERS IN CHILDREN

Hypothyroidism in children can be classified as primary or secondary (central) and can be either congenital or acquired, transient or permanent. Primary hypothyroidism is characterized by the production of thyroid hormones in the thyroid gland that are inadequate to meet the organism's needs. Insufficient secretion and action of hypothalamic thyrotropin-releasing hormone (TRH) and pituitary TSH causes secondary or central hypothyroidism (Segni, 2000a).

- **Proteomic Profiling of Thyroid Dysfunction:** Thyroid hormones (THs) play a critical role in regulating a wide range of metabolic functions in both central and peripheral systems. They influence the homeostasis, metabolism and regulatory activities of primary target organs, as well as the hematopoietic system (Masood et al., 2020; Segni, 2000b).

Figure 6.2 illustrates some of the pediatric endocrine disorders.

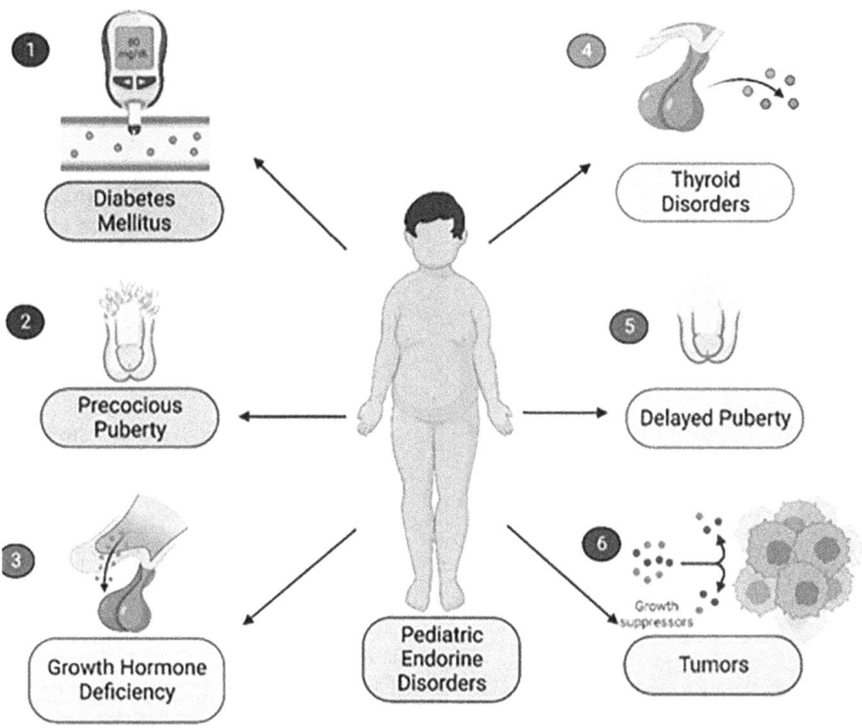

FIGURE 6.2 Endocrine disorders in children. This figure illustrates a comprehensive overview of pediatric metabolic disorders in children. Each category is colour-coded for clarity, and specific examples within each group are highlighted with accompanying symbols. The figure also emphasises the interconnectedness of endocrine pathways and the potential for crosstalk between different endocrine processes. Understanding these disorders is crucial for clinicians and researchers alike, as it provides insights into the underlying biochemical mechanisms, aiding in early diagnosis, intervention, and the development of targeted therapies for affected paediatric patients.

6.4 PAEDIATRIC METABOLIC DISORDERS

Metabolism refers to the biochemical reactions within cells to maintain life. These reactions are responsible for converting food into energy, eliminating waste products, and building and repairing tissues. The pathophysiology of metabolic disorders mainly includes – impaired Feedback inhibition, alteration in binding sites of a cofactor, and deficient enzyme activity, as shown in Figure 6.3. As a result, the affected individual may

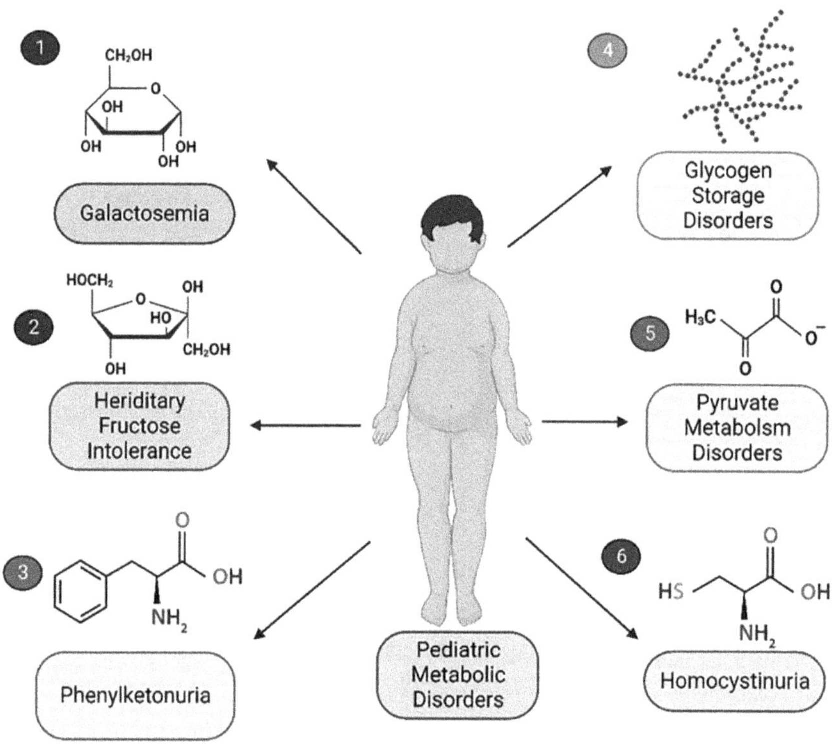

FIGURE 6.3 Metabolic disorders in children. This figure illustrates a comprehensive overview of pediatric metabolic disorders, encompassing a diverse range of genetic and acquired conditions affecting metabolic pathways in children. Each category is colour-coded for clarity, and specific examples within each group are highlighted with accompanying symbols. The figure also emphasises the interconnectedness of metabolic pathways and the potential for crosstalk between different metabolic processes. Understanding these disorders is crucial for clinicians and researchers alike, as it provides insights into the underlying biochemical mechanisms, aiding in early diagnosis, intervention, and the development of targeted therapies for affected paediatric patients.

have difficulty breaking down certain substances or producing essential compounds. Thus, leading to the accumulation of toxic metabolites or a deficiency of the needed end product (Zakir et al., 2022). Metabolic disorders can lead to symptoms like fatigue, nausea, muscle pain, and low appetite. It can also result in Developmental delays in infants and children. Diseases related to endocrine dysfunction, imbalance of electrolytes, or inborn errors of metabolism can be correlated to metabolic disorders. Often, infants with metabolic abnormalities exhibit symptoms that are comparable to those of neurological, infectious, and toxicological emergencies. Examples of Metabolic disorders include – Obesity, Diabetes Mellitus, Maple syrup urine disease (MSUD), and Tay-Sachs disease (Kwon and Tsai, 2007).

6.4.1 INBORN ERRORS OF METABOLISM (IEM)

IEMs are a class of hereditary illnesses caused by abnormalities in the structure or activity of enzymes that are vital for carrying out metabolic processes. Gene mutations encoding for transporters, enzymes, or other metabolism-related proteins, which result in transmembrane mobility, cell signaling, and cell differentiation, typically constitute the primary cause of IEM (Smith and Harding, 2011). These mutations can cause an enzyme to become absent or malfunction, interfering with normal metabolism and accumulating harmful compounds or a shortage of vital chemicals. It can result in the alteration of the primary structure of proteins. Hereditary metabolic diseases, which result from the inborn errors of metabolism, are genetic mutations in the enzymatic loci, which further affect enzymatic co-factors, transportation of proteins, and particular recognition markers. IEM are mainly Autosomal recessive disorders, whereas some are X-linked recessive conditions like – Fabry's disease, Hunter's syndrome, and Lesch-Nyhan syndrome. A few inherited Autosomal dominant traits include – Porphyria, Hyperlipidaemia, and hereditary angioedema (Ezgu, 2016).

The classification of IEM is shown in Table 6.1. It is done based on the following factors: the particular organ affected, symptoms shown, and the nature of the disease, that is, acute or chronic. Category 1 disorders are characterized by a single organ or a persistent symptom detected by specific laboratory tests. Since the underlying cause of the biochemical problem includes the specified outcome, making an accurate diagnosis usually becomes straightforward. Disorders in category 2 include a single metabolic pathway shared by many cells or organs and are affected by biochemical factors. It shows more erratic symptoms and multiple illnesses involving different organ systems (Martins, 1999).

TABLE 6.1 Classification of IEM Under Category 2

Group	Type of Metabolic Defect	Examples of Disorders
Group 1	Defects in the synthesis or breakdown of complex compounds	Fabry disease, Gaucher disease, Nieman disease, Krabbe disease, Tay-Sachs disease, Pompe disease, and Zellweger syndrome.
Group 2	Abnormalities in the intermediate metabolism pathways	Disorders based on Amino acid metabolism: Cystinuria, Phenylketonuria, Tyrosinemia, Homocystinuria, Maple syrup urine disease.
		Disorders based on Urea cycle defects: Carbamoyl phosphate synthetase deficiency, Ornithine transcarbamylase deficiency.
		Disorders due to sugar intolerances: Galactokinase deficiency, Epimerase deficiency, fructose-1,6-biphosphatase deficiency.
Group 3	Deficiencies in the generation or utilisation of energy	Phosphoenolpyruvate carboxykinase deficiency, Pyruvate dehydrogenase complex deficiency, and Carnitine plasma transport defect.

6.4.1.1 PROTEOMICS IN THE DIAGNOSIS OF INBORN ERRORS

Analysis of many molecules is done in proteomics with the help of Mass spectroscopy. Thus, proteomics has been used to diagnose genetic illnesses related to metabolism by identifying specific proteins or peptides (Proteomic biomarkers), encouraging the timely implementation of therapeutic interventions. By quantifying proteins and determining the chemical changes (based on their interactions and post-translational modifications) that regulate them, these modern methods have comprehensively been used to characterise pathogenic biochemical processes involved in metabolic disorders. Proteomics is an effective technique that can indicate new or unannotated proteins and biomarkers involved and analyse interrupted pathways, which are the primary cause of diseases (Costanzo et al., 2017). Proteomics-based molecular profiling of gene products enables the prioritisation of causative genes based on aberrantly expressed gene products and reclassifies possible splice or unclear missense variants. Thus, in addition to DNA analysis and RNA sequencing, proteomics offers direct protein level quantification, making it a useful tool that leads to the validation of transcriptomic data and increases the perspective of diagnostic rates of metabolic disorders. Proteomics increases the evidence of measured proteins and identifies additional downstream signaling consequences resulting from pathogenic variations. Thus, it boosts the evidence for protein deficiencies that have not been identified or for which interpretation is challenging (Smirnov et al., 2023). Table 6.2 shows various inborn errors of metabolism along with the analytical technique and specific proteomic biomarkers (involved in the metabolic disorder).

TABLE 6.2 Inborn Errors of Metabolism with Specific Proteomic Biomarkers and Analytical Techniques Used for Their Detection

Disorders	Specific Proteomic Biomarkers	Analytical Techniques
Lysosomal diseases: Fabry disease Gaucher disease Niemann-Pick disease	Transferrin, α2 – HS glycoprotein, α2- antiplasmin, Vit. D binding protein. Cathepsin. 24 – dehydrocholesterol reductase 4, acid alpha-glucosidase, Superoxide dismutase 2.	LC-MS/MS and MALDI-TOF-MS analysis.
Organic acidemias: Methylmalonic-acidemia	Cytoskeleton organisation, cellular detoxification and oxidative stress.	2D-DIGE electrophoresis followed by MS.
Congenital disorders of glycosylation (CDG): Defects in O- glycosylation CDG type–1 disorder	Apolipoprotein C-III Serum transferrin	MALDI-TOF or MALDI-MS SELDI-TOF-MS

Proteomics has provided new comprehensive insights into various pediatric endocrine illnesses, including inborn metabolic abnormalities (Kosteria et al., 2018b). If intellectual disability is identified early, diagnosis and treatment with focused therapies can be initiated, and the overall prognosis can be better determined, thus leading to efficient management of the associated disorder (Tein, 2023).

6.4.1.2 MONITORING TREATMENT EFFICACY THROUGH PROTEOMICS

The genetic material contained in genes is translated into messenger RNA (mRNA), which is further subjected to additional processing, modification, splicing, and translation to yield several proteins. The protein products produced from an individual's genetic code are collectively called the proteome. Expression proteomics reveals the differences in protein expression between the healthy and pathological states. Since metabolites are operational indicators of a cellular state, they are more directly associated with phenotype than proteins and genes, which are influenced by post-translational modification and epigenetic control (MacMillan et al., 2019). A wide range of therapeutic options for therapy have been made in managing IEM and enzymatic disorders due to the substantial advancements in our understanding of these conditions' biochemical and molecular bases. Simultaneously, advancing increasingly complex and sensitive diagnostic techniques frequently integrated into prenatal screening programs have enabled earlier and more precise diagnoses before the onset of disease symptoms. Clinically, all of these metabolic Disorders show some similarities; that is, they do not impair fetal or embryonic growth, and patients experience a variable period of symptom-free time after birth before experiencing the acute or chronic manifestations of the particular disorder. Proteomics aids in the early detection of this class of diseases, which is crucial for providing treatment options to patients. Table 6.3 shows some metabolic disorders, the defective enzymes involved, and the treatment procedures for curing the disease.

TABLE 6.3 Enzymatic Disorders and Their Treatment Procedures

Disorders	Defective enzyme	Treatment	Supplementary Cofactors (That Can Be Added)
Homocystinuria	Cystathionine-β-synthase	Restriction of methionine	Pyridoxine
Aciduria type 1	Glutaryl-CoA dehydrogenase	Restriction of tryptophan and lysine	Riboflavin
Maple syrup urine disease	Alpha-keto acid dehydrogenase	Limiting the consumption of leucine, valine and isoleucine	Thiamine
Methylmalonic aciduria	methyl malonyl-CoA carboxylase	Restriction of isoleucine, valine, methionine, threonine	Hydroxocobalamin
Ornithine transcarbamylase deficiency	Ornithine transcarbamylase	Limiting arginine intake	Pyridoxine

Even though treatment options remain limited for many illnesses, either due to the lack of understanding of the underlying abnormality or the inability to intervene in the disease progression (Schwartz et al., 2008), signatures derived from histopathology provide information about the specific protein network which helps select the best therapeutic medication. Due to all these factors, researchers are trying to implement proteomics on samples undergoing clinical trials (Liotta et al., 2001).

6.4.2 CHILDHOOD OBESITY

Obesity occurs when the body fat percentage of a person rises to the point that they become more susceptible to health issues. Excess body fat in children and adolescents is a significant public health concern known as childhood obesity. It may have both short-term and long-term health effects, such as a high chance of developing several chronic illnesses such as type 2 diabetes, heart disease, dyslipidaemia, polycystic ovarian disease, and mental health problems like obstructive sleep apnoea and pseudotumor cerebri(Sahoo et al., 2015). The most frequent side effects of obesity also include an increased risk of psychological morbidity, symptoms of asthma, and orthopaedic issues. Adverse effects on the cardiovascular system, including elevated blood pressure, persistent low-grade inflammation, and an altered blood lipid profile, are also associated with childhood obesity. Childhood obesity is also associated with a high risk of developing non–insulin–dependent or Type 1 diabetes. Childhood obesity can result when there is a sustained deficit in calories burned over an extended period. When people get obese, they require a lot more calories to maintain that state than people who are not obese. Fat bodies require significantly more energy than non-obese bodies to continue functioning (Reilly, 2007). Genetics is considered one of the most researched parameters contributing to obesity. According to specific research, a 25–40% BMI is heritable. However, genetic susceptibility must frequently be combined with relevant environmental, nutritional, and behavioral factors to influence weight (Sahoo et al., 2015). Body mass index (BMI) is a simple calculation that correlates well with direct measures of Fatness. It is calculated by dividing weight (kilograms) by square height (meters). For this reason, BMI is widely used to define obesity in clinical care. For a specific BMI, adiposity will be affected by age, sex, and ethnicity. Henceforth, the risks of obesity-associated illnesses can be determined. Since it is challenging to pinpoint the precise amount of body fat, BMI is typically used to identify and monitor obesity in children. Childhood obesity is currently the most prevalent disorder, and its prevalence is continually rising. From the standpoint of public health, paediatric obesity is significant because it results in poor health in both childhood and adulthood (Aycan, 2009).

6.4.2.1 ROLE OF PROTEOMICS IN UNDERSTANDING OBESITY

Fat plays a vital role in the development of Obesity by secreting many molecules that coordinate essential physiological functions. Numerous animal and cell-cultured models have been studied using various proteomic techniques. However, the protein composition of human adipose tissue and the identification of the adipose tissue Secretome have not been examined widely (Peral et al., 2009). Once a disease is initiated, pharmacological treatment may be helpful; however, the available therapies have significant drawbacks and can only marginally reduce body weight. To support the development and implementation of new treatments at all levels, scientific communities are trying to study the molecular mechanisms causing obesity by comprehending their aetiology. Nearly every organ in the body is involved in the complicated pathways that lead to obesity. Most proteomic research has been done on the peripheral organs, specifically on adipose tissue and adipocyte primary cultures or cell lines. Genetic and environmental factors influence human physiology and behavior, impacting energy balance and obesity. In reality, the susceptibility of the genes constitutes the basis for the hereditary contribution to the illness. In recent years, several monogenic candidate genes have been discovered. The ob gene encodes for the hormone leptin and its receptor (Lepr); pro-opiomelanocortin (POMC) codes for melanocortin stimulating hormone (*a-MSH*), melanocortin receptor 4 (*MCR4*), and the fat mass and obesity-associated (*FTO*) gene. These genes are primarily involved in appetite and body weight regulation. Given the complex nature of obesity and the fact that environmental factors and genetic predisposition play a significant role in its development, there are high chances that protein activity and the functional final product of a gene play a substantial role in determining the mechanisms underlying the disease.

Several researchers have used quantitative gel and gel-free methods alongside MS to explore various facets of the obesity issue in humans, animals, and cellular models for treatments by protein profiling and target identification in lean and obese models of obesity (Barceló-Batllori and Gomis, 2009). The existence of different protein magnitudes and the enormous complexity of the biological Materials may obscure the detection of low-abundance proteins. Thereby reducing the effectiveness of MS proteome analysis. Thus, to simplify the analyte for more focused detection, gel-based techniques like 2-dimensional gel electrophoresis (2D PAGE) and gel-free technologies like HPLC are also frequently employed (Brockman and Chen, 2012).

6.4.2.2 IDENTIFICATION OF BIOMARKERS FOR OBESITY-RELATED COMPLICATIONS

Obesity and chronic diseases have been linked biologically to the endocrine function of adipose tissue (incredibly visceral adipose tissue) concerning the cytokines and adipokines released. Thus, based on disease-causing biomarkers, the identification of an obese phenotype can be made, and patients susceptible to the development of the disease can be identified (Aleksandrova et al., 2020). Measurements of the obesity-related biomarkers in epidemiological studies by linking obesity to the risk of chronic diseases may provide crucial information about the pathophysiologic pathways and aetiology of obesity-related diseases. Here, we will focus on the prospective studies that link pre-diagnostic levels of biomarkers to disease because in case-control studies, when blood samples are collected after diagnosis, the required biomarker may get altered by the existing disease. Some of the well-known Obesity biomarkers are discussed below:

i. **Biomarkers Under Insulin/ IGF axis:**

   a. **Insulin/C-peptide:** Research has been done on IGF-1, IGF-binding proteins, and C-peptide, which is cleaved from proinsulin and is thought to indicate endogenous insulin production having a longer half-life concerning insulin itself. It has been demonstrated that C-peptide and fasting insulin strongly correlate with BMI. Evidence suggests that in non-diabetic persons, C-peptide can predict cardiovascular mortality.

   b. **IGF-1:** It has been linked to the emergence of cancer because it controls the growth, differentiation, migration, and survival of cells in healthy and genetically damaged tissues. There has been limited research on the relationship between obesity and BMI and free IGF-1. However, a small cross-sectional investigation found that free IGF-1 was higher in obese than normal-weight people.

ii. **Biomarkers Under inflammation:**

   a. **C-reactive protein (CRP):** It has been proposed that low-grade chronic inflammation associated with obesity promotes cell migration, survival, and proliferation, which may contribute to cancer development. Due to CRP genetic variations, patients with higher lifetime CRP concentrations were at a greater risk of colorectal cancer.

iii. **Adipokines as Biomarkers:**

   a. **Adiponectin:** It is an anti-inflammatory sensitiser of Insulin released from adipocytes. Persons with obesity have lower adiponectin concentrations than those with average weight because adiponectin expression gets downregulated in adipose tissue in these individuals.

   b. **Leptin:** Adipocytes secrete leptin and regulate energy expenditure and appetite. It is also a measure of adipose tissue mass; obese people have higher leptin concentrations than people of average weight, suggesting that obesity may cause leptin resistance.

   c. **Resistin:** It contributes to insulin resistance linked to obesity and contains pro-inflammatory qualities. It is secreted from white adipose tissues.

iv. Adipokines act as mediators between the risk of disease and obesity by mediating the metabolic and inflammatory effects. Other examples of Adipokines include Apelin, IL-6, Visfatin, Chemerin, and Omentin (Katsareli and Dedoussis, 2014; Nimptsch et al., 2019).

6.5 APPLICATIONS OF PROTEOMICS IN CLINICAL PRACTICE

The scientific method of identifying every protein species found in a cell or tissue is known as proteomics. Even though the name "proteomics" was just introduced (Huber, 2003), it was not long before the techniques used in proteomic analysis were taken from classical biochemistry. This is because proteome analysis looks at changes in all proteins expressed by a genome. While proteomic technology is widely used to characterise all protein species within a given cell, many researchers also use it to understand protein changes between healthy and pathological states. Like any other new technique, proteomics was initially hailed with great promise. This new technology is ironing out all the kinks (Colantonio and Chan, 2005). In the complex and poorly understood subject of inborn errors of metabolism, proteomics has been widely used to understand better the pathophysiologic mechanisms involved and, consequently, extrapolate panels of biomarkers for early diagnosis and therapy response monitoring. Tandem mass spectrometry, first used in the 1990s, has completely changed screening procedures by enabling the simultaneous identification of numerous Metabolic diseases with a single test (Kosteria et al., 2018b). Figure 6.4 depicts all the proteomic applications in clinical practice.

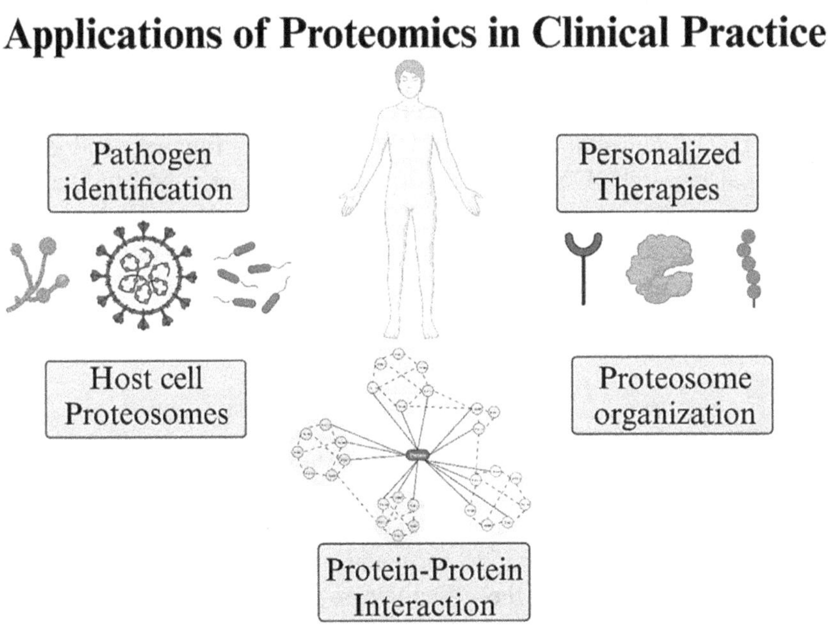

FIGURE 6.4 Application of proteomics in clinical practice. Proteomics is a broad field with applications in Pathogen identification, Host cell Proteosome analysis, protein-protein interaction, proteasomal organisation, and personalized therapies.

6.5.1 EARLY DIAGNOSIS AND PREDICTIVE BIOMARKERS

Early diagnosis and discovering predictive biomarkers are crucial to prompt intervention and successful treatment of these problems for paediatric endocrine and metabolic diseases. Early diagnosis enables timely treatment, which may avert issues and enhance the affected children's long-term prognosis. Predictive biomarkers are essential in identifying individuals at risk or likely to develop certain conditions to allow a proactive approach to healthcare. Before symptoms manifest, biomarkers can identify youngsters genetically prone to endocrine and metabolic diseases. This makes early intervention possible and may even stop the illness or its complications from developing. Hormone production and function problems are associated with pediatric endocrine diseases. Measurable indications that can be used to identify people at risk of getting a specific ailment are known as predictive biomarkers. Many biomarkers may indicate the likelihood of developing a disease or its course in pediatric endocrine and metabolic diseases. Specific metabolites may have elevated levels that indicate metabolic problems. For instance, poor glucose control in diabetes is linked to elevated glycated haemoglobin levels (HbA1c). Early detection of many endocrine issues can be facilitated by measuring hormone levels, including insulin, cortisol, and thyroid hormones (Mehta et al., 2021). Unusual levels could indicate a malfunction and direct additional research (Cho and Suh, 2016). Finding universal biomarkers for pediatric endocrine disorders is difficult because these conditions are frequently heterogeneous. Long-term research is required to confirm the predictive power of biomarkers and comprehend their temporal trajectory. Developments in hormone assays, metabolomics, and genetic testing present novel approaches to enhance early diagnosis and intervention.

6.5.2 MONITORING TREATMENT RESPONSES

Due to the dynamic nature of growth and development, pediatric endocrine and metabolic disorders provide particular problems regarding diagnosis and therapy. Determining the effectiveness of interventions, enhancing therapeutic approaches, and improving long-term results for paediatric patients is essential to track treatment responses. Protein expression patterns can be systematically achieved before and after therapy using mass spectrometry and quantitative proteomics. By identifying treatment-induced modifications in the proteome, researchers and clinicians can gather insight into the underlying molecular mechanisms of therapeutic interventions (Kosteria et al., 2018b). Changes in protein abundance can be measured using quantitative proteomics methods like tandem mass spectrometry (MS/MS). Clinicians can determine how treatment affects the total protein expression profile by comprehensively analysing the pre-and post-treatment data (Gygi et al., 1999). Phosphorylation is one of the most critical post-translational modifications in signaling cascades. By observing alterations in phosphorylation patterns throughout a treatment, phosphoproteomics can predict how biological functions are dynamically regulated (Cirillo and Valencia., 2019). Early decision-making of treatment outcomes is made possible by identifying particular proteins or protein signatures that can function as reliable markers of therapeutic efficacy (Rifai et al., 2006). Proteogenomics, integrating proteomic and genomic data, facilitates more knowledge of personalized therapy responses. This method enables customised therapeutic approaches by considering individual differences in the genomic and protein-level landscapes (Mertins et al., 2016). Using longitudinal monitoring, proteomics helps medical professionals monitor changes in the proteome over time. This continuous assessment is crucial in determining potential relapse markers, assessing how long treatment responses last, and modifying treatment plans as essential (Wang et al., 2017). These applications help to benefit researchers with knowledge of treatment dynamics and open avenues to more individualized and successful therapeutic approaches for paediatric patients.

6.5.3 PERSONALIZED TREATMENT RESPONSES:

Personalized medicine has gained popularity as it can significantly transform the treatment of paediatric endocrine and metabolic disorders by customising each patient's specific genetic, molecular, and clinical profile. Genomic profiling is a standardised step to identify genetic variants linked to conditions in personalized medicine. Mass spectrometry is one proteomic approach that complements genomic data by revealing the precise protein expression and changes affecting disease outcomes (Collins and Varmus, 2015). Proteomic analysis simplified how protein biomarkers linked to various paediatric endocrine and metabolic disease subtypes or stages were found. These indicators enable therapies based on the disease's unique biological features (Mertins et al., 2016). Proteogenomics integrates genomic and proteomic data to provide a more comprehensive picture of the molecular basis of diseases. This approach enables the identification of novel therapeutic targets, drug responses, and potential biomarkers that can guide personalized treatment strategies (Mertins et al., 2016). Pharmaco-proteomics is the study of how pharmaceuticals affect proteins at the level of individual molecules, offering insights into differences in therapeutic efficacy and metabolism. By predicting a patient's unique response to medication, pharmacoproteomic techniques in paediatric endocrine diseases can optimise treatment outcomes (Zhang et al., 2014). Personalized medicine focuses on the necessity of ongoing evaluations and modifications to treatment regimens. Clinicians can monitor dynamic changes in the protein Landscape over time with longitudinal proteome monitoring, making it easier to promptly identify therapeutic responses, resistance, or possible side effects (Bai et al., 2020). A patient-centric approach is emphasised by personalized medicine, which integrates the patient's values and preferences into treatment choices. Proteomic data aids in well-informed decision-making by enabling medical professionals to customise interventions according to young patients and their families' distinct biological traits and preferences (Trusheim et al., 2011). Personalized medicine techniques for paediatric endocrine and metabolic diseases incorporating proteomics allow for a more comprehensive understanding of the molecular details underlying these problems.

6.5.4 INTEGRATION WITH GENOMICS AND OTHER OMICS TECHNOLOGIES

Complex interactions at the genetic, proteomic, and other omics levels characterise paediatric endocrine and metabolic diseases. Proteomics, other omics technologies, and genomics are integrated to provide an integrative framework for studying the molecular pathways underlying various illnesses. Understanding the genetic basis of paediatric endocrine diseases is based on genomics, which identifies DNA polymorphisms linked to disease susceptibility, severity, and progression. Next-generation sequencing technology advancements have expedited the process of identifying the genetic components causing these illnesses (Kwak et al., 2016). Proteomics enhances genomics by shedding light on the functional aspects of genomic data. Proteins can be identified and quantified using mass spectrometry-based proteomic approaches, showing dynamic changes in protein expression, post-translational modifications, and protein-protein interactions linked to paediatric endocrine and metabolic diseases (Zhang et al., 2014). By combining proteomic and genomic data, proteogenomics provides a more comprehensive understanding of the molecular environment. With the help of this method, new peptides, fusion proteins, and non-coding RNAs can be identified, leading to a better comprehension of the functional effects of genetic changes in paediatric endocrine and metabolic disorders (Mertins et al., 2016). Integrating metabolomics and lipidomics enhances genomics and proteomics by identifying the subsequent impacts on metabolites and lipids. The altered biochemical processes in paediatric endocrine and metabolic disorders can be better understood because of the insights these omics technologies provide into metabolic pathways (Fiehn, 2002). By examining the whole RNA transcriptome, Transcriptomics can identify gene expression patterns linked to paediatric endocrine diseases. A more comprehensive understanding of the mechanisms behind the disease can be achieved by combining transcriptome and proteomics data to understand better the regulatory mechanisms controlling protein expression (Wang et al., 2009). Clinical practice is directly affected by integrative omics techniques. Clinicians can now provide paediatric patients with endocrine and metabolic problems with more individualized and accurate care using genomes, proteomics, and other omics data to customise therapeutic and diagnostic approaches (Hasin et al., 2017). Integrating genomics, proteomics, and other omics technologies provides a multidimensional understanding of paediatric endocrine and metabolic disorders. This holistic approach enhances our ability to unravel the molecular complexity of these disorders, paving the way for more targeted diagnostics, personalized treatment strategies, and a deeper understanding of the underlying pathophysiology.

6.6 CHALLENGES AND FUTURE DIRECTIONS

Despite several challenges, proteomics has enormously contributed to understanding the concept of pediatric endocrine and metabolic disorders. Limitations in current proteomic approaches, such as sensitivity, specificity, and quantification accuracy, pose a significant struggle for the comprehensive profiling of the pediatric proteome. However, advanced technologies, including novel mass spectrometry techniques, enhanced sample preparation methods, and improved bioinformatics tools, pave the way to overcome these limitations. As we delve deep into these cutting-edge technologies, addressing ethical considerations associated with pediatric proteomics research is essential. Safeguarding the privacy and well-being of young participants, obtaining informed consent, and ensuring responsible data usage are critical features to uphold in this advancing landscape. Culminating the future directions of proteomics applications in pediatric endocrine and metabolic disorders and integrating technological progress with ethical considerations will be crucial for advancing scientific knowledge and ethical research practices.

6.7 CONCLUSION

This deep dive into how proteomics helps us understand and treat children's hormone and metabolism issues brings to light the critical molecular insights we need to tackle these complex health challenges. By exploring vital proteomic techniques like gel electrophoresis, mass spectrometry, and protein microarrays, we have looked closely at specific conditions affecting kids, such as diabetes, growth hormone issues, thyroid problems, genetic metabolism errors, and obesity. This discussion has opened a multi-layered view on the subject, highlighting how proteomics can be a game-changer in clinical settings. It is about catching diseases early, finding biomarkers predicting health issues, tracking how well treatments work, and tailoring medical care to each child's needs. As we consider the hurdles, like the current limits of proteomics, the exciting future tech on the horizon, and the ethical questions around research with kids, this conversation emphasises the need to marry scientific advances with a solid moral compass. Adding real-life stories into the mix shows how impactful proteomics can be, making diagnoses more accurate and treatments more effective for our kids. This exploration broadens our understanding and highlights the vast potential for ongoing research and breakthroughs in this area, setting the stage for better health outcomes for our youngest.

KEYWORDS

- **disease diagnosis**
- **endocrine disorders**
- **metabolic disorders**
- **paediatric research**
- **protein profiling**
- **proteomic analysis**
- **proteomics**

REFERENCES

Aleksandrova, K., Egea Rodrigues, C., Floegel, A., & Ahrens, W. (2020). Omics biomarkers in obesity: Novel etiological insights and targets for precision prevention. *Current Obesity Reports, 9*(3), 219–230. https://doi.org/10.1007/s13679-020-00393-y (accessed on 28th June 2025).

Ashique, S., De Rubis, G., Sirohi, E., Mishra, N., Rihan, M., Garg, A., Reyes, R. J., Manandhar, B., Bhatt, S., Jha, N. K., Singh, T. G., Gupta, G., Singh, S. K., Chellappan, D. K., Paudel, K. R., Hansbro, P. M., Oliver, B. G., & Dua, K. (2022). Short chain fatty acids: Fundamental mediators of the gut-lung axis and their involvement in pulmonary diseases. *Chemico-Biological Interactions, 368*, 110231. https://doi.org/10.1016/j.cbi.2022.110231 (accessed on 28th June 2025).

Aslam, B., Basit, M., Nisar, M. A., Khurshid, M., & Rasool, M. H. (2017). Proteomics: Technologies and their applications. *Journal of Chromatographic Science, 55*(2), 182–196. https://doi.org/10.1093/chromsci/bmw167 (accessed on 28th June 2025).

Aycan, Z. (2009). Obesity in childhood: Definition and epidemiology. *Journal of Clinical Research in Pediatric Endocrinology, 1*(1). https://doi.org/10.4008/jcrpe.v1i1.25 (accessed on 28th June 2025).

Bai, B., Wang, X., Li, Y., Chen, P.-C., Yu, K., Dey, K. K., Yarbro, J. M., Han, X., Lutz, B. M., Rao, S., Jiao, Y., Sifford, J. M., Han, J., Wang, M., Tan, H., Shaw, T. I., Cho, J.-H., Zhou, S., Wang, H., … Peng, J. (2020). Deep multilayer brain proteomics identifies molecular networks in Alzheimer's disease progression. *Neuron, 105*(6), 975–991.e7. https://doi.org/10.1016/j.neuron.2019.12.015 (accessed on 28th June 2025).

Bantscheff, M., Schirle, M., Sweetman, G., Rick, J., & Kuster, B. (2007). Quantitative mass spectrometry in proteomics: A critical review. *Analytical and Bioanalytical Chemistry, 389*(4), 1017–1031. https://doi.org/10.1007/s00216-007-1486-6 (accessed on 28th June 2025).

Barceló-Batllori, S., & Gomis, R. (2009). Proteomics in obesity research. *Proteomics – Clinical Applications, 3*(2), 263–278. https://doi.org/10.1002/prca.200800178 (accessed on 28th June 2025).

Barsnes, H., & Vaudel, M. (2018). SearchGUI: A highly adaptable common interface for proteomics search and de novo engines. *Journal of Proteome Research, 17*(7), 2552–2555. https://doi.org/10.1021/acs.jproteome.8b00175 (accessed on 28th June 2025).

Biomarkers and surrogate endpoints: Preferred definitions and conceptual framework. (2001). *Clinical Pharmacology & Therapeutics, 69*(3), 89–95. https://doi.org/10.1067/mcp.2001.113989 (accessed on 28th June 2025).

Bradford, M. (1976). A rapid and sensitive method for the quantitation of microgram quantities of protein utilizing the principle of protein-dye binding. *Analytical Biochemistry, 72*(1–2), 248–254. https://doi.org/10.1006/abio.1976.9999 (accessed on 28th June 2025).

Brockman, D., & Chen, X. (2012). Proteomics in the characterisation of adipose dysfunction in obesity. *Adipocyte, 1*(1), 25–37. https://doi.org/10.4161/adip.19129 (accessed on 28th June 2025).

Brunelle, J. L., & Green, R. (2014). One-dimensional SDS-polyacrylamide gel electrophoresis (1D SDS-PAGE) (pp. 151–159). https://doi.org/10.1016/B978-0-12-420119-4.00012-4 (accessed on 28th June 2025).

Buchberger, A. R., DeLaney, K., Johnson, J., & Li, L. (2018). Mass spectrometry imaging: A review of emerging advancements and future insights. *Analytical Chemistry, 90*(1), 240–265. https://doi.org/10.1021/acs.analchem.7b04733 (accessed on 28th June 2025).

Chandramouli, K., & Qian, P.-Y. (2009). Proteomics: Challenges, techniques and possibilities to overcome biological sample complexity. *Human Genomics and Proteomics, 1*(1). https://doi.org/10.4061/2009/239204 (accessed on 28th June 2025).

Chen, Z.-T., Liang, Z.-G., & Zhu, X.-D. (2015). A review: Proteomics in nasopharyngeal carcinoma. *International Journal of Molecular Sciences, 16*(12), 15497–15530. https://doi.org/10.3390/ijms160715497 (accessed on 28th June 2025).

Cho, W. K., & Suh, B.-K. (2016). Catch-up growth and catch-up fat in children born small for gestational age. *Korean Journal of Pediatrics, 59*(1), 1. https://doi.org/10.3345/kjp.2016.59.1.1 (accessed on 28th June 2025).

Cirillo, D., & Valencia, A. (2019). Big data analytics for personalised medicine. *Current Opinion in Biotechnology, 58*, 161–167. https://doi.org/10.1016/j.copbio.2019.03.004 (accessed on 28th June 2025).

Colantonio, D. A., & Chan, D. W. (2005). The clinical application of proteomics. *Clinica Chimica Acta, 357*(2), 151–158. https://doi.org/10.1016/j.cccn.2005.03.020 (accessed on 28th June 2025).

Collins, F. S., & Varmus, H. (2015). A new initiative on precision medicine. *New England Journal of Medicine, 372*(9), 793–795. https://doi.org/10.1056/NEJMp1500523 (accessed on 28th June 2025).

Costanzo, M., Zacchia, M., Bruno, G., Crisci, D., Caterino, M., & Ruoppolo, M. (2017). Integration of proteomics and metabolomics in exploring genetic and rare metabolic diseases. *Kidney Diseases, 3*(2), 66–77. https://doi.org/10.1159/000477493 (accessed on 28th June 2025).

Domon, B., & Aebersold, R. (2006). Mass spectrometry and protein analysis. *Science, 312*(5771), 212–217. https://doi.org/10.1126/science.1124619 (accessed on 28th June 2025).

Ezgu, F. (2016). Inborn errors of metabolism (pp. 195–250). https://doi.org/10.1016/bs.acc.2015.12.001 (accessed on 28th June 2025).

Fiehn, O. (2002). Metabolomics–the link between genotypes and phenotypes. *Plant Molecular Biology, 48*(1/2), 155–171. https://doi.org/10.1023/A:1013713905833 (accessed on 28th June 2025).

Finoulst, I., Pinkse, M., Van Dongen, W., & Verhaert, P. (2011). Sample preparation techniques for the untargeted LC-MS-based discovery of peptides in complex biological matrices. *Journal of Biomedicine and Biotechnology, 2011*, 1–14. https://doi.org/10.1155/2011/245291 (accessed on 28th June 2025).

Garg, C., Kaur, A., Singh, T. G., Sharma, V. K., & Singh, S. K. (2022). Therapeutic implications of sonic hedgehog pathway in metabolic disorders: Novel target for effective treatment. *Pharmacological Research, 179*, 106194. (accessed on 28th June 2025).

Golubnitschaja, O., Baban, B., Boniolo, G., Wang, W., Bubnov, R., Kapalla, M., Krapfenbauer, K., Mozaffari, M. S., & Costigliola, V. (2016). Medicine in the early twenty-first century: Paradigm and anticipation – EPMA position paper 2016. *EPMA Journal, 7*(1), 23. https://doi.org/10.1186/s13167-016-0072-4 (accessed on 28th June 2025).

Golubnitschaja, O., Kinkorova, J., & Costigliola, V. (2014). Predictive, preventive and personalised medicine as the hardcore of 'Horizon 2020': EPMA position paper. *EPMA Journal, 5*(1), 6. https://doi.org/10.1186/1878-5085-5-6 (accessed on 28th June 2025).

Görg, A., Obermaier, C., Boguth, G., Harder, A., Scheibe, B., Wildgruber, R., & Weiss, W. (2000). The current state of two-dimensional electrophoresis with immobilised pH gradients. *Electrophoresis, 21*(6), 1037–1053. https://doi.org/10.1002/(SICI)1522-2683(20000401)21:6<1037::AID-ELPS1037>3.0.CO;2-V (accessed on 28th June 2025).

Guerrasio, R., Haberhauer-Troyer, C., Steiger, M., Sauer, M., Mattanovich, D., Koellensperger, G., & Hann, S. (2013). Measurement uncertainty of isotopologue fractions in fluxomics determined via mass spectrometry. *Analytical and Bioanalytical Chemistry, 405*(15), 5133–5146. https://doi.org/10.1007/s00216-013-6910-5 (accessed on 28th June 2025).

Gygi, S. P., Rist, B., Gerber, S. A., Turecek, F., Gelb, M. H., & Aebersold, R. (1999). Quantitative analysis of complex protein mixtures using isotope-coded affinity tags. *Nature Biotechnology, 17*(10), 994–999. https://doi.org/10.1038/13690 (accessed on 28th June 2025).

Haag, A. M. (2016). Mass analyzers and mass spectrometers (pp. 157–169). https://doi.org/10.1007/978-3-319-41448-5_7 (accessed on 28th June 2025).

Hasin, Y., Seldin, M., & Lusis, A. (2017). Multi-omics approaches to disease. *Genome Biology, 18*(1), 83. https://doi.org/10.1186/s13059-017-1215-1 (accessed on 28th June 2025).

Holman, J. D., Dasari, S., & Tabb, D. L. (2013). Informatics of protein and posttranslational modification detection via shotgun proteomics (pp. 167–179). https://doi.org/10.1007/978-1-62703-360-2_14 (accessed on 28th June 2025).

Hoving, S., Voshol, H., & van Oostrum, J. (2000). Towards high-performance two-dimensional gel electrophoresis using ultrazoom gels. *Electrophoresis, 21*(13), 2617–2621. https://doi.org/10.1002/1522-2683(20000701)21:13<2617::AID-ELPS2617>3.0.CO;2-C (accessed on 28th June 2025).

Huber, L. A. (2003). Is proteomics heading in the wrong direction? *Nature Reviews Molecular Cell Biology, 4*(1), 74–80. https://doi.org/10.1038/nrm1007 (accessed on 28th June 2025).

Katsareli, E. A., & Dedoussis, G. V. (2014). Biomarkers in the field of obesity and its related comorbidities. *Expert Opinion on Therapeutic Targets, 18*(4), 385–401. https://doi.org/10.1517/14728222.2014.882321 (accessed on 28th June 2025).

Kaur, P., Khan, H., Grewal, A., Dua, K., Singh, S., & Singh, T. G. (2023). Correlation of metabolic disorders and FOXO signaling in AD: A therapeutic approach. *Authorea Preprints.* (accessed on 28th June 2025).

Khan, H., Tiwari, P., Kaur, A., & Singh, T. G. (2021). Sirtuin acetylation and deacetylation: A complex paradigm in neurodegenerative disease. *Molecular Neurobiology, 58*, 3903–3917. (accessed on 28th June 2025).

Király, M., Dalmadiné Kiss, B., Vékey, K., Antal, I., & Ludányi, K. (2016). [Mass spectrometry: Past and present]. *Acta Pharmaceutica Hungarica, 86*(1), 3–11. (accessed on 28th June 2025).

Knoppers, B. M., & Chadwick, R. (2005). Human genetic research: Emerging trends in ethics. *Nature Reviews Genetics, 6*(1), 75–79. https://doi.org/10.1038/nrg1505 (accessed on 28th June 2025).

Kosteria, I., Kanaka-Gantenbein, C., Anagnostopoulos, A. K., Chrousos, G. P., & Tsangaris, G. Th. (2018a). Pediatric endocrine and metabolic diseases and proteomics. *Journal of Proteomics, 188*, 46–58. https://doi.org/10.1016/j.jprot.2018.03.011 (accessed on 28th June 2025).

Kosteria, I., Kanaka-Gantenbein, C., Anagnostopoulos, A. K., Chrousos, G. P., & Tsangaris, G. Th. (2018b). Pediatric endocrine and metabolic diseases and proteomics. *Journal of Proteomics, 188*, 46–58. https://doi.org/10.1016/j.jprot.2018.03.011 (accessed on 28th June 2025).

Kwak, S. H., Jung, C., Ahn, C. H., Park, J., Chae, J., Jung, H. S., Cho, Y. M., Lee, D. H., Kim, J.-I., & Park, K. S. (2016). Clinical whole exome sequencing in early-onset diabetes patients. *Diabetes Research and Clinical Practice, 122*, 71–77. https://doi.org/10.1016/j.diabres.2016.10.005 (accessed on 28th June 2025).

Kwon, K. T., & Tsai, V. W. (2007). Metabolic emergencies. *Emergency Medicine Clinics of North America, 25*(4), 1041–1060. https://doi.org/10.1016/j.emc.2007.07.009 (accessed on 28th June 2025).

Laemmli, U. K. (1970). Cleavage of structural proteins during the assembly of the head of bacteriophage T4. *Nature, 227*(5259), 680–685. https://doi.org/10.1038/227680a0 (accessed on 28th June 2025).

Liotta, L. A., Espina, V., Mehta, A. I., Calvert, V., Rosenblatt, K., Geho, D., Munson, P. J., Young, L., Wulfkuhle, J., & Petricoin, E. F. (2003). Protein microarrays: Meeting analytical challenges for clinical applications. *Cancer Cell, 3*(4), 317–325. https://doi.org/10.1016/S1535-6108(03)00086-2 (accessed on 28th June 2025).

Liotta, L. A., Kohn, E. C., & Petricoin, E. F. (2001). Clinical proteomics. *JAMA, 286*(18), 2211. https://doi.org/10.1001/jama.286.18.2211 (accessed on 28th June 2025).

MacBeath, G., & Schreiber, S. L. (2000). Printing proteins as microarrays for high-throughput function determination. *Science, 289*(5485), 1760–1763. https://doi.org/10.1126/science.289.5485.1760 (accessed on 28th June 2025).

MacMullan, M. A., Dunn, Z. S., Graham, N., Yang, L., & Wang, P. (2019). Quantitative proteomics and metabolomics reveal biomarkers of disease as potential immunotherapy targets and indicators of therapeutic efficacy. *Theranostics, 9*(25), 7872–7888. https://doi.org/10.7150/thno.37373 (accessed on 28th June 2025).

Martins, A. M. (1999). Inborn errors of metabolism: A clinical overview. *São Paulo Medical Journal, 117*(6), 251–265. https://doi.org/10.1590/S1516-31801999000600006 (accessed on 28th June 2025).

Masood, A., Benabdelkamel, H., Ekhzaimy, A. A., & Alfadda, A. A. (2020). Plasma-based proteomics profiling of patients with hyperthyroidism after antithyroid treatment. *Molecules, 25*(12), 2831. https://doi.org/10.3390/molecules25122831 (accessed on 28th June 2025).

Matthiesen, R., & Bunkenborg, J. (2013). Introduction to mass spectrometry-based proteomics (pp. 1–45). https://doi.org/10.1007/978-1-62703-392-3_1 (accessed on 28th June 2025).

Mehta, S., Nain, P., Agrawal, B. K., & Singh, R. P. (2022). Vitamin D with calcium supplementation managing glycemic control with HbA1c and improve quality of life in patients with diabetes. *Turkish Journal of Pharmaceutical Sciences, 19*(2), 161–167. https://doi.org/10.4274/tjps.galenos.2021.62357 (accessed on 28th June 2025).

Mehta, S., Nain, P., Agrawal, B. K., Singh, R. P., Kaur, J., Maity, S., Bhattacharjee, A., Peela, J., Nauhria, S., & Nauhria, S. (2021). Effectiveness of empagliflozin with vitamin D supplementation in peripheral neuropathy in type 2 diabetic patients. *Cureus, 13*(12), e20208. https://doi.org/10.7759/cureus.20208 (accessed on 28th June 2025).

Mertins, P., Mani, D. R., Ruggles, K. V., Gillette, M. A., Clauser, K. R., Wang, P., Wang, X., Qiao, J. W., Cao, S., Petralia, F., Kawaler, E., Mundt, F., Krug, K., Tu, Z., Lei, J. T., Gatza, M. L., Wilkerson, M., Perou, C. M., Yellapantula, V., Carr, S. A. (2016). Proteogenomics connects somatic mutations to signalling in breast cancer. *Nature, 534*(7605), 55–62. https://doi.org/10.1038/nature18003 (accessed on 28th June 2025).

Nimptsch, K., Konigorski, S., & Pischon, T. (2019). Diagnosis of obesity and use of obesity biomarkers in science and clinical medicine. *Metabolism, 92*, 61–70. https://doi.org/10.1016/j.metabol.2018.12.006 (accessed on 28th June 2025).

Nowakowski, A. B., Wobig, W. J., & Petering, D. H. (2014). Native SDS-PAGE: High-resolution electrophoretic separation of proteins with retention of native properties, including bound metal ions. *Metallomics, 6*(5), 1068–1078. https://doi.org/10.1039/C4MT00033A (accessed on 28th June 2025).

Olshina, M. A., & Sharon, M. (2016). Mass spectrometry: A technique of many faces. *Quarterly Reviews of Biophysics, 49*, e18. https://doi.org/10.1017/S0033583516000160 (accessed on 28th June 2025).

Paweletz, C. P., Charboneau, L., Bichsel, V. E., Simone, N. L., Chen, T., Gillespie, J. W., Emmert-Buck, M. R., Roth, M. J., Petricoin III, E. F., & Liotta, L. A. (2001). Reverse-phase protein microarrays that capture disease progression show activation of pro-survival pathways at the cancer invasion front. *Oncogene, 20*(16), 1981–1989. https://doi.org/10.1038/sj.onc.1204265 (accessed on 28th June 2025).

Peral, B., Camafeita, E., Fernández-Real, J.-M., & López, J. A. (2009). Tackling the human adipose tissue proteome to gain insight into obesity and related pathologies. *Expert Review of Proteomics, 6*(4), 353–361. https://doi.org/10.1586/epr.09.53 (accessed on 28th June 2025).

Pergande, M., & Cologna, S. (2017). Isoelectric point separations of peptides and proteins. *Proteomes, 5*(4), 4. https://doi.org/10.3390/proteomes5010004 (accessed on 28th June 2025).

Rabilloud, T., & Lelong, C. (2011). Two-dimensional gel electrophoresis in proteomics: A tutorial. *Journal of Proteomics, 74*(10), 1829–1841. https://doi.org/10.1016/j.jprot.2011.05.040 (accessed on 28th June 2025).

Ranke, M. B. (2021). Short and long-term effects of growth hormone in children and adolescents with GH deficiency. *Frontiers in Endocrinology, 12*, 720419. https://doi.org/10.3389/fendo.2021.720419 (accessed on 28th June 2025).

Reilly, J. J. (2007). Childhood obesity: An overview. *Children & Society, 21*(5), 390–396. https://doi.org/10.1111/j.1099-0860.2007.00092.x (accessed on 28th June 2025).

Rifai, N., Gillette, M. A., & Carr, S. A. (2006). Protein biomarker discovery and validation: The long and uncertain path to clinical utility. *Nature Biotechnology, 24*(8), 971–983. https://doi.org/10.1038/nbt1235 (accessed on 28th June 2025).

Rihal, V., Kaur, A., Singh, T. G., & Abdel-Daim, M. M. (2022). Therapeutic and mechanistic intervention of vitamin D in neuropsychiatric disorders. *Psychiatry Research, 317*, 114782. (accessed on 28th June 2025).

Sabbagh, B., Mindt, S., Neumaier, M., & Findeisen, P. (2016). Clinical applications of MS-based protein quantification. *PROTEOMICS – Clinical Applications, 10*(4), 323–345. https://doi.org/10.1002/prca.201500116 (accessed on 28th June 2025).

Sahoo, K., Sahoo, B., Choudhury, A., Sofi, N., Kumar, R., & Bhadoria, A. (2015). Childhood obesity: Causes and consequences. *Journal of Family Medicine and Primary Care, 4*(2), 187. https://doi.org/10.4103/2249-4863.154628 (accessed on 28th June 2025).

Schena, M., Shalon, D., Davis, R. W., & Brown, P. O. (1995). Quantitative monitoring of gene expression patterns with a complementary DNA microarray. *Science, 270*(5235), 467–470. https://doi.org/10.1126/science.270.5235.467 (accessed on 28th June 2025).

Schwartz, I. V., Souza, C. F. M. de, & Giugliani, R. (2008). Treatment of inborn errors of metabolism. *Jornal de Pediatria, 0*(0). https://doi.org/10.2223/JPED.1801 (accessed on 28th June 2025).

Segni, M. (2000a). Disorders of the thyroid gland in infancy, childhood and adolescence.

Segni, M. (2000b). Disorders of the thyroid gland in infancy, childhood and adolescence.

Sharma, T., Kaur, D., Grewal, A. K., & Singh, T. G. (2021). Therapies modulating insulin resistance in Parkinson's disease: A cross talk. *Neuroscience Letters, 749*, 135754. (accessed on 28th June 2025).

Sharma, V. K., & Singh, T. G. (2020). Insulin resistance and bioenergetic manifestations: Targets and approaches in Alzheimer's disease. *Life Sciences, 262*, 118401. (accessed on 28th June 2025).

Singh, R., Rao, H. K., & Singh, T. G. (2020). Advanced glycated end products (AGEs) in diabetes and its complications: An insight. *Plant Arch, 20*(1), 3838–3841.

Singh, S., Singh, T. G., Mahajan, K., & Dhiman, S. (2020). Medicinal plants used against various inflammatory biomarkers for the management of rheumatoid arthritis. *Journal of Pharmacy and Pharmacology, 72*(10), 1306–1327.

Smirnov, D., Konstantinovskiy, N., & Prokisch, H. (2023). Integrative omics approaches to advance rare disease diagnostics. *Journal of Inherited Metabolic Disease, 46*(5), 824–838. https://doi.org/10.1002/jimd.12663 (accessed on 28th June 2025).

Smith, L., & Harding, C. O. (2011). Inborn errors of metabolism. In *Pediatric Critical Care* (pp. 1089–1104). Elsevier. https://doi.org/10.1016/B978-0-323-07307-3.10076-X (accessed on 28th June 2025).

Sood, S., Devi, S., Singh, T. G., & Mittal, N. (2023). Pathogenesis of obesity-associated cardiovascular diseases: Key role of biomolecules. *Health Sciences Review*, 100098.

Sugai, T. (2017). Mass and charge measurements on heavy ions. *Mass Spectrometry, 6*(3), S0074–S0074. https://doi.org/10.5702/massspectrometry.S0074 (accessed on 28th June 2025).

Tein, I. (2023). Recent advances in neurometabolic diseases: The genetic role in the modern era. *Epilepsy & Behavior, 145*, 109338. https://doi.org/10.1016/j.yebeh.2023.109338 (accessed on 28th June 2025).

Trusheim, M. R., Burgess, B., Hu, S. X., Long, T., Averbuch, S. D., Flynn, A. A., Lieftucht, A., Mazumder, A., Milloy, J., Shaw, P. M., Swank, D., Wang, J., Berndt, E. R., Goodsaid, F., & Palmer, M. C. (2011). Quantifying factors for the success of stratified medicine. *Nature Reviews Drug Discovery, 10*(11), 817–833. https://doi.org/10.1038/nrd3557 (accessed on 28th June 2025).

Tsangaris, G. T. (2009). From proteomics research to clinical practice. *Expert Review of Proteomics, 6*(3), 235–238. https://doi.org/10.1586/epr.09.14 (accessed on 28th June 2025).

Urban, P. L. (2016). Quantitative mass spectrometry: An overview. *Philosophical Transactions of the Royal Society A: Mathematical, Physical and Engineering Sciences, 374*(2079), 20150382. https://doi.org/10.1098/rsta.2015.0382 (accessed on 28th June 2025).

Veenstra, T. D., Prieto, D. A., & Conrads, T. P. (2004). Proteomic patterns for early cancer detection. *Drug Discovery Today, 9*(20), 889–897. https://doi.org/10.1016/S1359-6446(04)03246-5 (accessed on 28th June 2025).

Vercauteren, F. G. G., Bergeron, J. J. M., Vandesande, F., Arckens, L., & Quirion, R. (2004). Proteomic approaches in brain research and neuropharmacology. *European Journal of Pharmacology, 500*(1–3), 385–398. https://doi.org/10.1016/j.ejphar.2004.07.039 (accessed on 28th June 2025).

Vilbaste, M., Tammekivi, E., & Leito, I. (2020). Uncertainty contribution of derivatisation in gas chromatography/mass spectrometric analysis. *Rapid Communications in Mass Spectrometry, 34*(16). https://doi.org/10.1002/rcm.8704 (accessed on 28th June 2025).

Wang, J., Chang, S., Li, G., & Sun, Y. (2017). Application of liquid biopsy in precision medicine: Opportunities and challenges. *Frontiers of Medicine, 11*(4), 522–527. https://doi.org/10.1007/s11684-017-0526-7 (accessed on 28th June 2025).

Wang, Z., Gerstein, M., & Snyder, M. (2009). RNA-Seq: A revolutionary tool for transcriptomics. *Nature Reviews Genetics, 10*(1), 57–63. https://doi.org/10.1038/nrg2484 (accessed on 28th June 2025).

Weiss, R. H., & Kim, K. (2012). Metabolomics in the study of kidney diseases. *Nature Reviews Nephrology, 8*(1), 22–33. https://doi.org/10.1038/nrneph.2011.152 (accessed on 28th June 2025).

Wilkins, M. R., Sanchez, J.-C., Gooley, A. A., Appel, R. D., Humphery-Smith, I., Hochstrasser, D. F., & Williams, K. L. (1996). Progress with proteome projects: Why all proteins expressed by a genome should be identified and how to do it. *Biotechnology and Genetic Engineering Reviews, 13*(1), 19–50. https://doi.org/10.1080/02648725.1996.10647923 (accessed on 28th June 2025).

Wilschefski, S., & Baxter, M. (2019). Inductively coupled plasma mass spectrometry: Introduction to analytical aspects. *Clinical Biochemist Reviews, 40*(3), 115–133. https://doi.org/10.33176/AACB-19-00024 (accessed on 28th June 2025).

Yau, M., Maclaren, N. K., & Sperling, M. A. (2000). Etiology and pathogenesis of diabetes mellitus in children and adolescents.

Zakir, F., Mohapatra, S., Farooq, U., Mirza, Mohd. A., & Iqbal, Z. (2022). Introduction to metabolic disorders. In *Drug Delivery Systems for Metabolic Disorders* (pp. 1–20). Elsevier. https://doi.org/10.1016/B978-0-323-99616-7.00001-3 (accessed on 28th June 2025).

Zhang, B., Wang, J., Wang, X., Zhu, J., Liu, Q., Shi, Z., Chambers, M. C., Zimmerman, L. J., Shaddox, K. F., Kim, S., Davies, S. R., Wang, S., Wang, P., Kinsinger, C. R., Rivers, R. C., Rodriguez, H., Townsend, R. R., Ellis, M. J. C., Carr, S. A., … Liebler, D. C. (2014). Proteogenomic characterisation of human colon and rectal cancer. *Nature, 513*(7518), 382–387. https://doi.org/10.1038/nature13438 (accessed on 28th June 2025).

Zhang, G., Annan, R. S., Carr, S. A., & Neubert, T. A. (2010). Overview of peptide and protein analysis by mass spectrometry. *Current Protocols in Protein Science, 62*(1). https://doi.org/10.1002/0471140864.ps1601s62 (accessed on 28th June 2025).

Zhu, H., Bilgin, M., & Snyder, M. (2003). Proteomics. *Annual Review of Biochemistry, 72*(1), 783–812. https://doi.org/10.1146/annurev.biochem.72.121801.161511 (accessed on 28th June 2025).

Zhu, H., Bilgin, M., Bangham, R., Hall, D., Casamayor, A., Bertone, P., Lan, N., Jansen, R., Bidlingmaier, S., Houfek, T., Mitchell, T., Miller, P., Dean, R. A., Gerstein, M., & Snyder, M. (2001). Global analysis of protein activities using proteome chips. *Science, 293*(5537), 2101–2105. https://doi.org/10.1126/science.1062191 (accessed on 28th June 2025).

CHAPTER 7

Dietary Alteration of Gut Microbiota in Epigenetics of Colorectal Cancer

SHUBHAM SINGH BARTWAL,[1] TEESHYO BHATTACHARYA,[2] CHANCHAL MITTAL,[2] SUBHASH CHANDER,[3,*] and TEREZINHA DE JESUS ANDREOLI PINTO[4]

[1]*National Institute of Pharmaceutical Education and Research (NIPER), Hyderabad, Telangana, India*

[2]*National Institute of Pharmaceutical Education and Research (NIPER), Kolkata, West Bengal, India*

[3]*Amity Institute of Phytochemistry and Phytomedicine (AIP&P), Amity University Uttar Pradesh, Noida, Uttar Pradesh, India*

[4]*Department of Pharmacy, Faculty of Pharmaceutical Sciences, University of São Paulo, São Paulo, Brazil*

*Corresponding author

ABSTRACT

Over the past few years, there has been an intricate interplay between diet, gut microbiota, epigenetics, and their collective influence. Progression of colorectal neoplasia within the context of metabolic disorders has emerged as a prominent area of scientific investigation. A healthy metabolism is essential for a higher quality of life and well-being. Gut microbes act as a critical conduit in the metabolism of food and other Xenobiotics. Metabolic defects and harmful metabolites often become the root cause of various diseases. In multiple instances, gut microbes also either start such diseases by negatively impacting the epigenetic with chemicals and

Precision Nutrition and Endocrine Health: Synthesis, Characterization, and Applications.
Thakur Gurjeet Singh and Sanjana Mehta (Eds.)

DOI: 10.1201/9781998511877-7

toxins, leading to improper release of metabolic enzymes, or they produce harmful metabolites from the Inappropriate diet intake, which can also lead to diverse types of metabolic defects. Colorectal cancer is a disease from metabolic defects due to various epigenetic alterations. Various studies have elucidated the involvement of gut microbes in promoting the situation. This book chapter explores the dynamic crosstalk between dietary components, gut microbial composition, and epigenetic modifications, providing a comprehensive overview of the molecular pathways implicated in colorectal carcinogenesis within the context of metabolic disorders. Furthermore, critical updates of various diagnostic and prognostic approaches based on gut microflora alteration are also discussed. The chapter will also shed light on the different therapeutic approaches targeting these intricate molecular interactions, focusing on personalized dietary interventions, innovative approaches like probiotic-based therapies, and immunotherapies to mitigate colorectal cancer risk in individuals with metabolic disorders.

7.1 INTRODUCTION

Colorectal neoplasia is counted among the rampant malignancies, contributing to a significant Cosmopolitan Health Challenge. Globally, CRC ranks second in mortality and third in incidence. Depending on the stage of diagnosis, colorectal cancer has varying prognoses. The etiology of CRC is highly complicated and involves environmental and genetic factors. Environmental variables that contribute significantly to the progression of sporadic colorectal cancer (CRC) include smoking, Western food habits, diabetes, weight gain and obesity, and heavy alcohol usage (Mehta et al., 2021). The gut microbiota has a significant role in environmental risk factors. A growing body of research indicates that gut microbiota is essential for the development, spread, and metastasis of colorectal cancer (Chaitanya et al., 2022; Cheng et al., 2020; Mehta et al., 2022). Gut microbes typically benefit our digestive system by digesting dietary materials that our digestive system is otherwise unable to digest. Dysregulation of these microbes has been implicated in many inflammatory diseases, including colorectal cancer. One key aspect of gut microbiota alteration is the epigenetic modification of the host genes by the gut microbiota by protein regulators of DNA methylation (e.g., DNA methyltransferases) and histone acetylation (e.g., HDACs, HATs) play a crucial role in gene expression modulation, which in turn alters Nucleosome architecture, and post-transcriptional regulation by undertaking ncRNAs Fellows et al., 2018; Thapa et al., 2023; Ye et al., 2017). In this chapter, we will discuss the microbes that are the critical drivers of colorectal carcinogenesis, the mechanistic and pathophysiological cycles orchestrated by the gut microbes in advancing colorectal neoplasia, and the identification, cure and challenges.

7.2 COLORECTAL CANCER AND GUT MICROBIOTA

The human intestinal host, around 1013 to 1014 microorganisms, has >100 times as many genes as the human genome, and the total number of bacterial cells is around 10 times that of human cells (Gill et al., 2006; Tsai et al., 2019; Sharma et al., 2021). Although fungi and viruses are also present, bacteria make up most of the microorganisms that reside in the gastrointestinal tract. The gut microbiota is essential to human health because it establishes a symbiotic relationship with the host marked by advantages, interdependencies, and limits for both sides. The primary determinants influencing the makeup and functioning of gut microbiota dysbiosis include age, food, medications, and way of living (Kim and Jazwinski, 2018; Zmora et al., 2019; Weersma et al., 2020). There is a substantial link between host gene changes and dysbiosis of the gut microbiome; according to recent studies (Liang et al., 2020), infection and inflammation result from an imbalance in the gut flora, which encourages bacterial translocation and compromises the intestinal mucosal barrier (Wang et al., 2019). Some studies have revealed a connection between problems of the gut microbiota and an array of ailments, such as neurological conditions, heart disease, diabetes, and several cancers. (Ashique et al., 2022; Franzosa et al., 2019; Gubert et al., 2020; Gurung et al., 2020; Jin et al., 2019; Son and Kim, 2022).

7.2.1 CARCINOGENIC GUT MICROBES

Enterotoxigenic *Bacteroides fragilis* and *Streptococcus bovis* have been found in recent investigations, while other pathogens reported being associated with CRC include *Fusobacterium nucleatum*, *Escherichia coli*, *Enterococcus faecalis*, and *Peptostreptococusanaerobius* (Dalal et al., 2021). These bacterial communities are formed since birth, and humans provide nutrients as they develop a lifetime symbiotic relationship. In CRC patients, the numbers of Bifidobacterium, *Faecalibacterium*, and *Blautia* are reduced, but elevated levels of bacteria like *Porphyromonas* and *Mogibacteriumare* reported. Analysis of gut microbiota revealed an elevated abundance of *Erysipelotrichaceae*, *Prevotellaceae*, and *Coriobacteriaceae* in the intestinal lumen of colorectal cancer patients. This implies that Encounter between the lumen bacteria and the host may raise the risk of colorectal cancer (Dalal et al., 2021).

7.2.2 PATHOPHYSIOLOGICAL OUTLOOK

Epigenetic interaction is a critical driver in CRC carcinogenesis; in this segment, we will delve into how food and environmental factors affect the gut microbiota epigenetically, leading to altered metabolism and colorectal cancer, as shown in Table 7.1.

TABLE 7.1 Risks of Colorectal Cancer by Various Microbes

S. No.	Name of bacteria	Level of Risk Associated with Colorectal Cancer	Mechanisms	References
1.	SCFA producing bacteria	Low	Altering metabolic and immunological regulation that guards against CRC	Donohoe et al. (2014); Makki et al. (2018)
2.	Enterotoxigenic Bacteroides fragilis (ETBF)	High	Damage to DNA	Chung et al. (2018)
3.	*Escherichia coli*	High	Promotion of intestinal inflammation	Wilson et al. (2019)
4.	*Fusobacterium* nucleatum	High	Myeloid-derived cells and suppressor cells recruitment	Wilson et al. (2019)
			NK or T-cell inhibition of anti-tumor defense; E-cadherin/β-catenin modulation	

7.2.2.1 IMPACT OF FOOD AND ENVIRONMENTAL FACTORS

The potential impact of diet on gut flora formation is particularly significant during early development, potentially shaping its influence on health throughout life (Chu et al., 2016; Singh et al., 2020). It has long been understood that a fetus's intestines are sterile and that microbiological growth starts once the baby is exposed to germs from the surrounding environment (Aagaard et al., 2014). Adults with vegetarian vs. omnivorous diets have been discovered to have different gut flora compositions and functions. Compared to omnivores, long-term vegetarians had higher percentages of *Bacteroides Prevotella and Clostridium clostridia forme in their feces but lower percentages of Clostridium coccidia* (Mannan et al., 2023; Matijašić et al., 2014). Vegan diets, which exclude all animal products, also encourage the growth of Bacteriodaceae more than omnivorous diets do, though not as much as vegetarian diets do, as indicated by the abundance of OTU counts. Compared to omnivores, vegans and vegetarians consumed less protein (Losasso et al., 2018). Intestinal bacteria break down a variety of food components; specific nutritional elements, including fiber-rich carbohydrates, plant-based Sulphur metabolites (mustard oil glycosides), diverse lipid profiles, and a spectrum of bioactive polyphenols that influence host epigenetics and act as crucial drivers of CRC carcinogenesis (Wirbel et al., 2019). Red meat produces much choline, which is a precursor to the formation of TMA, later implicated in CRC formation; genetic analysis of fecal samples of CRC has shown upregulation of (*cutC*) and (*cutD*) genes secreting choline TMA-lyase and choline TMA -lyase-activating enzyme respectively (Nitter et al., 2014).

7.2.2.2 EPIGENETIC CROSSTALK BETWEEN HOST AND MICROBIOME

Genetically modified cells can exhibit inducible or conditional gene expression patterns in response to environmental stimuli through targeted changes in DNA regulatory regions while preserving their genomic integrity. Consequently, alterations in the amounts of luminal nutrients, including SCFAs generated by the resident microbial community, further influence the host's physiological processes. DNA methyltransferases (DNMTs) methylate CpG islands on DNA, and acetyl, methyl, or crotonyl groups can be added or removed from lysine residues on histones, which are examples of epigenetic alterations. Comparing germ-free (GF) mice to traditionally grown (ConvR) mice or conventionalized (ConvD, GF animals that had cecal content transfer from conventional mice), GF mice exhibit substantially less methylation and acetylation at several histones. This suggests that the gut bacteria regulate histone methylation and acetylation. The gut microbiota modifies histones and alters DNA's epigenetic makeup (*H. pylori* infection is a prominent example). A potential outcome of abnormal DNA methylation is alterations in miRNA profiles, which have been linked to a higher risk of gastric cancer (elevated miR-129-2 methylation) (Joshi et al., 2022; Watari et al., 2019).

It has been demonstrated that the host's genetic modification impacts the host and the host's microbial composition (Alenghat et al., 2013). In a model of neonatal necrotizing enterocolitis (NEC), an inflammatory bowel disease affecting premature babies, Cortese et al. (2016) investigated the host-microbe crosstalk. They discovered that prenatal administration of the glucocorticoid dexamethasone changed the host's epigenome and the microbiota's composition, decreasing *Bacteroides* and increasing *Firmicutes*. Furthermore, probiotic and pathogenic bacteria were added to IECs, causing DNA alterations in more than 200 locations. The reciprocal interactions between the gut microbiota regions and the host epigenome are highlighted in these studies. These findings demonstrate the mutual relationships between the gut microbiota and the host epigenome (Cortese et al., 2016).

7.2.2.3 GENERAL DISEASE PATHWAY

Numerous bacteria have a role in the pathophysiology of colorectal cancer; however, recently, anaerobic gram-negative rods called fusobacteria have been reported for causing severe human diseases, which is still an area of investigation. Some research reports frequently linked these bacteria to colorectal cancer. The two *Fusobacterium* species that are most frequently observed are *F. necrophorum* and *F. nucleatum* (Fn) (Afra et al., 2013; Kumar et al., 2023). Both bacterial strains frequently live in the oral cavity and can occasionally lead to gingiva and periodontal tissue infections, as reported in two studies published in 2011 (Castellarin et al., 2012; Kostic et al., 2012; Thapa et al., 2021).

The gastrointestinal tract's inflammatory process can be influenced by gut microbiota. Stool from CRC patients was given to germ-free, carcinogen-fed mice, which increased histological inflammation and expression of inflammatory gene markers. This is because gut microorganisms can induce chemotactic factors, attracting T cells into tumors. These factors include CXCL9 and CXCL10 for cytotoxic T lymphocytes, type 1

T helper (TH1), and CCL17 and CCL20 for TH cells that produce IL-17 (Cremonesi et al., 2018).

Through its virulence factor, B. fragilis toxin, enterotoxigenic B. fragilis, a strain abundant in patients with CRC, can initiate an inflammatory cascade involving IL-17, nuclear factor-κB signaling, and signal transducer and activator of transcription 3. This occurs in colonic epithelial cells (Boleij et al., 2015; Wu et al., 2009).

Regarding specific bacterial species, research has shown that *F. nucleatum* can stimulate the nuclear factor-κB pathway and promote myeloid cell infiltration in tumors, creating a pro-inflammatory environment that helps colorectal neoplasia progress in ApcMin mice, a standard rodent model of colorectal cancer. These signaling pathways are reported to produce CXC chemokines, which attract polymorphonuclear immature in ApcMin animals (Kostic et al., 2013; Tomkovich et al., 2017).

The activities of other bacteria, such as the CRC-enriched genotoxic polyketide synthase (pks) + *E. coli* (Arthur et al., 2012, 2014; Bonnet et al., 2014), *E. faecalis* (Wang et al., 2012) and *A. finegoldii*, (Moschen et al., 2016) are also documented for the promotion of cancer, depending upon inflammation. Interactions between the gut microbiota and the human immune system occur through pattern recognition receptors (PRRs). PRRs trigger the gut immune system by identifying microbial antigens and initiating a series of signaling molecules downstream. Toll-like receptors (TLRs) (Kesselring et al., 2016), nucleotide-binding oligomerization-like receptors (Couturier-Maillard et al., 2013), RIG-I-like receptors (Zhu et al., 2017), and missing in melanoma 2-like receptors (Man et al., 2015) are among the PRRs linked in animal models to colitis-associated carcinogenesis. *Peptostreptococcus anaerobius*, another bacterium linked to CRC, may induce tumor formation in mice by activating TLR4 signaling, while *F. nucleatum* can only do this by activating the TLR2 or TLR4 pathways (Tsoi et al., 2017; Wu et al., 2018; Yang et al., 2017).

A critical area of interaction between the microbiota and the host is metabolism. There is proof that several dietary elements, such as red and processed meat, are linked to colorectal cancer (Alexander et al., 2011; O'Keefe, 2016). Numerous harmful substances have been documented, encompassing carcinogenic substances such as N-nitroso compounds and hydrogen sulphide, produced by microbial metabolism (Louis et al., 2014). Research in mice has also shown that the gut microbiota can worsen haem-induced epithelial hyperproliferation by impairing mucus barrier function (Ijssennagger et al., 2015).

Butyrate and propionate are short-chain fatty acids (SCFAs) among the metabolites generated by microorganisms upon the breakdown of food ingredients. Consuming nondigestible carbs like fiber and digestion-resistant starch causes the colon to produce SCFAs by microbial fermentation (Louis et al., 2014). Documented as an anti-inflammatory chemical, Butyrate can cause CRC cell lines to undergo apoptosis and downregulate pro-inflammatory cytokines by blocking histone deacetylases in immune cells and colonocytes (Buda et al., 2003; Chang et al., 2014; Singh et al., 2014). Moreover, it has been demonstrated in animal models that butyrate and propionate alter colonic regulatory T cells to have a strong anti-inflammatory impact (Furusawa et al., 2013; Smith et al., 2013). Populations at high risk of colorectal cancer have been associated with lower levels of SCFAs. Another class of metabolites that are intimately associated with gut microbiota and nutrition is bile acids. These are steroid acids produced by the liver; later, these are converted into secondary forms by intestinal bacteria (de Aguiar Vallim et al., 2013). Those who ate high-fat diets had higher levels of secondary bile acids, such as deoxycholic acid, in their colonic contents, which was associated with a higher risk of colorectal cancer (Ou et al., 2012, 2013). In one study, the carcinogen azoxymethane was found to cause a higher incidence of colonic tumors in rats when colons were subjected to elevated levels of bile acids through diversion surgery (Chomchai et al., 1974). These findings strengthened the theory that bile acids could promote the growth of colon tumors. Moreover, it has been demonstrated that deoxycholic acid stimulates the growth of tumors *in vivo* and causes oxidative DNA damage *in vitro* (Bernstein et al., 2009). Toxins that cause damage to DNA (genotoxicity) are produced by the microbiota and are linked to another carcinogenic process. Two distinct genotoxins produced by bacteria are colibactin and CDT. Enteric infections like Escherichia and Campylobacter species create CDT, which is carcinogenic because it causes double-strand DNA breaks through its deoxyribonuclease activity (Cuevas-Ramos et al., 2010; He et al., 2019). Figure 7.1. provides an overview of the suggested paths connecting gut microbes to colorectal cancer.

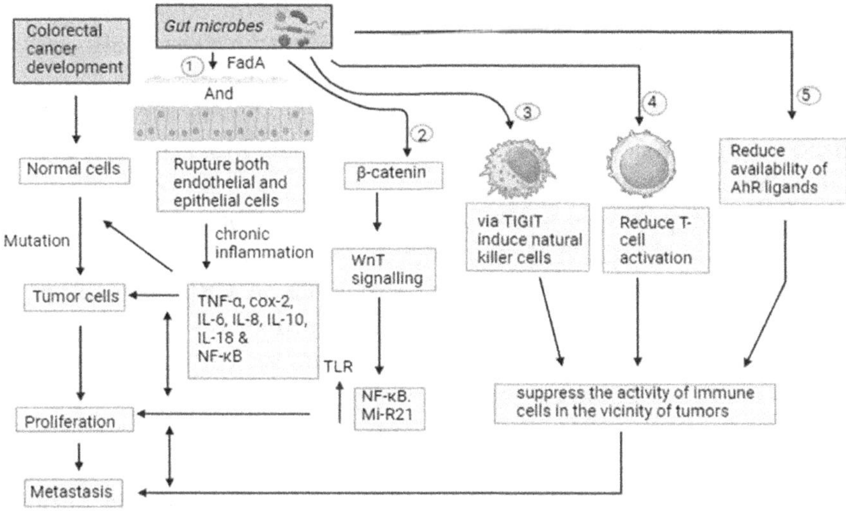

FIGURE 7.1 An overview of potential routes of gut microbes in progression of colorectal cancer development.

7.3 DIAGNOSIS

Treatment of any disease is always preceded by diagnosis to confirm the disease and followed prognosis to see whether the therapy is properly functioning. It becomes quintessential when it comes to CRC caused by gut microbiota. The gold standard is the analysis of the fecal matter for microbes and metabolites. Gut microbiome composition is significantly altered in colorectal cancer, and looking deeply into gut bacteria's genetic alteration is the crucial driver of carcinogenesis. In a routine diagnostic approach, DNA is extracted from the patient's stool. Various techniques like shotgun sequencing, 16S sequencing and qPCR are often employed for judging these alterations via various studies. In studies carried out on colorectal cancer patients, some of these genes in bacteria are upregulated (Goedert et al., 2014). A marker called afa-C1 operon was highly upregulated in diffusely adherent *E. coli* (DAEC) in CRC patients, as shown by Eklof et al. (2017). A similar study showed that a particular gene, *m3*, was highly upregulated in various bacterial strains like *Fusobacterium* and *Clostridium symbiosum* in the stool samples of CRC patients.

In previous sections, we mentioned how metabolites from microbiota promote CRC, so metabolite profiling from patients' stools can also serve diagnostic and prognostic purposes. Various techniques, such as mass spectroscopy, LC-MS, and HPLC, can detect various metabolites. Lyophilized samples of stool can also be subjected to GC-MS/TOF (Wei et al., 2016; Wang et al., 2020).

The techniques specifically detect SCFAs like butyrate and amino acids like proline, which are implicated in CRC. Yang et al. conducted extensive metabolic profiling of stool samples of CRC patients, and GC-MS data revealed a high amount of proline in CRC patients compared to regular patients (Yang et al., 2019). CRC is a complex disorder, so investigations are required beyond stool tests. Numerous studies have shown links between oral microbiota, including Streptococcus and *Prevotella* species, with colorectal cancer (CRC), and research is underway to predict CRC possibility by investing in oral bacterial profiles (Amitay et al., 2018; Mannan et al., 2023). Researchers can create an oral microbiota-based classifier that distinguishes the cases from healthy controls in a study examining the oral microbiota of patients with colorectal adenoma, colorectal cancer, and healthy individuals.

7.4 THERAPEUTIC OUTLOOK

Therapy in microbiota-related colorectal cancer is by no means a straightforward proposition. Gut microbes modulate the anticancer drug action. Shreds of evidence indicate that microbes modulate the action of chemotherapy or immunotherapy, and in many instances, microbiota decreases the efficacy of anti-cancer therapeutics. In this view, the first treatment is the cause leading to the formation of CRC (Iida et al., 2013; Sepich-Poore et al., 2021). In this view, we try to alleviate the obesity responsible for CRC by using probiotics and prebiotics. This section will discuss how these methods mechanistically impact therapy in microbiota-related CRC.

7.4.1 OBESITY REDUCTION

Adipokines, sex hormones, insulin or insulin-like growth factor 1 signaling, and systemic inflammation are crucial components linked with obesity and colorectal cancer (CRC). The gut microbiota has become a key player in these mechanisms by modifying pro-inflammatory molecules and metabolites derived from microorganisms (Ciofi et al., 2006). Reduced microbial diversity and a shift in gut microbiota composition are linked to obesity. Obesity brought on by diet can cause widespread histone methylation and acetylation linked to a downstream transcriptome pattern that mimics the progression of cancer in animals in a gut microbiota-dependent manner. Due to these connections, controlling weight in obese people can significantly alter their gut microbiota (Li et al., 2014; Qin et al., 2018).

7.4.2 PREBIOTIC APPLICATION

Prebiotics can be defined as indigestible food matter that stimulates the formation of a particular microorganism. As far as colorectal cancer is concerned, prebiotics have a significant contribution in preventing carcinogenesis (Gibson et al., 2017). Prebiotics impart their anti-carcinogenic indirectly by supporting the growth of those bacteria that provide anticancer effects by modulating the immune environment in the gut (Calderon et al., 2022). The prebiotics also imparts indirect action by getting selectively fermented by the probiotics in the gut to SCFAs. Butyrate and other SCFAs impart anti-tumorigenic action by acting as a histone deacetylase inhibitor, and their beneficial effects are reducing inflammation, inducing apoptosis, and improving epithelial barrier function (Fukuda et al., 2011; Rakoff-Nahoum et al., 2016; Tong et al., 2016).

Prebiotics have direct action wherein they directly impact the tumor microenvironment. Prebiotic oligosaccharides can interact with the bacterial receptor and inhibit pathogen colonization by imitating the microvillus glycoconjugates and preventing pathogens from attaching to epithelial cells (Monteagudo-Mera et al., 2019). Additionally, prebiotics may enter intestinal cells directly and change the profile gene expression. One study that used oligosaccharides with varying degrees of polymerization (DP) showed that only prebiotics with DP could enhance IFN-γ and IL-production in $CD4^+$ T cells, indicating that it can be fully absorbed through the intestine and, after that, modulate the intestinal immune response (Belcheva et al., 2014).

7.4.3 PROBIOTIC THERAPY

Probiotics are live microorganisms that benefit the host's health when given in sufficient amounts (Martin et al., 2022). They mediate their therapeutic effect in three ways. The first one interferes with the growth of microbes in the gut. Reduced growth can result from various microbes competing for nutrients to survive, as in the case of Clostridium difficile, or their secretions can also result in a hostile environment detrimental to the growth of other microbes (Mills et al., 2018; Piewngam et al., 2018).

The second way by which probiotics impart their therapeutic efficiency is by immunomodulation in the gut, sometimes by decreasing inflammation like by inhibiting STAT3 and NF-κB signaling, or certain probiotic bacteria, including *Lactobacillus rhamnosus* GG and *Lactobacillus acidophilus*, reduce the expression of Th17 cells and the secretion of IL23 and IL17 (Klaenhammer et al., 2012). Immunomodulation also occurs by reducing inflammation, as in CRC mice models induced by DMH, Lactobacillus casei, which has demonstrated antitumor properties. Splenocyte analysis has revealed a decreased Treg level and an increased Th17 population at the systemic level despite the intestinal content showing downregulation of proinflammatory cytokines (MCP-1, TNF-α) and upregulation of IL-10 (Chen et al., 2015; Konieczna et al., 2012).

The third way of therapeutic effect is by improving gut barrier function. Increased tight junction permeability, or gut barrier dysfunction, has been linked to CRC. Cachexia develops due to endotoxemia and microbial translocation, both facilitated by a leaky gut (Miller et al., 2017). The induction of the epithelial-mesenchymal transition (EMT) and metastasis in colorectal cancer (CRC) is also linked to the loss of tight junction protein. *Lactobacillus rhamnosus, Lactobacillus plantarum*, and *Escherichia coli* are among the probiotic strains that have been demonstrated to enhance the function of the gut barrier by either upregulating or normalizing the expression of tight junction proteins (claudin-1, occludin, ZO-1, ZO-2) (Rocha-Ramírez et al., 2017; Wang et al., 2014), the therapeutic effects of probiotics are illustrated in the given Figure 7.2.

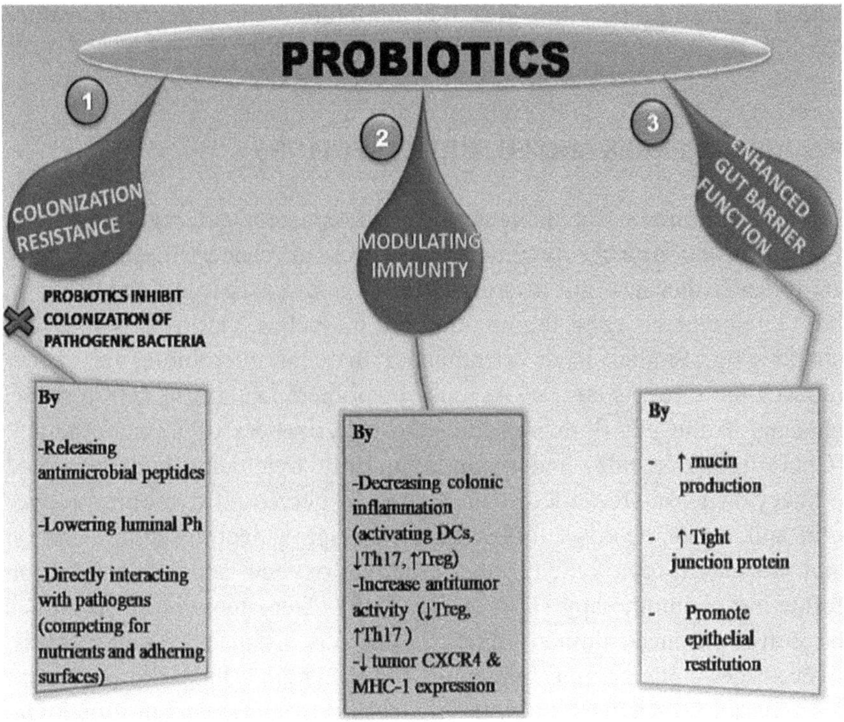

FIGURE 7.2 Showing therapeutic effects of probiotics.

7.4.4 *ANTIBIOTIC*

Deviation from the standard community of microbes in the gut has been associated with compromised gut barrier function, inflammation, and, ultimately, cancer and tumor growth. Treatment with antibiotics to reduce gut microbiome and reverse harmful dysbiosis is a logical avenue for research in the treatment of cancer (Cao et al., 2017). Antibiotics are frequently used *in vivo* models to investigate the effects of gut microbiome on cancer or other inflammatory diseases (Zackular et al., 2016). Antibiotic-mediated depletion of the microbiome has been shown in multiple studies to reduce the development of colorectal cancer. Antibiotic treatment has also been linked to inhibiting tumor growth, invasion, and proliferation. Metronidazole treatment eliminates *Fusobacterium* colonization and decreases CRC growth in mice with CRC xenografts, indicating the potential use of antibiotics for *Fusobacterium*-enriched CRC patients (Bullman et al., 2017).

These studies support the idea that antibiotics can potentially reduce harmful microbiomes and the proliferation of tumor cells.

7.5 CHALLENGES AND FUTURE DIRECTIONS

There are numerous challenges when we consider gut microbe-related CRC. In one aspect, treating these types of cancers becomes very complicated because gut microbes can alter the activity of the drug, so both chemotherapy and immunotherapy in such scenarios become very challenging. Studies have documented that gut microbiota very often reduces the effectiveness of various chemotherapeutic drugs. In a study, changes in the gut flora impacted the effectiveness of immunotherapy (CpG-oligonucleotide) and oxaliplatin. Both treatments had decreased efficacy in germ-free mice, which showed decreased cytokine production and tumor necrosis following CpG-oligonucleotide administration and decreased cytotoxicity and reactive oxygen species production following chemotherapy (Iida et al., 2013). Treatments with probiotics have also produced limited effects. Numerous instances of endocarditis, liver abscess, pneumonia, fungemia, and bacteremia linked to probiotics are reported, particularly with their excessive use (Doron and Snydman, 2015). Furthermore, there are reports of antibiotic resistance transmission via these probiotics. The above-reported approaches are often documented for beneficial effects on the disease, but we still have no microbiota-based biomarkers. Given this gap, more clinical studies are needed to identify patients who suffer from CRC, and a thorough microbial analysis needs to be done to identify microbial prognostic markers.

7.6 CONCLUSION

The complex connection between the gut microbiota and colorectal cancer (CRC) has been the subject of extensive research. This chapter explores essential aspects of gut microbial communities that can trigger long-term inflammation and create an environment favorable for the development of colorectal cancer. It discusses the current therapeutic approaches and ongoing challenges and suggests potential future research directions. To fully understand the complex relationship between CRC and gut microbiota, more detailed research is needed to uncover the exact mechanisms and causal pathways involved in this intricate interplay.

KEYWORDS

- **colorectal**
- **dietary**
- **epigenetic**
- **metabolic disorders**
- **microbiota**
- **therapeutics**

REFERENCES

Aagaard, K., Ma, J., Antony, K. M., Ganu, R., Petrosino, J., & Versalovic, J. (2014). The placenta harbours a unique microbiome. *Science Translational Medicine, 6*(237). https://doi.org/10.1126/SCITRANSLMED.3008599/SUPPL_FILE/6-237RA65_SM.PDF (accessed on 28th June 2025).

Afra, K., Laupland, K., Leal, J., Lloyd, T., & Gregson, D. (2013). Incidence, risk factors, and outcomes of *Fusobacterium* species bacteremia. http://www.biomedcentral.com/1471-2334/13/264 (accessed on 28th June 2025).

Alenghat, T., Osborne, L. C., Saenz, S. A., Kobuley, D., Ziegler, C. G. K., Mullican, S. E., Choi, I., Grunberg, S., Sinha, R., Wynosky-Dolfi, M., Snyder, A., Giacomin, P. R., Joyce, K. L., Hoang, T. B., Bewtra, M., Brodsky, I. E., Sonnenberg, G. F., Bushman, F. D., Won, K. J., … Artis, D. (2013). Histone deacetylase three coordinates commensal-bacteria-dependent intestinal homeostasis. *Nature, 504*(7478), 153–157. https://doi.org/10.1038/nature12687 (accessed on 28th June 2025).

Alexander, D. D., Weed, D. L., Cushing, C. A., & Lowe, K. A. (2011). Meta-analysis of prospective studies of red meat consumption and colorectal cancer. *European Journal of Cancer Prevention, 20*(4), 293–307. https://doi.org/10.1097/CEJ.0b013e328345f985 (accessed on 28th June 2025).

Amitay, E. L., Krilaviciute, A., & Brenner, H. (2018). Systematic review: Gut microbiota in fecal samples and detection of colorectal neoplasms. *Gut Microbes, 9*(4), 293–307. https://doi.org/10.1080/19490976.2018.1445957 (accessed on 28th June 2025).

Arthur, J. C., Gharaibeh, R. Z., Mühlbauer, M., Perez-Chanona, E., Uronis, J. M., McCafferty, J., Fodor, A. A., & Jobin, C. (2014). Microbial genomic analysis reveals the essential role of inflammation in bacteria-induced colorectal cancer. *Nature Communications, 5*, 4724. https://doi.org/10.1038/ncomms5724 (accessed on 28th June 2025).

Arthur, J. C., Perez-Chanona, E., Mühlbauer, M., Tomkovich, S., Uronis, J. M., Fan, T. J., Campbell, B. J., Abujamel, T., Dogan, B., Rogers, A. B., Rhodes, J. M., Stintzi, A., Simpson, K. W., Hansen, J. J., Keku, T. O., Fodor, A. A., & Jobin, C. (2012). Intestinal inflammation targets cancer-inducing activity of the microbiota. *Science (New York, N.Y.), 338*(6103), 120–123. https://doi.org/10.1126/science.1224820 (accessed on 28th June 2025).

Ashique, S., De Rubis, G., Sirohi, E., Mishra, N., Rihan, M., Garg, A., Reyes, R. J., Manandhar, B., Bhatt, S., Jha, N. K., Singh, T. G., Gupta, G., Singh, S. K., Chellappan, D. K., Paudel, K. R., Hansbro, P. M., Oliver, B. G., & Dua, K. (2022). Short chain fatty acids: Fundamental mediators of the gut-lung axis and their involvement in pulmonary diseases. *Chemico-Biological Interactions, 368*, 110231. https://doi.org/10.1016/j.cbi.2022.110231 (accessed on 28th June 2025).

Belcheva, A., Irrazabal, T., Robertson, S. J., Streutker, C., Maughan, H., Rubino, S., Moriyama, E. H., Copeland, J. K., Kumar, S., Green, B., Geddes, K., Pezo, R. C., Navarre, W. W., Milosevic, M., Wilson, B. C., Girardin, S. E., Wolever, T. M. S., Edelmann, W., Guttman, D. S., … Martin, A. (2014). Gut microbial metabolism drives the transformation of msh2-deficient colon epithelial cells. *Cell, 158*(2), 288–299. https://doi.org/10.1016/J.CELL.2014.04.051 (accessed on 28th June 2025).

Bernstein, H., Bernstein, C., Payne, C. M., & Dvorak, K. (2009). Bile acids as endogenous etiologic agents in gastrointestinal cancer. In *World Journal of Gastroenterology, 15*(27), 3329–3340. https://doi.org/10.3748/wjg.15.3329 (accessed on 28th June 2025).

Boleij, A., Hechenbleikner, E. M., Goodwin, A. C., Badani, R., Stein, E. M., Lazarev, M. G., Ellis, B., Carroll, K. C., Albesiano, E., Wick, E. C., Platz, E. A., Pardoll, D. M., & Sears, C. L. (2015). The *Bacteroides fragilis* toxin gene is prevalent in the colon mucosa of colorectal cancer patients. *Clinical Infectious Diseases, 60*(2), 208–215. https://doi.org/10.1093/cid/ciu787 (accessed on 28th June 2025).

Bonnet, M., Buc, E., Sauvanet, P., Darcha, C., Dubois, D., Pereira, B., Dechelotte, P., Bonnet, R., Pezet, D., & Darfeuille-Michaud, A. (2014). Colonization of the human gut by *E. coli* and colorectal cancer risk. *Clinical Cancer Research, 20*(4), 859–867. https://doi.org/10.1158/1078-0432.CCR-13-1343 (accessed on 28th June 2025).

Buda, A., Qualtrough, D., Jepson, M. A., Martines, D., Paraskeva, C., & Pignatelli, M. (2003). Butyrate downregulates alpha2beta1 integrin: A possible role in the induction of apoptosis in colorectal cancer cell lines. *Gut, 52*(5), 729–734. https://doi.org/10.1136/gut.52.5.729 (accessed on 28th June 2025).

Calderon, G., Patel, C., Camilleri, M., James-Stevenson, T., Bohm, M., Siwiec, R., Rogers, N., Wo, J., Lockett, C., Gupta, A., Xu, H., & Shin, A. (2022). Associations of habitual dietary intake with fecal short-chain fatty acids and bowel functions in irritable bowel syndrome. *Journal of Clinical Gastroenterology, 56*(3), 234–242. https://doi.org/10.1097/MCG.0000000000001521 (accessed on 28th June 2025).

Cao, H., Xu, M., Dong, W., Deng, B., Wang, S., Zhang, Y., Wang, S., Luo, S., Wang, W., Qi, Y., Gao, J., Cao, X., Yan, F., & Wang, B. (2017). Secondary bile acid-induced dysbiosis promotes intestinal carcinogenesis. *International Journal of Cancer, 140*(11), 2545–2556. https://doi.org/10.1002/IJC.30643 (accessed on 28th June 2025).

Castellarin, M., Warren, R. L., Freeman, J. D., Dreolini, L., Krzywinski, M., Strauss, J., Barnes, R., Watson, P., Allen-Vercoe, E., Moore, R. A., & Holt, R. A. (2012). *Fusobacterium nucleatum* infection is prevalent in human colorectal carcinoma. *Genome*

Research, 22(2), 299–306. https://doi.org/10.1101/gr.126516.111 (accessed on 28th June 2025).

Chaitanya, M. V. N. L., Ramanunny, A. K., Babu, M. R., Gulati, M., Vishwas, S., Singh, T. G., Chellappan, D. K., Adams, J., Dua, K., & Singh, S. K. (2022). Journey of rosmarinic acid as biomedicine to nano-biomedicine for treating cancer: Current strategies and future perspectives. *Pharmaceutics, 14*(11), 2401. https://doi.org/10.3390/pharmaceutics14112401 (accessed on 28th June 2025).

Chang, P. V., Hao, L., Offermanns, S., & Medzhitov, R. (2014). The microbial metabolite butyrate regulates intestinal macrophage function via histone deacetylase inhibition. *Proceedings of the National Academy of Sciences of the United States of America, 111*(6), 2247–2252. https://doi.org/10.1073/pnas.1322269111 (accessed on 28th June 2025).

Chen, L., Zou, Y., Peng, J., Lu, F., Yin, Y., Li, F., & Yang, J. (2015). *Lactobacillus acidophilus* suppresses colitis-associated activation of the IL-23/Th17 axis. *Journal of Immunology Research, 2015*, Article 909514. https://doi.org/10.1155/2015/909514 (accessed on 28th June 2025).

Cheng, Y., Ling, Z., & Li, L. (2020). The intestinal microbiota and colorectal cancer. *Frontiers in Immunology, 11*, 615056. https://doi.org/10.3389/fimmu.2020.615056 (accessed on 28th June 2025).

Chomchai, C., Bhadrachari, N., & Nigro, N. D. (1974). The effect of bile on the induction of experimental intestinal tumors in rats. *Diseases of the Colon and Rectum, 17*(3), 310–312. https://doi.org/10.1007/BF02586971 (accessed on 28th June 2025).

Chu, D. M., Meyer, K. M., Prince, A. L., & Aagaard, K. M. (2016). Impact of maternal nutrition in pregnancy and lactation on offspring gut microbial composition and function. *Gut Microbes, 7*(6), 459–470. https://doi.org/10.1080/19490976.2016.1241357 (accessed on 28th June 2025).

Chung, L., Orberg, E. T., Geis, A. L., Wu, S., Sears, C. L., & Housseau, F. (2018). *Bacteroides fragilis* toxin coordinates a pro-carcinogenic inflammatory cascade via targeting of colonic epithelial cells. *Cell Host & Microbe, 23*, 203–214. https://doi.org/10.1016/j.chom.2018.01.007 (accessed on 28th June 2025).

Chung, L., Thiele Orberg, E., Geis, A. L., Chan, J. L., Fu, K., DeStefano Shields, C. E., Dejea, C. M., Fathi, P., Chen, J., Finard, B. B., Tam, A. J., McAllister, F., Fan, H., Wu, X., Ganguly, S., Lebid, A., Metz, P., Van Meerbeke, S. W., Huso, D. L., … Housseau, F. (2018). *Bacteroides fragilis* toxin coordinates a pro-carcinogenic inflammatory cascade via targeting of colonic epithelial cells. *Cell Host and Microbe, 23*(2), 203–214.e5. https://doi.org/10.1016/j.chom.2018.01.007 (accessed on 28th June 2025).

Ciofi, C., De Boer, M., Bruford, M. W., Hecht, M. K., Wallace, B., Macintyre, R. J., Lenk, P., Eidenmueller, B., Staudter, H., Wicker, R., & Wink, M. (2006). Human gut microbes associated with obesity. *Nature, 444*(7122), 1022–1023. https://doi.org/10.1038/4441022a (accessed on 28th June 2025).

Cortese, R., Lu, L., Yu, Y., Ruden, D., & Claud, E. C. (2016). Epigenome-microbiome crosstalk: A potential new paradigm influencing neonatal susceptibility to disease. *Epigenetics, 11*(3), 205–215. https://doi.org/10.1080/15592294.2016.1155011 (accessed on 28th June 2025).

Cuevas-Ramos, G., Petit, C. R., Marcq, I., Boury, M., Oswald, E., & Nougayrède, J. P. (2010). *Escherichia coli* induces DNA damage in vivo and triggers genomic instability in mammalian cells. *Proceedings of the National Academy of Sciences of the United*

States of America, 107(25), 11537–11542. https://doi.org/10.1073/pnas.1001261107 (accessed on 28th June 2025).

Dalal, N., Jalandra, R., Bayal, N., Yadav, A. K., Harshulika, Sharma, M., Makharia, G. K., Kumar, P., Singh, R., Solanki, P. R., & Kumar, A. (2021). Gut microbiota-derived metabolites in CRC progression and causation. *Journal of Cancer Research and Clinical Oncology, 147*(11), 3141–3155. https://doi.org/10.1007/S00432-021-03729-W (accessed on 28th June 2025).

De Aguiar Vallim, T. Q., Tarling, E. J., & Edwards, P. A. (2013). Pleiotropic roles of bile acids in metabolism. *Cell Metabolism, 17*(5), 657–669. https://doi.org/10.1016/J.CMET.2013.03.013 (accessed on 28th June 2025).

Doll, R., & Peto, R. (1981). The causes of cancer: Quantitative estimates of avoidable cancer risks in the United States today. *Journal of the National Cancer Institute, 66*(6), 1192–1308. https://doi.org/10.1093/jnci/66.6.1192 (accessed on 28th June 2025).

Donohoe, D. R., Holley, D., Collins, L. B., Montgomery, S. A., Whitmore, A. C., Hillhouse, A., Curry, K. P., Renner, S. W., Greenwalt, A., Ryan, E. P., Godfrey, V., Heise, M. T., Threadgill, D. S., Han, A., Swenberg, J. A., Threadgill, D. W., & Bultman, S. J. (2014). A gnotobiotic mouse model demonstrates that dietary fibre protects against colorectal tumorigenesis in a microbiota- and butyrate-dependent manner. *Cancer Discovery, 4*(12), 1387–1397. https://doi.org/10.1158/2159-8290.CD-14-0501/42418/AM/A-GNOTOBIOTIC-MOUSE-MODEL-DEMONSTRATES-THAT (accessed on 28th June 2025).

Doron, S., & Snydman, D. R. (2015). Risk and safety of probiotics. *Clinical Infectious Diseases, 60*(suppl_2), S129–S134. https://doi.org/10.1093/CID/CIV085 (accessed on 28th June 2025).

Eklöf, V., Löfgren-Burström, A., Zingmark, C., Edin, S., Larsson, P., Karling, P., Alexeyev, O., Rutegård, J., Wikberg, M. L., & Palmqvist, R. (2017). Cancer-associated fecal microbial markers in colorectal cancer detection. *International Journal of Cancer, 141*(12), 2528–2536. https://doi.org/10.1002/IJC.31011 (accessed on 28th June 2025).

Fellows, R., Denizot, J., Stellato, C., Cuomo, A., Jain, P., Stoyanova, E., Balázsi, S., Hajnády, Z., Liebert, A., Kazakevych, J., Blackburn, H., Corrêa, R. O., Fachi, J. L., Sato, F. T., Ribeiro, W. R., Ferreira, C. M., Perée, H., Spagnuolo, M., Mattiuz, R., … Varga-Weisz, P. (2018). Microbiota-derived short-chain fatty acids promote histone crotonylation in the colon through histone deacetylases. *Nature Communications, 9*(1), 1–15. https://doi.org/10.1038/s41467-017-02651-5 (accessed on 28th June 2025).

Franzosa, E. A., Sirota-Madi, A., Avila-Pacheco, J., Fornelos, N., Haiser, H. J., Reinker, S., Vatanen, T., Hall, A. B., Mallick, H., McIver, L. J., Sauk, J. S., Wilson, R. G., Stevens, B. W., Scott, J. M., Pierce, K., Deik, A. A., Bullock, K., Imhann, F., Porter, J. A., … Xavier, R. J. (2018). Gut microbiome structure and metabolic activity in inflammatory bowel disease. *Nature Microbiology, 4*(2), 293–305. https://doi.org/10.1038/s41564-018-0306-4 (accessed on 28th June 2025).

Fukuda, S., Toh, H., Hase, K., Oshima, K., Nakanishi, Y., Yoshimura, K., Tobe, T., Clarke, J. M., Topping, D. L., Suzuki, T., Taylor, T. D., Itoh, K., Kikuchi, J., Morita, H., Hattori, M., & Ohno, H. (2011). *Bifidobacteria* can protect from enteropathogenic infection through the production of acetate. *Nature, 469*(7331), 543–547. https://doi.org/10.1038/nature09646 (accessed on 28th June 2025).

Gibson, G. R., Hutkins, R., Sanders, M. E., Prescott, S. L., Reimer, R. A., Salminen, S. J., Scott, K., Stanton, C., Swanson, K. S., Cani, P. D., Verbeke, K., & Reid, G. (2017). Expert consensus document: The International Scientific Association for Probiotics and Prebiotics (ISAPP) consensus statement on the definition and scope of prebiotics. *Nature Reviews Gastroenterology & Hepatology, 14*(8), 491–502. https://doi.org/10.1038/nrgastro.2017.75 (accessed on 28th June 2025).

Gill, S. R., Pop, M., DeBoy, R. T., Eckburg, P. B., Turnbaugh, P. J., Samuel, B. S., Gordon, J. I., Relman, D. A., Fraser-Liggett, C. M., & Nelson, K. E. (2006). Metagenomic analysis of the human distal gut microbiome. *Science, 312*(5778), 1355–1359. https://doi.org/10.1126/SCIENCE.1124234/SUPPL_FILE/GILL.SOM.PDF (accessed on 28th June 2025).

Goedert, J. J., Sampson, J. N., Moore, S. C., Xiao, Q., Xiong, X., Hayes, R. B., Ahn, J., Shi, J., & Sinha, R. (2014). Fecal metabolomics: Assay performance and association with colorectal cancer. *Carcinogenesis, 35*(9), 2089–2096. https://doi.org/10.1093/CARCIN/BGU131 (accessed on 28th June 2025).

Gubert, C., Kong, G., Renoir, T., & Hannan, A. J. (2020). Exercise, diet and stress as modulators of gut microbiota: Implications for neurodegenerative diseases. *Neurobiology of Disease, 134*, 104621. https://doi.org/10.1016/J.NBD.2019.104621 (accessed on 28th June 2025).

Gurung, M., Li, Z., You, H., Rodrigues, R., Jump, D. B., Morgun, A., & Shulzhenko, N. (2020). Role of gut microbiota in type 2 diabetes pathophysiology. *EBioMedicine, 51*, 102590. https://doi.org/10.1016/j.ebiom.2019.11.051 (accessed on 28th June 2025).

Iida, N., Dzutsev, A., Stewart, C. A., Smith, L., Bouladoux, N., Weingarten, R. A., Molina, D. A., Salcedo, R., Back, T., Cramer, S., Dai, R. M., Kiu, H., Cardone, M., Naik, S., Patri, A. K., Wang, E., Marincola, F. M., Frank, K. M., Belkaid, Y., Trinchieri, G., … Goldszmid, R. S. (2013). Commensal bacteria control cancer response to therapy by modulating the tumor microenvironment. *Science, 342*(6161), 967–970. https://doi.org/10.1126/science.1240527 (accessed on 28th June 2025).

Iida, N., Dzutsev, A., Stewart, C. A., Smith, L., Bouladoux, N., Weingarten, R. A., Molina, D. A., Salcedo, R., Back, T., Cramer, S., Dai, R.-M., Kiu, H., Cardone, M., Naik, S., Patri, A. K., Wang, E., Marincola, F. M., Frank, K. M., Belkaid, Y., & Goldszmid, R. S. (2013). Commensal bacteria control cancer response to therapy by modulating the tumor microenvironment. *Science, 342*(6161), 967–970. https://doi.org/10.1126/science.1240527 (accessed on 28th June 2025).

Jin, M., Qian, Z., Yin, J., Xu, W., & Zhou, X. (2019). The role of intestinal microbiota in cardiovascular disease. *Journal of Cellular and Molecular Medicine, 23*(4), 2343–2350. https://doi.org/10.1111/JCMM.14195 (accessed on 28th June 2025).

Joshi, D., Khursheed, R., Gupta, S., Wadhwa, D., Singh, T. G., Sharma, S., Porwal, S., Gauniyal, S., Vishwas, S., Goyal, S., Gupta, G., Eri, R. D., Williams, K. A., Dua, K., & Singh, S. K. (2022). Biosimilars in oncology: Latest trends and regulatory status. *Pharmaceutics, 14*(12), 2721. https://doi.org/10.3390/pharmaceutics14122721 (accessed on 28th June 2025).

Kho, Z. Y., & Lal, S. K. (2018). The human gut microbiome – A potential controller of wellness and disease. *Frontiers in Microbiology, 9*(AUG), 356589. https://doi.org/10.3389/FMICB.2018.01835/BIBTEX (accessed on 28th June 2025).

Kim, S., & Jazwinski, S. M. (2018). The gut microbiota and healthy aging: A mini-review. *Gerontology, 64*(6), 513–520. https://doi.org/10.1159/000490615 (accessed on 28th June 2025).

Klaenhammer, T. R., Kleerebezem, M., Kopp, M. V., & Rescigno, M. (2012). The impact of probiotics and prebiotics on the immune system. *Nature Reviews Immunology, 12*(10), 728–734. https://doi.org/10.1038/nri3312 (accessed on 28th June 2025).

Konieczna, P., Groeger, D., Ziegler, M., Frei, R., Ferstl, R., Shanahan, F., Quigley, E. M. M., Kiely, B., Akdis, C. A., & O'Mahony, L. (2012). *Bifidobacterium infantis* 35624 administration induces Foxp3 T regulatory cells in human peripheral blood: A potential role for myeloid and plasmacytoid dendritic cells. *Gut, 61*(3), 354–366. https://doi.org/10.1136/GUTJNL-2011-300936 (accessed on 28th June 2025).

Kostic, A. D., Chun, E., Robertson, L., Glickman, J. N., Gallini, C. A., Michaud, M., Clancy, T. E., Chung, D. C., Lochhead, P., Hold, G. L., El-Omar, E. M., Brenner, D., Fuchs, C. S., Meyerson, M., & Garrett, W. S. (2013). *Fusobacterium nucleatum* potentiates intestinal tumorigenesis and modulates the tumor-immune microenvironment. *Cell Host and Microbe, 14*(2), 207–215. https://doi.org/10.1016/j.chom.2013.07.007 (accessed on 28th June 2025).

Kostic, A. D., Gevers, D., Pedamallu, C. S., Michaud, M., Duke, F., Earl, A. M., Ojesina, A. I., Jung, J., Bass, A. J., Tabernero, J., Baselga, J., Liu, C., Shivdasani, R. A., Ogino, S., Birren, B. W., Huttenhower, C., Garrett, W. S., & Meyerson, M. (2012). Genomic analysis identifies the association of *Fusobacterium* with colorectal carcinoma. *Genome Research, 22*(2), 292–298. https://doi.org/10.1101/gr.126573.111 (accessed on 28th June 2025).

Kumar, M., Nguyen, T. P. N., Kaur, J., Singh, T. G., Soni, D., Singh, R., & Kumar, P. (2023). Opportunities and challenges in application of artificial intelligence in pharmacology. *Pharmacological Reports: PR, 75*(1), 3–18. https://doi.org/10.1007/s43440-022-00445-1 (accessed on 28th June 2025).

Li, R., Grimm, S. A., Chrysovergis, K., Kosak, J., Wang, X., Du, Y., Burkholder, A., Janardhan, K., Mav, D., Shah, R., Eling, T. E., & Wade, P. A. (2014). Obesity, rather than diet, drives epigenomics alterations in colonic epithelium resembling cancer progression. *Cell Metabolism, 19*(4), 702. https://doi.org/10.1016/J.CMET.2014.03.012 (accessed on 28th June 2025).

Li, T., Nakatsu, G., Chen, Y. X., Yau, T. O., Chu, E., Wong, S., Szeto, C. H., Ng, S. C., Chan, F. K. L., Fang, J. Y., Sung, J. J. Y., & Yu, J. (2020). A novel faecal *Lachnoclostridium* marker for the non-invasive diagnosis of colorectal adenoma and cancer. *Gut, 69*(7), 1248–1257. https://doi.org/10.1136/GUTJNL-2019-318532 (accessed on 28th June 2025).

Liang, S., Mao, Y., Liao, M., Xu, Y., Chen, Y., Huang, X., Wei, C., Wu, C., Wang, Q., Pan, X., & Tang, W. (2020). Gut microbiome associated with *APC* gene mutation in patients with intestinal adenomatous polyps. *International Journal of Biological Sciences, 16*(1), 135. https://doi.org/10.7150/IJBS.37399 (accessed on 28th June 2025).

Makki, K., Deehan, E. C., Walter, J., & Bäckhed, F. (2018). *Cell Host & Microbe*: The impact of dietary fiber on gut microbiota in host health and disease. https://doi.org/10.1016/j.chom.2018.05.012 (accessed on 28th June 2025).

Mannan, A., Dhiamn, S., Garg, N., & Singh, T. G. (2023). Pharmacological modulation of Sonic Hedgehog signaling pathways in angiogenesis: A mechanistic perspective.

Developmental Biology, 504, 58–74. https://doi.org/10.1016/j.ydbio.2023.09.009 (accessed on 28th June 2025).

Mannan, A., Kakkar, C., Dhiman, S., & Singh, T. G. (2023). Advancing the frontiers of adaptive cell therapy: A transformative mechanistic journey from preclinical to clinical settings. *International Immunopharmacology, 125*, 111095. https://doi.org/10.1016/j.intimp.2023.111095 (accessed on 28th June 2025).

Martin, Z., Spry, G., Hoult, J., Maimone, I. R., Tang, X., Crichton, M., & Marshall, S. (2022). What is the efficacy of dietary, nutraceutical, and probiotic interventions for managing symptoms of gastroesophageal reflux disease? A systematic literature review and meta-analysis. *Clinical Nutrition ESPEN, 52*, 340–352. https://doi.org/10.1016/J.CLNESP.2022.09.015 (accessed on 28th June 2025).

Matijašić, B. B., Obermajer, T., Lipoglavšek, L., Grabnar, I., Avguštin, G., & Rogelj, I. (2014). Association of dietary type with fecal microbiota in vegetarians and omnivores in Slovenia. *European Journal of Nutrition, 53*(4), 1051–1064. https://doi.org/10.1007/s00394-013-0607-6 (accessed on 28th June 2025).

Mehta, S., Nain, P., Agrawal, B. K., & Singh, R. P. (2022). Vitamin D with calcium supplementation managing glycemic control with HbA1c and improve quality of life in patients with diabetes. *Turkish Journal of Pharmaceutical Sciences, 19*(2), 161–167. https://doi.org/10.4274/tjps.galenos.2021.62357 (accessed on 28th June 2025).

Mehta, S., Nain, P., Agrawal, B. K., Singh, R. P., Kaur, J., Maity, S., Bhattacharjee, A., Peela, J., Nauhria, S., & Nauhria, S. (2021). Effectiveness of empagliflozin with vitamin D supplementation in peripheral neuropathy in type 2 diabetic patients. *Cureus, 13*(12), e20208. https://doi.org/10.7759/cureus.20208 (accessed on 28th June 2025).

Miller, L. E., Lehtoranta, L., & Lehtinen, M. J. (2017). The effect of *Bifidobacterium animalis* ssp. *lactis* HN019 on cellular immune function in healthy elderly subjects: Systematic review and meta-analysis. *Nutrients, 9*(3), 191. https://doi.org/10.3390/NU9030191 (accessed on 28th June 2025).

Mills, J. P., Rao, K., & Young, V. B. (2018). Probiotics for prevention of *Clostridium difficile* infection. *Current Opinion in Gastroenterology, 34*(1), 3. https://doi.org/10.1097/MOG.0000000000000410 (accessed on 28th June 2025).

Monteagudo-Mera, A., Rastall, R. A., Gibson, G. R., Charalampopoulos, D., & Chatzifragkou, A. (2019). Adhesion mechanisms mediated by probiotics and prebiotics and their potential impact on human health. *Applied Microbiology and Biotechnology, 103*(16), 6463–6472. https://doi.org/10.1007/S00253-019-09978-7 (accessed on 28th June 2025).

Nitter, M., Norgård, B., de Vogel, S., Eussen, S. J. P. M., Meyer, K., Ulvik, A., Ueland, P. M., Nygård, O., Vollset, S. E., Bjørge, T., Tjønneland, A., Hansen, L., Boutron-Ruault, M., Racine, A., Cottet, V., Kaaks, R., Kühn, T., Trichopoulou, A., Bamia, C., … Riboli, E. (2014). Plasma methionine, choline, betaine, and dimethylglycine about colorectal cancer risk in the European Prospective Investigation into Cancer and Nutrition (EPIC). *Annals of Oncology, 25*(8), 1609–1615. https://doi.org/10.1093/ANNONC/MDU185 (accessed on 28th June 2025).

Piewngam, P., Zheng, Y., Nguyen, T. H., Dickey, S. W., Joo, H. S., Villaruz, A. E., Glose, K. A., Fisher, E. L., Hunt, R. L., Li, B., Chiou, J., Pharkjaksu, S., Khongthong, S., Cheung, G. Y. C., Kiratisin, P., & Otto, M. (2018). Pathogen elimination by probiotic *Bacillus* via signalling interference. *Nature, 562*(7728), 532–537. https://doi.org/10.1038/s41586-018-0616-y (accessed on 28th June 2025).

Qin, Y., Roberts, J. D., Grimm, S. A., Lih, F. B., Deterding, L. J., Li, R., Chrysovergis, K., & Wade, P. A. (2018). An obesity-associated gut microbiome reprograms the intestinal epigenome, leading to altered colonic gene expression. *Genome Biology, 19*(1), 1–14. https://doi.org/10.1186/S13059-018-1389-1/FIGURES/6 (accessed on 28th June 2025).

Rakoff-Nahoum, S., Foster, K. R., & Comstock, L. E. (2016). The evolution of cooperation within the gut microbiota. *Nature, 533*(7602), 255–259. https://doi.org/10.1038/nature17626 (accessed on 28th June 2025).

Rocha-Ramírez, L. M., Pérez-Solano, R. A., Castañón-Alonso, S. L., Moreno Guerrero, S. S., Ramírez Pacheco, A., García Garibay, M., & Eslava, C. (2017). Probiotic *Lactobacillus* strains stimulate the inflammatory response and activate human macrophages. *Journal of Immunology Research, 2017*, Article 4607491. https://doi.org/10.1155/2017/4607491 (accessed on 28th June 2025).

Ruan, W., Engevik, M. A., Spinler, J. K., & Versalovic, J. (2020). Healthy human gastrointestinal microbiome: Composition and function after a decade of exploration. *Digestive Diseases and Sciences, 65*(3), 695–705. https://doi.org/10.1007/S10620-020-06118-4/METRICS (accessed on 28th June 2025).

Ruan, W., Engevik, M. A., Spinler, J. K., & Versalovic, J. (2020). Healthy human gastrointestinal microbiome: Composition and function after a decade of exploration. In *Digestive Diseases and Sciences, 65*(3), 695–705. https://doi.org/10.1007/s10620-020-06118-4 (accessed on 28th June 2025).

Sánchez Y Sánchez de la Barquera, B., Martínez Carrillo, B. E., Aguirre Garrido, J. F., Martínez Méndez, R., Benítez Arciniega, A. D., Valdés Ramos, R., & Soto Piña, A. E. (2022). Emerging evidence on the use of probiotics and prebiotics to improve the gut microbiota of older adults with frailty syndrome: A narrative review. *The Journal of Nutrition, Health & Aging, 26*(10), 926–935. https://doi.org/10.1007/s12603-022-1842-4 (accessed on 28th June 2025).

Schumacher, A., & Petronis, A. (2006). Epigenetics of complex diseases: From general theory to laboratory experiments. *Current Topics in Microbiology and Immunology, 310*, 81–115. https://doi.org/10.1007/3-540-31181-5_6/COVER (accessed on 28th June 2025).

Sepich-Poore, G. D., Zitvogel, L., Straussman, R., Hasty, J., Wargo, J. A., & Knight, R. (2021). The microbiome and human cancer. *Science, 371*(6536). https://doi.org/10.1126/science.abc4552 (accessed on 28th June 2025).

Sharma, A., Khan, H., Singh, T. G., Grewal, A. K., Najda, A., Kawecka-Radomska, M., Kamel, M., Altyar, A. E., & Abdel-Daim, M. M. (2021). Pharmacological modulation of ubiquitin-proteasome pathways in oncogenic signaling. *International Journal of Molecular Sciences, 22*(21), 11971. https://doi.org/10.3390/ijms222111971 (accessed on 28th June 2025).

Shock, T., Badang, L., Ferguson, B., & Martinez-Guryn, K. (2021). The interplay between diet, gut microbes, and host epigenetics in health and disease. In *Journal of Nutritional Biochemistry, 95*. https://doi.org/10.1016/j.jnutbio.2021.108631 (accessed on 28th June 2025).

Singh, M., Sharma, P., Singh, P. K., Singh, T. G., & Saini, B. (2020). Medicinal potential of heterocyclic compounds from diverse natural sources for the management of cancer.

Mini Reviews in Medicinal Chemistry, 20(11), 942–957. https://doi.org/10.2174/1389557520666200212104742 (accessed on 28th June 2025).

Son, Y. M., & Kim, J. (2022). The microbiome-immune axis therapeutic effects in cancer treatments. *Journal of Microbiology and Biotechnology, 32*(9), 1086–1097. https://doi.org/10.4014/jmb.2208.08002 (accessed on 28th June 2025).

Thapa, K., Khan, H., Kaur, G., Kumar, P., & Singh, T. G. (2023). Therapeutic targeting of angiopoietins in tumor angiogenesis and cancer development. *Biochemical and Biophysical Research Communications, 687*, 149130. https://doi.org/10.1016/j.bbrc.2023.149130 (accessed on 28th June 2025).

Thapa, K., Khan, H., Sharma, U., Grewal, A. K., & Singh, T. G. (2021). Poly (ADP-ribose) polymerase-1 as a promising drug target for neurodegenerative diseases. *Life Sciences, 267*, 118975. https://doi.org/10.1016/j.lfs.2020.118975 (accessed on 28th June 2025).

Tomkovich, S., Yang, Y., Winglee, K., Gauthier, J., Mühlbauer, M., Sun, X., Mohamadzadeh, M., Liu, X., Martin, P., Wang, G. P., Oswald, E., Fodor, A. A., & Jobin, C. (2017). Locoregional effects of microbiota in a preclinical model of colon carcinogenesis. *Cancer Research, 77*(10), 2620–2632. https://doi.org/10.1158/0008-5472.CAN-16-3472 (accessed on 28th June 2025).

Tong, L. C., Wang, Y., Wang, Z. B., Liu, W. Y., Sun, S., Li, L., Su, D. F., & Zhang, L. C. (2016). Propionate ameliorates dextran sodium sulphate-induced colitis by improving intestinal barrier function and reducing inflammation and oxidative stress. *Frontiers in Pharmacology, 7*(AUG), Article 202262. https://doi.org/10.3389/FPHAR.2016.00253/BIBTEX (accessed on 28th June 2025).

Tsai, Y. L., Lin, T. L., Chang, C. J., Wu, T. R., Lai, W. F., Lu, C. C., & Lai, H. C. (2019). Probiotics, prebiotics and amelioration of diseases. *Journal of Biomedical Science, 26*(1), 1–8. https://doi.org/10.1186/S12929-018-0493-6/METRICS (accessed on 28th June 2025).

Wang, J., Zhang, C., Guo, C., & Li, X. (2019). Chitosan ameliorates DSS-induced ulcerative colitis mice by enhancing intestinal barrier function and improving microflora. *International Journal of Molecular Sciences, 20*(22), 5751. https://doi.org/10.3390/IJMS20225751 (accessed on 28th June 2025).

Wang, L., Cao, H., Liu, L., Wang, B., Walker, W. A., Acra, S. A., & Yan, F. (2014). The epidermal growth factor receptor activation mediates mucin production stimulated by p40, a *Lactobacillus rhamnosus* GG-derived protein. *Journal of Biological Chemistry, 289*(29), 20234–20244. https://doi.org/10.1074/jbc.M114.553800 (accessed on 28th June 2025).

Wang, Q., Yu, C., Yue, C., & Liu, X. (2020). *Fusobacterium nucleatum* produces cancer stem cell characteristics via EMT-resembling variations. *International Journal of Clinical and Experimental Pathology, 13*(7), 1819–1828. (accessed on 28th June 2025).

Watari, J., Ito, C., Shimoda, T., Tomita, T., Oshima, T., Fukui, H., Das, K. M., & Miwa, H. (2019). DNA methylation silencing of microRNA gene methylator in the precancerous background mucosa with and without gastric cancer: Analysis of the effects of *H. pylori* eradication and long-term aspirin use. *Scientific Reports, 9*(1), 1–10. https://doi.org/10.1038/s41598-019-49069-1 (accessed on 28th June 2025).

Weersma, R. K., Zhernakova, A., & Fu, J. (2020). Interaction between drugs and the gut microbiome. *Gut, 69*(8), 1510–1519. https://doi.org/10.1136/gutjnl-2019-320204 (accessed on 28th June 2025).

Wei, Z., Cao, S., Liu, S., Yao, Z., Sun, T., Li, Y., Li, J., Zhang, D., & Zhou, Y. (2016). Could gut microbiota be a prognostic biomarker associated with colorectal cancer patients' survival? A pilot study on relevant mechanisms. *Oncotarget, 7*(29), 46158. https://doi.org/10.18632/ONCOTARGET.10064 (accessed on 28th June 2025).

Wilson, M. R., Jiang, Y., Villalta, P. W., Stornetta, A., Boudreau, P. D., Carrá, A., Brennan, C. A., Chun, E., Ngo, L., Samson, L. D., Engelward, B. P., Garrett, W. S., Balbo, S., & Balskus, E. P. (2019). The human gut bacterial genotoxin colibactin alkylates DNA. *Science (New York, N.Y.), 363*(6428), eaar7785. https://doi.org/10.1126/science.aar7785 (accessed on 28th June 2025).

Wirbel, J., Pyl, P. T., Kartal, E., Zych, K., Kashani, A., Milanese, A., Fleck, J. S., Voigt, A. Y., Palleja, A., Ponnudurai, R., Sunagawa, S., Coelho, L. P., Schrotz-King, P., Vogtmann, E., Habermann, N., Niméus, E., Thomas, A. M., Manghi, P., Gandini, S., … Zeller, G. (2019). Meta-analysis of fecal metagenomes reveals global microbial signatures that are specific for colorectal cancer. *Nature Medicine, 25*(4), 679–689. https://doi.org/10.1038/s41591-019-0406-6 (accessed on 28th June 2025).

Wu, S., Rhee, K. J., Albesiano, E., Rabizadeh, S., Wu, X., Yen, H. R., Huso, D. L., Brancati, F. L., Wick, E., McAllister, F., Housseau, F., Pardoll, D. M., & Sears, C. L. (2009). A human colonic commensal promotes colon tumorigenesis via activation of T helper type 17 T cell responses. *Nature Medicine, 15*(9), 1016–1022. https://doi.org/10.1038/nm.2015 (accessed on 28th June 2025).

Yang, Y., Misra, B. B., Liang, L., Bi, D., Weng, W., Wu, W., Cai, S., Qin, H., Goel, A., Li, X., & Ma, Y. (2019). Integrated microbiome and metabolome analysis reveal a novel interplay between commensal bacteria and metabolites in colorectal cancer. *Theranostics, 9*(14), 4101. https://doi.org/10.7150/THNO.35186 (accessed on 28th June 2025).

Ye, J., Wu, W., Li, Y., & Li, L. (2017). Influences of the gut microbiota on DNA methylation and histone modification. *Digestive Diseases and Sciences, 62*(5), 1155–1164. https://doi.org/10.1007/S10620-017-4538-6 (accessed on 28th June 2025).

Zackular, J. P., Baxter, N. T., Chen, G. Y., & Schloss, P. D. (2016). Manipulation of the gut microbiota reveals role in colon tumorigenesis. *mSphere, 1*(1). https://doi.org/10.1128/MSPHERE.00001-15/ASSET/701E2E68-C14B-4046-8D43-60B866B50118/ASSETS/GRAPHIC/SPH0011600090005.JPEG (accessed on 28th June 2025).

Zmora, N., Suez, J., & Elinav, E. (2018). You are what you eat: Diet, health and the gut microbiota. *Nature Reviews Gastroenterology & Hepatology, 16*(1), 35–56. https://doi.org/10.1038/s41575-018-0061-2 (accessed on 28th June 2025).

Zmora, N., Suez, J., & Elinav, E. (2019). You are what you eat: Diet, health and the gut microbiota. *Nature Reviews. Gastroenterology & Hepatology, 16*(1), 35–56. https://doi.org/10.1038/s41575-018-0061-2 (accessed on 28th June 2025).

CHAPTER 8

Impact of Diet on Gut Microbiome and Metabolic Disorders

RAJWINDER KAUR,[1] RUPINDER KAUR,[1,*] SAPNA AHUJA,[1] UJJWAL KAUSHIK,[1] BALAKUMAR CHANDRASEKARAN,[2] THAKUR GURJEET SINGH,[1] and SANJANA MEHTA[1]

[1]*Chitkara College of Pharmacy, Chitkara University, Punjab, India*

[2]*Faculty of Pharmacy, Philadelphia University, Amman, Jordan*

*Corresponding author

ABSTRACT

Metabolic diseases, including obesity and type 2 diabetes mellitus, impose an alarming health concern due to the proceeding high prevalence of morbidity and mortality. Recent research indicates the role of the human gut microbiome and diet in initiating or remission of metabolic disorders. Diet is the most crucial factor that governs these pathological conditions through its impact on the gut microbiome, as it is a significant factor in maintaining the homeostasis of host metabolism processes. The millions of microorganisms living in the human gut are influenced by long-term food consumption. The microbiome can be more readily modified by diet, which may impact human physiological functions by interaction with the host's metabolic processes, further changing the mucosal immune response, absorption, and digestion and leading to metabolic diseases. A diet packed with fat and sugar causes insulin resistance, low-grade inflammation, and dyslipidemia; however, on the contrary, a diet abundant in fiber has been demonstrated to reduce inflammation, boost insulin sensitivity, and lower dyslipidemias. Thus, feeding an unhealthy diet might cause modifications in the gut microbiome makeup and lead to the pathophysiology

Precision Nutrition and Endocrine Health: Synthesis, Characterization, and Applications.
Thakur Gurjeet Singh and Sanjana Mehta (Eds.)

DOI: 10.1201/9781998511877-8

of metabolic syndrome/disorders by rupturing the intestinal barrier and inducing low-grade systemic inflammation. Maintaining a balanced diet can alter the microbiome, improve gut barrier physiology, and promote the generation of anti-inflammatory substances. Consequently, diet could potentially be beneficial in regulating the host's physiology and treating several metabolic ailments. While diet modifies the constitution and activity of the gut microbiome, the gut microbiome can also modulate the dietary metabolites in beneficial or harmful ways to the human host's metabolic processes. To improve human health, a deeper understanding of these interactions could prove helpful in suggesting individualized dietary programs and nutrition-based therapeutic approaches. The current book chapter focuses on the complex interactions among diet, gut microbiome, and various physiological mechanisms that affect the development of metabolic processes/disorders that might hold the potential as a therapeutic approach for various metabolic disorders.

8.1 INTRODUCTION

Metabolic disorders are metabolic syndromes that combine physiological, biochemical, and clinical variables, including insulin resistance, endothelial dysfunction, dyslipidemia, visceral fat accumulation, and so forth (Bhargava et al., 2022; Singh et al., 2022; Wang et al., 2023). Consuming more-calorie substances in diet and substituting sedentary activities during leisure time has contributed to a positive energy balance in recent decades. This imbalance is characterized by excess energy consumption over energy utilization; it is now the primary risk factor for obesity and its associated complications (Heymsfield and Wadden, 2017). Lipids leak into the bloodstream in this scenario because the adipose tissue cannot hold all the extra energy as triglycerides. Ectopic fat accumulation is caused by the overabundance of lipids supplemented to non-adipose tissues, which lack the metabolic flexibility necessary to enhance fat oxidation in response to elevated fatty acid supply (Wu et al., 2021). Adipocytes that have accumulated too much fat produce and secrete more proinflammatory adipokines, developing insulin resistance and the subsequent onset of Type 2 Diabetes Mellitus (T2DM) and Non-Alcoholic Fatty Liver Disease (NAFLD) (Bhargava et al., 2022; Reilly and Saltiel, 2017).

Over time, more emphasis has been placed on the possible role of the gut microbiome in developing several health complications.

Specifically, gut microbiota has been targeted as a vital player in the emergence of numerous metabolic diseases, namely obesity, T2DM, and NAFDL (Ekta et al., 2020; Wu et al., 2021).

The current worldwide obesity epidemic is associated with a shift in lifestyle that emphasizes low physical activity and increased caloric intake. Obesity brought on by a Western diet alters gut microbiome makeup; for example, the Mollicutes class of Firmicutes has considerably risen (Turnbaugh et al., 2008). Recently, the focus on the gut microbiome's potential role as a mechanism underlying obesity and its associated comorbidities has been enhanced. The ability of gut microbiota to transform food into human nutrition and the increased capacity of the gut microbiome linked to obesity to obtain energy from the diet makes it an essential interface for energy acquisition (Wu et al., 2021). The phylum Bacteroidetes is more prevalent in NAFLD patients, whereas the abundance of Firmicutes, producing short-chain fatty acids (SCFAs) and dehydroxylate seven alpha, is much lower (Da Silva et al., 2018; Wang et al., 2016).

Dietary macronutrients power the human gut microbiome, which generates bioactive substances such as bile acids, ammonia, phenols, SCFAs, and endotoxins generated from the microbiota function as mediators of microbe-host communication, which is critical for preserving host physiology. Metabolite profiles linked to the gut flora offer more information on how diet and lifestyle choices affect illness. Metagenomics, metaproteomic, and metabolomics are just a few of the many meta-omics techniques that have come to knowledge to study the role of metabolites originating from microbiota. (Vernocchi et al., 2016).

8.2 METABOLIC DISORDERS

8.2.1 DIABETES

DM is a metabolic disorder with hyperglycemia as its hallmark characteristic, a physiologically aberrant state marked by persistently increased blood glucose levels. Metabolic dysfunctions of carbohydrates, lipids, and proteins can be the chronic and heterogeneous manifestation of hyperglycemia, which is caused by defects in either insulin secretion, insulin action, or both (Garg et al., 2021; Kaur et al., 2023).

The metabolic irregularities of fats and carbohydrates assisting in hyperglycemia distress the normal physiology of several human systems. The disturbances above develop moderately and are primarily due to the detrimental impact of hyperglycemia and the related metabolic disorders on the typical configuration and operation of the micro- and microvasculature, which are fundamental to the structure and functionality of all organs in the body. Microvascular and macrovascular problems are caused by structural and physiological anomalies in the vasculature, leading to harmful effects on the kidneys, eyes, heart, and nerves. They are distinguished by damage to organs, progressively leading to organ failure. Eye-associated problems give rise to retinopathy, which can lead to blindness. Kidney-related issues can result in nephropathy, further leading to the progression of kidney failure. Heart-related complaints comprise an increase in blood pressure (hypertension) and coronary artery disease. Nerve-linked issues cause neuropathy, which can cause alterations in the peripheral and autonomic nervous system (Banday et al., 2020; Najar et al., 2022). Atherosclerotic cardiovascular disease (CVD) is a prevalent condition in people with diabetes and is one of the major etiological factors of morbidity and death related to the disease (Devi et al., 2023; Sharma and Singh, 2020). Table 8.1 classifies the types of diabetes.

TABLE 8.1 Types of Diabetes

Classification	Definition	References
Type 1 Diabetes	It is an autoimmune illness mediated by T cells; death of pancreatic beta-cells results in insufficient insulin, which in turn produces hyperglycemia and a predisposition to ketoacidosis.	Kahanovitz et al. (2017)
	Exogenous insulin injections must be administered daily to control elevated blood glucose levels.	
Type 2 Diabetes	Persistent hyperglycemia is the hallmark of this chronic metabolic illness, which is caused by decreased insulin secretion, resistance to insulin's peripheral effects, or both.	Zheng et al. (2018)
Gestational Diabetes	Glucose intolerance that is developed or initially identified during pregnancy is known as gestational diabetes.	Coustan (2013)
	It falls into the A1GDM and A2GDM categories.	
	Diabetes treated with A1GDM responds well to dietary therapy and is not medication-controlled. Conversely, A2GDM is gestational diabetes treated with medication to attain appropriate glycemic control.	
Other Types	Hormonal imbalances, genetic defects, drugs, infections, etc. characterize different types of diabetes.	Banday et al. (2020)

8.2.2 OBESITY

Obesity is a long-term illness with enhanced buildup of body fat as its hallmark feature. Obesity is generally defined by a body mass index (BMI), computed as the weight in kilograms divided by the square of the height in meters (kg/m^2) (Singh et al., 2020; Ward et al., 2019). Table 8.2 describes the classification of obesity-based BMI as per WHO. According to the World Health Organization (WHO), obesity on the basis of BMI can be classified as in Table 8.2

TABLE 8.2 Classification of Obesity based on Body Mass Index (BMI) according to the World Health Organization (WHO)

Body Mass Index	Persisting Condition
< 25 kg/m^2	Underweight or normal weight
= 25 to <30 kg/m^2	Overweight
= 30 to <35 kg/m^2	Moderate Obesity
> 35 kg/m^2	Severe Obesity

Numerous genetic and environmental factors, including sex, race, physical activity, food, overnutrition and socioeconomic position, influence the occurrence of obesity (Hales et al., 2018). Furthermore, obesity is linked to social and personal factors such as marital status and present economic situation. (Asahara et al., 2020). The start and progression of obesity are attributed to many genes such as encoding leptin, melanocortin four receptor, proprotein convertase subtilisin/kexin type 1, proopiomelanocortin, kinase suppressor of RAS 2, and others (Loos and Yeo, 2022). Numerous other metabolic problems, such as T2D, NAFLD, CVD, chronic renal diseases, and malignancies, are frequently linked to obesity. Aside from adipose tissues, obesity's other difficulties include vascular epithelial cell malfunction and lipid buildup in other organs (Yang et al., 2022).

8.2.3 METABOLIC SYNDROME

Metabolic syndrome is a combination of metabolic disorders such as insulin resistance, obesity, atherogenic dyslipidemia, and increased blood pressure. The exponential rise in obesity cases worldwide in recent years has made metabolic syndrome increasingly relevant. Early diagnosis is crucial to properly implementing lifestyle and risk factor modification. Metformin, statins, and antihypertensives are a few examples of the medications used in pharmaceutical therapy for metabolic syndrome (Goyal et al., 2022; Soiza et al., 2018).

8.3 GUT MICROBIOME AND METABOLIC DISORDERS

8.3.1 GUT MICROBIOME

The gastrointestinal tract (GIT) of humans is one of the most significant interfaces (250–400 m^2) in the human system between the host, ambient variables, and antigens. The group of bacteria, archaea, and eukarya that inhabit the GIT system is known as the "gut microbiota." (Thursby and Juge, 2017). Gut bacteria support the host's digestive defenses and aid in the gut's regular operations. Numerous processes carried out by gut bacteria help the host, including controlling gut motility, generating vitamins, changing bile acid and steroids, breaking down xenobiotics, absorbing minerals, and activating and eliminating toxins, genotoxins, and mutagens (Macfarlane et al., 2009). For natural substances, such as lignans, gut bacteria are necessary to carry out their bioactivities (Zhang et al., 2015). The human gut contains a diversified microbiota population, and its symbiotic interaction with the host facilitates the digestion and metabolism of food components (Goldsmith and Sartor, 2014).

8.3.1.1 CARBOHYDRATE METABOLISM

Carbohydrates and simple sugars are rich in diet and serve as substrates for the metabolism of bacteria in the human stomach. In healthy people, the amount of carbohydrates consumed affects how the human microbiota is used and functions. The proportion of bacteria in the phylum Bacteroidetes increases when diets high in carbohydrates are consumed; many of these bacteria have an increased number of genes encoding for carbohydrate-active enzymes (glycosyltransferases, polysaccharide lyases, glycoside hydrolases) (Andoh, 2016). Regarding phylum Bacteroidetes, people who feed diets abundant in plant carbohydrates contain more significant *Prevotella* species. However, those who ingest animal fat and protein have more significant percentages of the Bacteroides species. Therefore, the metabolism of dietary carbohydrates primarily depends on the gut bacteria rather than the genetic material of humans. The gut microbiota's various roles in the metabolism of different meals may offer methods for dietary adjustments and microbiome functional enhancement (Wu et al., 2011).

8.3.1.2 GENERATION OF SHORT-CHAIN FATTY ACIDS

Anaerobic bacteria convert indigestible carbohydrates or resistant starch to SCFAs through fermentation. The phyla Firmicutes and Bacteroidetes work together in species specialized in oligosaccharide fermentation to generate SCFAs from indigestible carbohydrates in the small intestine. (e.g., *Bifidobacteria*) (Andoh, 2016). Mainly in acetate, propionate, and butyrate, SCFAs make up around two-thirds of colonic anion content. SCFAs, especially butyrate, are thought to account for 10% of the energy that individuals obtain from their food and are an essential source of colonic epithelial cells. Acetate is a substrate for lipogenesis and gluconeogenesis, whereas butyrate and propionate can control immunological response and intestinal physiology (Ashique et al., 2022; Macfarlane and Macfarlane, 2011). Most fermentation takes place in the proximal colon. However, because carbohydrates are used in the distal colon, gut microbiota utilizes different substrates (such as protein or amino acids). Therefore, the proximal colon, where fermentation is highest, has a lower colonic pH (pH5.5–6.5) than the distal colon (pH 6.5–7.0) (Simpson and Campbell, 2015). Various potentially dangerous substances, including ammonia, phenols, certain amines, and hydrogen sulphide, are produced when amino acids ferment. Certain substances could have a role in digestive disorders, including colon cancer or intestinal bowel illness (Andoh, 2016).

8.3.2 ROLE IN METABOLIC DISORDERS

8.3.2.1 OBESITY

Chronic disorders such as metabolic syndrome, T2DM, CVD, dyslipidemia, sudden death, osteoarthritis, and other conditions are more likely to occur in obese people due to the variations in energy consumption and utilization, resulting in an energy imbalance (Kobyliak et al., 2016).

The literature has demonstrated that obesity and its complications are associated with variations in the intestinal microbiota (Al-Assal et al., 2018). In particular, extended exposure to a high-fat diet is directly linked to a drop in *Bacteroides* and a rise in *Bacillaeceae, Clostridiaceae,* and other representatives of the *Firmicutes* phylum in the stomach of obese individuals. It is thought that this changed microbial makeup causes the synthesis of energy and calories from the undigested food to be upregulated, which modifies metabolic homeostasis (Pascale et al., 2018).

8.3.2.2 DIABETES

In a study comparing individuals with diabetes to those without the disease, it was found that there were significantly fewer *Firmicutes* and more *Bacteroidetes* and *Proteobacteria.* Consequently, there was a strong and positive correlation between decreased glucose tolerance and the ratios of *Bacteroidetes* to *Firmicutes* (Ríos-Covián et al., 2016). Metabolic disturbances linked to increased insulin resistance are caused by an elevation in acetate synthesis and a concurrent decrease in concentration (Gao et al., 2009; Care and Suppl, 2020). Furthermore, a distinct protective effect concerning T2D was noted in the instance of a particular bacteria, *Akkermansia muciniphila,* which has been demonstrated to diminish persistent subclinical inflammation and enhance insulin sensitivity (Duparc et al., 2017).

8.4 IMPACT OF DIETARY COMPONENTS ON GUT MICROBIOME

Diet is one of the main factors influencing an individual's microbial profile in humans, but age, exercise, and antibiotic use are also significant concerns (Cronin et al., 2021). The host benefits from several advantageous characteristics the gut microbiota provides because of its extensive genetic content and Metabolic complement. Among these bacteria' most significant functions are their assistance in preserving the mucosal barrier's integrity, their supply of nutrients, including vitamins, and their defense against infections. Furthermore, the connection between the mucosal immune system plays an integral part in working appropriate immune function (Thursby and Juge, 2017).

Because colonic bacteria produce active enzymes on carbohydrates, they can ferment complex carbs and produce metabolites like SCFAs (Musso et al., 2010). The most prevalent SCFAs in the colon are acetate, propionate, and butyrate, with a molar ratio of 3:1:1. Saturated carboxylic acids have a chain of one to six carbons (Caetano and Castelucci, 2022). The GI tract's epithelial cells quickly absorb these SCFAs, which signify a role in controlling various biological processes, namely gene expression, chemotaxis, differentiation, proliferation, and cell death (Corrêa-Oliveira et al., 2016).

8.4.1 MICROBIOTA HOST SIGNALING BY VARIOUS MECHANISMS

The host immune system and the gut microbiome interact from birth. The immune system develops in response to microbiota, and the microbiota, in turn, influences the immune system. Numerous signaling pathways involving numerous chemicals beyond the immune system communicate this cross-talk between the microorganisms and the host immune system. Various immune-mediated signaling pathways affect the gut, liver, muscles, and brain, among other organs, in addition to direct chemical interactions between the pathogen and host. These intricate relationships form a host-microbe metabolic axis (Schroeder and Bäckhed, 2016).

The host-microbe metabolic axis connects microbial species, sub-ecologies, and activities with specific host cellular pathways. It is an interactive, multidirectional chemical communication system. Multiple bacterial genomes can progressively modify metabolic pathways along these metabolic axes, leading to combinatorial metabolism of substrates by microbiome and host genome, as demonstrated by the synthesis of choline, SCFAs, and bile acids (Fischbach and Segre, 2016).

Mammals possess limited in-built capacity to digest polysaccharides but may absorb simple sugars in the small intestine. As a result, all undigested materials serve as the primary substrate for the growth and maintenance of the intestinal flora, which is the colon's primary energy source. This causes the host to extract energy and absorbable substrates and provides the resident bacterial species with energy and nutrients to multiply. The genetic and species diversity of the microbiota offers unique metabolic, biochemical, and enzymatic pathways associated with the hosts. Therefore, the microbiome is an active metabolic organ (Aoun et al., 2020).

8.4.2 SCFAS

Gut bacteria ferment indigestible food ingredients (soluble dietary fibers and prebiotics). Consuming prebiotics can cause microorganisms to produce SCFAs, with acetate, butyrate, and propionate being the primary end products. The metabolic products produced become a primary means of enabling prebiotics to have advantageous impacts on health (Blaak et al., 2020). The health benefits of elevated microbial SCFA production are enhanced gut barrier performance and decreased intestinal inflammation. Furthermore, SCFA may impact the motility and transit of the GIT. In addition to its impacts on digestive health, SCFA may influence the control of body weight through reaction to insulin sensitivity, energy intake, expenditure, and contribution to the pathophysiology of obesity and related disorders, including T2DM (Canfora et al., 2015; Ríos-Covián et al., 2016).

8.4.2.1 METABOLISM OF SCFAS

Anaerobic conditions in the proximal colon facilitate carbohydrate fermentation. Carbohydrates undergo microbial hydrolysis to become monosaccharides, which ferment via the Embden-Meyerhof pathway to produce phosphoenolpyruvate. Subsequently, the SCFA is produced via the phosphoenolpyruvate intermediate in various processes (Reichardt et al., 2014; Xiong et al., 2022).

8.4.3 ROLE OF PREBIOTICS AND PROBIOTICS

Prebiotics are typically indigestible food elements that explicitly enhance the growth and activity of specific bacterial strains in the digestive tract, whereas probiotics are a variety of beneficial microorganisms (da Silva et al., 2021). Probiotics and prebiotics have generally demonstrated alleviating effects on obesity, T2D, and other metabolic illnesses, as per the findings of experimental research and clinical trials; however, the situation may not be apparent for pregnant patients (Huang et al., 2021). Probiotics have been said to enhance specific metabolic markers and help with weight loss (Koutnikova et al., 2019; Wang et al., 2019).

8.4.3.1 IN OBESITY

Previous research has demonstrated a favorable link between eating habits and the human gut microbiota since dietary modifications can modify the microbiota's diversity and composition. Temporary dietary modifications have the potential to alter gut flora and may represent a viable therapy option for obesity (Al-Assal et al., 2018; John et al., 2018).

Gut microbiota and obesity are interlinked, and probiotic strains like *Lactobacillus pentosus* GSSK2 and *Lactobacillus plantarum* GS26A can help reduce obesity (Khanna et al., 2020). Probiotic use has been demonstrated to lower BMI and visceral fat. A clinical trial involving 20 healthy male participants fed a high-fat diet for four weeks revealed that probiotics avoided increased body weight and fat (Osterberg et al., 2015). A meta-analysis was done to investigate the impact of probiotics on body weight and glycemic control in individuals who are overweight or obese. Compared to adults in the control group, those who took probiotics experienced significant decreases in their body weight, BMI, waist circumference, and fat mass percentage. When probiotics were taken at higher dosages and lower ones, (1) there was a noticeable decrease in body fat; (2) probiotics with one strain as opposed to several strains; and (3) probiotics were given as food instead of as pills or powders.

8.4.3.1.1 Mechanism

- **Probiotics:** Probiotic supplementation may enhance the number of bacteria that make SCFA, reduce the number of LPS producers, and lessen the organic inflammation and tissue loss brought on by LPS. Probiotics also reduce opportunistic infections and their metabolites. Additionally, probiotics may lessen insulin resistance, inflammation, and fat storage (Sivamaruthi et al., 2019; Wang et al., 2019).
- **Prebiotics:** The prebiotic supplements that have been examined the most in recent studies include inulin, fructooligosaccharides, and galactooligosaccharides (Wiese et al., 2019). Fermentable carbohydrate inulin can enhance the treatment of obesity by decreasing food intake by 87%, as demonstrated by its capacity to raise cell density, making the hormone PYY, which lowers

hunger (Brooks et al., 2017). Giving GOS supplements to healthy people increases the amount of *Bifidobacterium* spp. and decreases the amount of *Bacteroides*. Subsequent research on prebiotics has revealed that these substances facilitate modifications in the makeup and functionality of the gut microbiome. Prebiotics improve metabolic results and the gut barrier's ability to fend off infections by increasing the amount of *Bifidobacterium* species and other butyrate makers (Beserra et al., 2015).

8.4.3.2 DIABETES

When diabetic rats were given *Bifidobacterium* probiotics for a month, their glucose metabolism returned to normal. This was demonstrated by an increase in the glucose turnover rate, a reduction in fasting insulin levels, and a decrease in glucose surges on the intraperitoneal glucose tolerance test. *Lactobacillus gasseri* probiotic given orally twice daily for 12 weeks significantly reduced fasting and postprandial glucose levels in a hereditary mouse model of T2D (Jayesh Shah and Swami, 2017).

Patients with T2D, particularly those not responding to traditional treatment, benefited from fermented foods like yoghurt. Prebiotic foods like *Lactobacillus plantarum*-fermented *Momordica charantia* juice possess anti-diabetic effects. Additionally, as managing gut metabolites is frequently involved in treating T2D, postbiotics may offer an alternate therapeutic option to probiotics, prebiotics, and fecal microbiota transplants (FMT) (Li et al., 2021).

8.4.4 DIETARY FIBERS

One of the planet's most intricate ecosystems is the human GIT, where various microorganisms coexist in a complex and evolving relationship over time. Particularly in developed countries, the rise of the low-fiber Western diet is linked to a higher prevalence of certain metabolic disease conditions. FMT is one of many techniques being investigated to modify the GIT's current microbial populations to provide health advantages and disease prevention tactics. Dietary fiber intervention is a further strategy for altering the microbiota and achieving better health outcomes. Fiber's significant contributions to the control of metabolism and the avoidance of chronic GI disorders have long been recognized (Cronin et al., 2021).

Dietary fiber comprises carbohydrates derived from plants indigestible to digestive enzymes encoded in the human genome, such as amylase. As an alternative, fiber can be digested through anaerobic fermentation by specific gut microbiota species, with SCFAs being the predominant byproduct (De Menezes et al., 2013).

Research has indicated that dietary fibers, specifically beta-glucans, might be advantageous in treating and preventing metabolic syndrome, T2D, obesity, and CVD. Numerous studies have shown that supplementing with beta-glucan lowers triglycerides and cholesterol in people (Bozbulut and Sanlier, 2019).

8.4.5 MICRONUTRIENTS AND MACRONUTRIENTS

8.4.5.1 MICRONUTRIENTS

- **Polyphenols:** Polyphenols from fruits, vegetables, cereals, tea, coffee, and wine, including flavonoids, phenolic acids, stilbenes, and lignans, have garnered attention in studies because of their possible anti-oxidative, anti-inflammatory, and anti-carcinogenic properties. In animal and clinical trials, polyphenols have been shown to affect microbial diversity, gut microorganisms, and the Firmicutes to Bacteroidetes (F/B) ratio. According to these and other research, polyphenols' prebiotic-like properties are primarily responsible for the health advantages they provide for people (Yang et al., 2020).
- **Vitamins:** Organic substances known as vitamins are necessary in tiny quantities to maintain their physiological role. They frequently perform several functions in the system, the most significant of which is acting as enzyme cofactors. Since our bodies cannot produce enough specific vitamins to meet our daily needs, diet is the primary source of these nutrients. However, the gut bacteria make other vitamins, such as K and B group vitamins. It is typical for patients to take one or more vitamin supplements that can deliver very high dosages of specific vitamins to address or worsen chronic health issues caused by vitamin deficiencies.

As a result, the upper gut's low absorption of these vitamins can impact the diversity and quantity of the gut microbiota (Yang et al., 2020)

- **Minerals and Trace Elements:** Minerals and trace elements are vital micronutrients for human metabolism and are also actively linked to the gut microbiota. Numerous human disorders are caused by an excess of trace elements and a dietary deficit. Examples are calcium, magnesium, iron, phosphorus, and zincsium, iron, phosphorus, zinc, etc.

The body's second-most prevalent inorganic element, phosphorus, is crucial for preserving the blood's systemic acid balance. Adults should ingest 700–1000 mg of phosphorus daily, although processed foods like baked goods and beverages with added sugar frequently cause excessive intake. Human dietary intervention research using a 1000 mg/day phosphorus supplement revealed improved fecal bacteria diversity and increased SCFA concentration (Yang et al., 2020).

Zinc is a necessary micronutrient that may help to preserve the epithelial cells' integrity by influencing the gut flora (Ohashi and Fukada, 2019). When broiler chickens suffer from a chronic zinc deficit, their gut microbiome is altered, leading to a notable rise in Proteobacteria and a fall in Firmicutes (Reed et al., 2015). According to animal research, adding 120 mg/kg of zinc to a "Salmonella typhimurium-challenged broiler" model increased *Lactobacillus* sp. It decreased the amount of *Salmonella* sp. and other harmful bacteria (Shao et al., 2014). Epidemiological research links a reduced prevalence of obesity to a high calcium intake. It states that a high calcium diet alters the gut flora in ways linked to a lean phenotype (Yang et al., 2020).

8.4.5.2 MACRONUTRIENTS

8.4.5.2.1 Carbohydrates

The body primarily uses carbohydrates as fuel, which remarkably affects how the gut microbiota is shaped and altered. Plant-based carbohydrates that do not break down in the upper GIT are categorized as dietary fiber. Composition affects how much the extensive intestinal microorganisms ferment them, in addition to other nutrients that remain undigested.

It has been mentioned in animal studies that the Western-style diet, which has comparatively lower fiber content, decreases the variety of the gut microbiota and the abundance of *Bifidobacterium* (Schroeder et al., 2018). Long-term ingestion of low-fiber diets may decrease the variety of gut bacteria (Yang et al., 2020).

Prebiotics, such as arabinoxylans (AX), arabinoxylan-oligosaccharides (AXOS), and xylo-oligosaccharides (XOS), are frequently present in wheat and are primarily known to enhance the population of beneficial bacteria, such as *Lactobacillus* and *Bifidobacterium*. In a dietary intervention, persons with metabolic syndrome who consumed an AX-enriched diet had elevated levels of *Bifidobacterium* sp. and reduced levels of microbial diversity. Enzymatic hydrolysis of AX may yield AXOS, composed of arabinoxylooligosaccharides and XOS. In healthy adults and children, it has been demonstrated that AXOS and XOS promote *Bifidobacterium* sp. and *Lactobacillus* sp. (Q. Yang et al., 2020).

8.4.5.2.2 Fat

A diet heavy in saturated and total fat negatively impacts gut microbiota. In 15 clinical reports (six randomised controlled interventional trials and nine observational studies), diets high in total and saturated fat were demonstrated to have a detrimental influence on the diversity and richness of gut microbiota (Wolters et al., 2019).

A recent randomized controlled-feeding clinical trial found that young adults in good health who consumed 40% fat were connected to unfavorable changes in their gut microbiota. Specifically, the intervention reduced the number of beneficial bacteria from the genus *Fecalibacterium*. It enhanced the number of harmful *Bacteroides* and *Alistipes* species, which are known to be prevalent in T2DM patients. On the other hand, 20% of fat consumption increased the amount of *Fecalibacterium* sp. and *Blautia* sp. in the gut microbiota. Restoring the gut microbiome in patients with metabolic illness and coronary heart disease required cutting their fat intake to less than 35% for two years. Since no change was shown in individuals not diagnosed with metabolic disorders, the study's findings revealed that the effectiveness of low-fat diet interventions on people relied on their level of metabolic dysfunction (Wan et al., 2019).

8.5 DIET-GUT MICROBIOME-METABOLIC DISORDER TRIADE

The function of the gut microbiome and its impact on human health is gaining attention, particularly in light of metabolic disorders that raise cardiovascular events and, consequently, the mortality impact in developed nations.

Gut Microbiome controls several metabolic processes in the host, such as those connected to glucose metabolism, lipid metabolism, and energy homeostasis (Dieterich et al., 2018). The Gut Microbiome is sometimes called "a new virtual metabolic organ" due to its wide range of metabolic activity (Evans et al., 2013). Previous research has demonstrated the significant functions that the gut microbiome contributes in the metabolism of bile acids, the bioavailability of minerals, the creation of vitamins B and K, amines, phenols, and sulphureous compounds, as well as in the degradation and absorption of nutrients. By maintaining cell-cell connections and repairing the epithelial barrier after disruption, the gut microbiome contributes to preserving gut integrity. Sustaining an appropriate microbiota composition is essential for defense against infections and is part of the host immune response. The gut Microbiome affects the CNS by controlling the secretion of neurotransmitters and other neuroactive chemicals (Moszak et al., 2020).

Diet's impact on human health is multifaceted. Poor dietary habits, such as a high-fat diet or a Western-style diet, are commonly associated with chronic diseases of the modern world, including obesity, T2D, and CVD (Ni et al., 2019). Long-term dietary practices are crucial for sustaining the high diversity and richness of microbial populations in the GI tract, a process known as "eubiosis," and assessing human health (Gentile and Weir, 2018). Diverse dietary patterns, namely the ratio of macro-to-micronutrients in the diet and the nutritional origins of macronutrients play a role in genetic modification. Dietary modifications, even brief ones, can actively amend host metabolism and modify the gut microbiota composition (David et al., 2014). Several other but equally important elements, such as the consumption of probiotics, the amount of bioactive compounds (e.g., polyphenols) in the diet, vitamin and mineral supplements, and excessive use of alcohol, tea, coffee, and salt, all have an impact on the healthful microbial population in the gut (Singh et al., 2019). Figure 8.1 illustrates the diet-gut microbiome-metabolic disorder tirade.

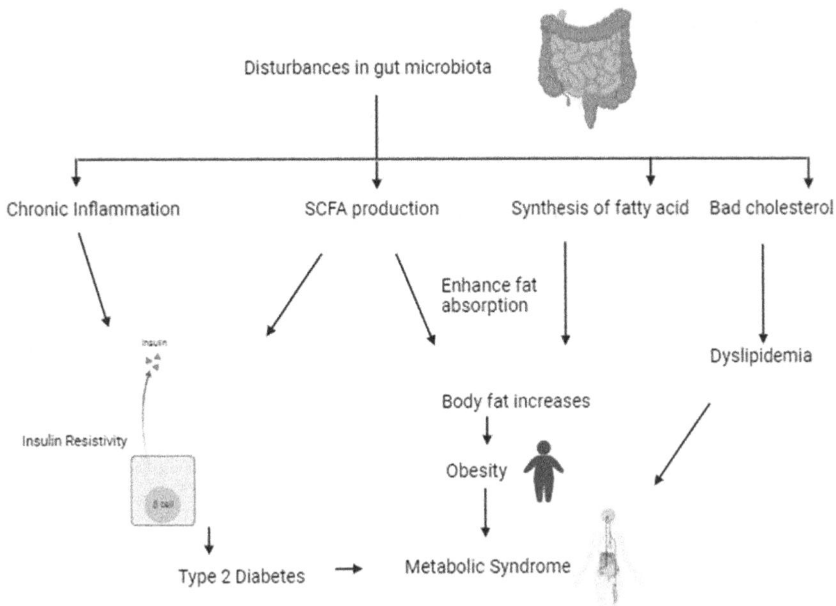

FIGURE 8.1 Diet-gut microbiome-metabolic disorder tirade.

Obesity is one of the most significant issues facing public health today. Although numerous factors contribute to obesity, an imbalance between energy expenditure and energy consumption from food and beverages is the most common cause. Emerging evidence shows that dysregulated gut flora could cause the imbalance (Turnbaugh et al., 2006). The bacterial microbiome played a significant character in the development of obesity by aiding in the digestion and absorption of nutrients, energy harvesting, preservation of intestinal epithelium tightness, metabolism of lipids, carbohydrates, and bile acids, regulation of intestinal motility, and immune and hormonal system regulation (Bäckhed et al., 2004).

Patients with T2D have dysregulated gut microbiome composition and functioning. It has been shown that people with T2D, a condition that may arise from obesity, have fewer fiber-degrading bacteria in their bodies (Arora, 2021; Karlsson, 2013). Additionally, it has been noted that one of the main contributors to insulin resistance and T2D was the dysregulation in gut microbiota make-up, which results in a reduction in gut integrity and metabolic endotoxemia (Zabarenko, 2007)

8.6 CONCLUSION

Trillions of bacteria make up the gut microbiome, which is essential to our general health. Diverse fibers in fruits, vegetables, and whole grains provide energy to the good bacteria in the stomach and support intestinal health. The SCFAs that these bacteria generate are involved in the control of metabolism. A microbial imbalance brought on by an unbalanced diet heavy in refined sugars and low in fiber may exacerbate metabolic illnesses, including T2D and obesity. It is crucial to make dietary decisions that maintain a vibrant and diversified microbial community in the gut because of the complex interactions between nutrition, gut microbiome, and metabolic health. Through the promotion of a balanced and healthy gut flora, this holistic approach can signify a pivotal role in the prevention or management of metabolic diseases.

8.7 FUTURE DIRECTIONS

Experts are progressively exploring the complex interplay among nutrition, gut microbiota, and metabolic well-being. The goal of personalized nutrition, fueled by developments in omics technologies, is to customize dietary recommendations according to each person's metabolic profile and microbiome makeup. To maximize dietary choices, this strategy considers variables such as genetics, lifestyle, and gut bacteria diversity.

Precision medicine also entails finding the biomarkers linked to particular food responses and microbiome configurations in the setting of metabolic illnesses. This may open the door for focused therapies, enabling medical practitioners to recommend highly customized eating regimens for improved metabolic results.

KEYWORDS

- **dietary fiber**
- **gut microbiome**
- **metabolic disorders**
- **personalized nutrition**
- **prebiotics**
- **probiotics**

REFERENCES

Al-Assal, K., Martinez, A. C., Torrinhas, R. S., Cardinelli, C., & Waitzberg, D. (2018). Gut microbiota and obesity. *Clinical Nutrition Experimental, 20*, 60–64. https://doi.org/10.1016/j.yclnex.2018.03.001 (accessed on 28th June 2025).

Andoh, A. (2016). Physiological role of gut microbiota for maintaining human health. *Digestion, 93*(3), 176–181. https://doi.org/10.1159/000444066 (accessed on 28th June 2025).

Aoun, A., Darwish, F., & Hamod, N. (2020). The influence of the gut microbiome on obesity in adults and the role of probiotics, prebiotics and synbiotics for weight loss. *Preventive Nutrition and Food Science, 25*(2), 113–123. https://doi.org/10.3746/pnf.2020.25.2.113 (accessed on 28th June 2025).

Asahara, S. I., Miura, H., Ogawa, W., & Tamori, Y. (2020). Sex difference in the association of obesity with personal or social background among urban residents in Japan. *PLoS ONE, 15*(11), 1–11. https://doi.org/10.1371/journal.pone.0242105 (accessed on 28th June 2025).

Ashique, S., De Rubis, G., Sirohi, E., Mishra, N., Rihan, M., Garg, A., Reyes, R.-J., Manandhar, B., Bhatt, S., Jha, N. K., Singh, T. G., Gupta, G., Singh, S. K., Chellappan, D. K., Paudel, K. R., Hansbro, P. M., Oliver, B. G., & Dua, K. (2022). Short chain fatty acids: Fundamental mediators of the gut-lung axis and their involvement in pulmonary diseases. *Chemico-Biological Interactions, 368*, 110231. https://doi.org/10.1016/j.cbi.2022.110231 (accessed on 28th June 2025).

Bäckhed, F., Ding, H., Wang, T., Hooper, L. V., Gou, Y. K., Nagy, A., Semenkovich, C. F., & Gordon, J. I. (2004). The gut microbiota as an environmental factor that regulates fat storage. *Proceedings of the National Academy of Sciences of the United States of America, 101*(44), 15718–15723. https://doi.org/10.1073/pnas.0407076101 (accessed on 28th June 2025).

Banday, M. Z., Sameer, A. S., & Nissar, S. (2020). Pathophysiology of diabetes: An overview. *Avicenna Journal of Medicine, 10*(4), 174–188. https://doi.org/10.4103/ajm.ajm_53_20 (accessed on 28th June 2025).

Beserra, B. T. S., Fernandes, R., do Rosario, V. A., Mocellin, M. C., Kuntz, M. G. F., & Trindade, E. B. S. M. (2015). A systematic review and meta-analysis of the prebiotics and synbiotics effects on glycaemia, insulin concentrations and lipid parameters in adult patients with overweight or obesity. *Clinical Nutrition, 34*(5), 845–858. https://doi.org/10.1016/j.clnu.2014.10.004 (accessed on 28th June 2025).

Bhargava, S. K., Singh, T. G., Mannan, A., Singh, S., & Gupta, S. (2022). Pharmacological evaluation of *Thuja occidentalis* for the attenuation of nephropathy in streptozotocin-induced diabetes rats. *Obesity Medicine, 31*, 100391. https://doi.org/10.1016/j.obmed.2022.100391 (accessed on 28th June 2025).

Bhargava, S. K., Singh, T. G., Mannan, A., Singh, S., Singh, M., & Gupta, S. (2022). Pharmacological evaluation of *Thuja occidentalis* for the attenuation of neuropathy via AGEs and TNF-α inhibition in diabetic neuropathic rats. *Environmental Science and Pollution Research International, 29*(40), 60542–60557. https://doi.org/10.1007/s11356-022-20106-3 (accessed on 28th June 2025).

Blaak, E. E., Canfora, E. E., Theis, S., Frost, G., Groen, A. K., Mithieux, G., Nauta, A., Scott, K., & Stahl, B. (2020). Short chain fatty acids in human gut and metabolic health. *Beneficial Microbes, 11*(1), 1–45. https://doi.org/10.3920/BM2020.0057 (accessed on 28th June 2025).

Bozbulut, R., & Sanlier, N. (2019). Promising effects of β-glucans on glycaemic control in diabetes. *Trends in Food Science and Technology, 83*, 159–166. https://doi.org/10.1016/j.tifs.2018.11.018 (accessed on 28th June 2025).

Brooks, L., Viardot, A., Tsakmaki, A., Stolarczyk, E., Howard, J. K., Cani, P. D., Everard, A., Sleeth, M. L., Psichas, A., Anastasovskaj, J., Bell, J. D., Bell-Anderson, K., Mackay, C. R., Ghatei, M. A., Bloom, S. R., Frost, G., & Bewick, G. A. (2017). Fermentable carbohydrate stimulates FFAR2-dependent colonic PYY cell expansion to increase satiety. *Molecular Metabolism, 6*(1), 48–60. https://doi.org/10.1016/j.molmet.2016.10.011 (accessed on 28th June 2025).

Caetano, M. A. F., & Castelucci, P. (2022). Role of short chain fatty acids in gut health and possible therapeutic approaches in inflammatory bowel diseases. *World Journal of Clinical Cases, 10*(28), 9985–10003. https://doi.org/10.12998/wjcc.v10.i28.9985 (accessed on 28th June 2025).

Canfora, E. E., Jocken, J. W., & Blaak, E. E. (2015). Short-chain fatty acids in control of body weight and insulin sensitivity. *Nature Reviews Endocrinology, 11*(10), 577–591. https://doi.org/10.1038/nrendo.2015.128 (accessed on 28th June 2025).

Care, D., & Suppl, S. S. (2020). Classification and diagnosis of diabetes: Standards of medical care in diabetes–2020. *Diabetes Care, 43*(Suppl. 1), S14–S31. https://doi.org/10.2337/dc20-S002 (accessed on 28th June 2025).

Corrêa-Oliveira, R., Fachi, J. L., Vieira, A., Sato, F. T., & Vinolo, M. A. R. (2016). Regulation of immune cell function by short-chain fatty acids. *Clinical and Translational Immunology, 5*(4), e73. https://doi.org/10.1038/cti.2016.17 (accessed on 28th June 2025).

Coustan, D. R. (2013). Gestational diabetes mellitus. *Clinical Chemistry, 59*(9), 1310–1321. https://doi.org/10.1373/clinchem.2013.203331 (accessed on 28th June 2025).

Cronin, P., Joyce, S. A., O'Toole, P. W., & O'Connor, E. M. (2021). Dietary fibre modulates the gut microbiota. *Nutrients, 13*(5), 1655. https://doi.org/10.3390/nu13051655 (accessed on 28th June 2025).

Da Silva, H. E., Teterina, A., Comelli, E. M., Taibi, A., Arendt, B. M., Fischer, S. E., Lou, W., & Allard, J. P. (2018). Nonalcoholic fatty liver disease is associated with dysbiosis independent of body mass index and insulin resistance. *Scientific Reports, 8*(1), 1466. https://doi.org/10.1038/s41598-018-19753-9 (accessed on 28th June 2025).

da Silva, T. F., Casarotti, S. N., de Oliveira, G. L. V., & Penna, A. L. B. (2021). The impact of probiotics, prebiotics, and synbiotics on the biochemical, clinical, and immunological markers, as well as on the gut microbiota of obese hosts. *Critical Reviews in Food Science and Nutrition, 61*(2), 337–355. https://doi.org/10.1080/10408398.2020.1733483 (accessed on 28th June 2025).

David, L. A., Maurice, C. F., Carmody, R. N., Gootenberg, D. B., Button, J. E., Wolfe, B. E., Ling, A. V., Devlin, A. S., Varma, Y., Fischbach, M. A., Biddinger, S. B., Dutton, R. J., & Turnbaugh, P. J. (2014). Diet rapidly and reproducibly alters the human gut microbiome. *Nature, 505*(7484), 559–563. https://doi.org/10.1038/nature12820 (accessed on 28th June 2025).

De Menezes, E. W., Giuntini, E. B., Dan, M. C. T., Sardá, F. A. H., & Lajolo, F. M. (2013). Codex dietary fibre definition—Justification for inclusion of carbohydrates from 3 to 9 degrees of polymerisation. *Food Chemistry, 140*(3), 581–585. https://doi.org/10.1016/j.foodchem.2013.02.075 (accessed on 28th June 2025).

Devi, S., Chauhan, S., Mannan, A., & Singh, T. G. (2023). Targeting cardiovascular risk factors with eugenol: An anti-inflammatory perspective. *Inflammopharmacology.* https://doi.org/10.1007/s10787-023-01392-w (accessed on 28th June 2025).

Dieterich, W., Schink, M., & Zopf, Y. (2018). Microbiota in the gastrointestinal tract. *Medical Sciences (Basel, Switzerland), 6*(4), 116. https://doi.org/10.3390/medsci6040116 (accessed on 28th June 2025).

Duparc, T., Plovier, H., Marrachelli, V. G., Van Hul, M., Essaghir, A., Ståhlman, M., Matamoros, S., Geurts, L., Pardo-Tendero, M. M., Druart, C., Delzenne, N. M., Demoulin, J. B., Van Der Merwe, S. W., Van Pelt, J., Bäckhed, F., Monleon, D., Everard, A., & Cani, P. D. (2017). Hepatocyte MyD88 affects bile acids, gut microbiota and metabolome contributing to regulate glucose and lipid metabolism. *Gut, 66*(4), 620–632. https://doi.org/10.1136/gutjnl-2015-310904 (accessed on 28th June 2025).

Ekta, Gupta, M., Kaur, A., Singh, T. G., & Bedi, O. (2020). Pathobiological and molecular connections involved in the high fructose and high fat diet induced diabetes associated nonalcoholic fatty liver disease. *Inflammation Research, 69*(9), 851–867. https://doi.org/10.1007/s00011-020-01373-7 (accessed on 28th June 2025).

Evans, J. M., Morris, L. S., & Marchesi, J. R. (2013). The gut microbiome: The role of a virtual organ in the endocrinology of the host. *Journal of Endocrinology, 218*(3), R37–R47. https://doi.org/10.1530/JOE-13-0131 (accessed on 28th June 2025).

Fischbach, M. A., & Segre, J. A. (2016). Signaling in host-associated microbial communities. *Cell, 164*(6), 1288–1300. https://doi.org/10.1016/j.cell.2016.02.037 (accessed on 28th June 2025).

Gao, Z., Yin, J., Zhang, J., Ward, R. E., Martin, R. J., Lefevre, M., Cefalu, W. T., & Ye, J. (2009). Butyrate improves insulin sensitivity and increases energy expenditure in mice. *Diabetes, 58*(7), 1509–1517. https://doi.org/10.2337/db08-1637 (accessed on 28th June 2025).

Garg, N., Singh, T. G., Khan, H., Arora, S., Kaur, A., & Mannan, A. (2021). Mechanistic interventions of selected *Ocimum* species in management of diabetes, obesity and liver disorders: Transformative developments from preclinical to clinical approaches. *Biointerface Research in Applied Chemistry, 12*(1), Article 1. https://doi.org/10.33263/BRIAC121.13041323 (accessed on 28th June 2025).

Gentile, C. L., & Weir, T. L. (2018). The gut microbiota at the intersection of diet and human health. *Science, 362*(6416), 776–780. https://doi.org/10.1126/science.aau5812 (accessed on 28th June 2025).

Goldsmith, J. R., & Sartor, R. B. (2014). The role of diet on intestinal microbiota metabolism: Downstream impacts on host immune function and health, and therapeutic implications. *Journal of Gastroenterology, 49*(5), 785–798. https://doi.org/10.1007/s00535-014-0953-z (accessed on 28th June 2025).

Goyal, S., Sood, A., Gautam, I., Pradhan, S., Mondal, P., Singh, G., Jaura, R. S., Singh, T. G., & Sibia, R. S. (2022). Serum protease-activated receptor (PAR-1) levels as a potential biomarker for diagnosis of inflammation in type 2 diabetic patients.

Inflammopharmacology, 30(5), 1843–1851. https://doi.org/10.1007/s10787-022-01049-0 (accessed on 28th June 2025).

Hales, C. M., Fryar, C. D., Carroll, M. D., Freedman, D. S., Aoki, Y., & Ogden, C. L. (2018). Differences in obesity prevalence by demographic characteristics and urbanization level among adults in the United States, 2013–2016. *JAMA, 319*(23), 2419–2429. https://doi.org/10.1001/jama.2018.7270 (accessed on 28th June 2025).

Heymsfield, S. B., & Wadden, T. A. (2017). Mechanisms, pathophysiology, and management of obesity. *New England Journal of Medicine, 376*(3), 254–266. https://doi.org/10.1056/nejmra1514009 (accessed on 28th June 2025).

Huang, L., Thonusin, C., Chattipakorn, N., & Chattipakorn, S. C. (2021). Impacts of gut microbiota on gestational diabetes mellitus: A comprehensive review. *European Journal of Nutrition, 60*(5), 2343–2360. https://doi.org/10.1007/s00394-021-02483-6 (accessed on 28th June 2025).

Jayesh Shah, N., & Swami, O. C. (2017). Role of probiotics in diabetes: A review of their rationale and efficacy. *EMJ Diabetes, October*, 104–110. https://doi.org/10.33590/emjdiabet/10310327 (accessed on 28th June 2025).

John, G. K., Wang, L., Nanavati, J., Twose, C., Singh, R., & Mullin, G. (2018). Dietary alteration of the gut microbiome and its impact on weight and fat mass: A systematic review and meta-analysis. *Genes, 9*(3), 167. https://doi.org/10.3390/genes9030167 (accessed on 28th June 2025).

Kahanovitz, L., Sluss, P. M., & Russell, S. J. (2017). Type 1 diabetes—a clinical perspective. *Point of Care, 16*(1), 37–40. https://doi.org/10.1097/POC.0000000000000125 (accessed on 28th June 2025).

Kaur, N., Kishore, L., Farooq, S. A., Kajal, A., Singh, R., Agrawal, R., Mannan, A., & Singh, T. G. (2023). *Cucurbita pepo* seeds improve peripheral neuropathy in diabetic rats by modulating the inflammation and oxidative stress in rats. *Environmental Science and Pollution Research International.* https://doi.org/10.1007/s11356-023-28339-6 (accessed on 28th June 2025).

Khanna, S., Walia, S., Kondepudi, K. K., & Shukla, G. (2020). Administration of indigenous probiotics modulate high-fat diet-induced metabolic syndrome in Sprague Dawley rats. *Antonie van Leeuwenhoek, 113*(9), 1345–1359. https://doi.org/10.1007/s10482-020-01445-y (accessed on 28th June 2025).

Kobyliak, N., Virchenko, O., & Falalyeyeva, T. (2016). Pathophysiological role of host microbiota in the development of obesity. *Nutrition Journal, 15*(1), 43. https://doi.org/10.1186/s12937-016-0166-9 (accessed on 28th June 2025).

Koutnikova, H., Genser, B., Monteiro-Sepulveda, M., Faurie, J. M., Rizkalla, S., Schrezenmeir, J., & Clement, K. (2019). Impact of bacterial probiotics on obesity, diabetes and non-alcoholic fatty liver disease related variables: A systematic review and meta-analysis of randomised controlled trials. *BMJ Open, 9*(3), e017995. https://doi.org/10.1136/bmjopen-2017-017995 (accessed on 28th June 2025).

Li, H. Y., Zhou, D. D., Gan, R. Y., Huang, S. Y., Zhao, C. N., Shang, A., Xu, X. Y., & Li, H. Bin. (2021). 益生菌、益生元、合成菌和后生物制剂对代谢性疾病的影响和机制. *Nutrients, 13*(9), 3199. (accessed on 28th June 2025).

Loos, R. J. F., & Yeo, G. S. H. (2022). The genetics of obesity: From discovery to biology. *Nature Reviews Genetics, 23*(2), 120–133. https://doi.org/10.1038/s41576-021-00414-z (accessed on 28th June 2025).

Macfarlane, G. T., & Macfarlane, S. (2011). Fermentation in the human large intestine: Its physiologic consequences and the potential contribution of prebiotics. *Journal of Clinical Gastroenterology, 45*(Suppl. 3), S120–S127. https://doi.org/10.1097/MCG.0b013e31822fecfe (accessed on 28th June 2025).

Macfarlane, S., Steed, H., & Macfarlane, G. T. (2009). Intestinal bacteria and inflammatory bowel disease. *Critical Reviews in Clinical Laboratory Sciences, 46*(1), 25–54. https://doi.org/10.1080/10408360802485792 (accessed on 28th June 2025).

Moszak, M., Szulińska, M., & Bogdański, P. (2020). You are what you eat—The relationship between diet, microbiota, and metabolic disorders—A review. *Nutrients, 12*(4), 1096. https://doi.org/10.3390/nu12041096 (accessed on 28th June 2025).

Musso, G., Gambino, R., & Cassader, M. (2010). Obesity, diabetes, and gut microbiota: The hygiene hypothesis expanded? *Diabetes Care, 33*(10), 2277–2284. https://doi.org/10.2337/dc10-0556 (accessed on 28th June 2025).

Najar, I. A., Bhat, M. H., Qadrie, Z. L., Amaldoss, M. J. N., Kushwah, A. S., Singh, T. G., Kabra, A., Khan, N., & Kumar, M. (2022). Cardioprotection by *Citrus grandis* (L.) peel ethanolic extract in alloxan-induced cardiotoxicity in diabetic rats. *BioMed Research International, 2022*, 2807337. https://doi.org/10.1155/2022/2807337 (accessed on 28th June 2025).

Ni, Y., Wu, L., Jiang, J., Yang, T., Wang, Z., Ma, L., Zheng, L., Yang, X., Wu, Z., & Fu, Z. (2019). Late-night eating-induced physiological dysregulation and circadian misalignment are accompanied by microbial dysbiosis. *Molecular Nutrition & Food Research, 63*(24), 1900867. https://doi.org/10.1002/mnfr.201900867 (accessed on 28th June 2025).

Ohashi, W., & Fukada, T. (2019). Contribution of zinc and zinc transporters in the pathogenesis of inflammatory bowel diseases. *Journal of Immunology Research, 2019*, 8396878. https://doi.org/10.1155/2019/8396878 (accessed on 28th June 2025).

Osterberg, K. L., Boutagy, N. E., McMillan, R. P., Stevens, J. R., Frisard, M. I., Kavanaugh, J. W., Davy, B. M., Davy, K. P., & Hulver, M. W. (2015). Probiotic supplementation attenuates increases in body mass and fat mass during high-fat diet in healthy young adults. *Obesity, 23*(12), 2364–2370. https://doi.org/10.1002/oby.21230 (accessed on 28th June 2025).

Pascale, A., Marchesi, N., Marelli, C., Coppola, A., Luzi, L., Govoni, S., Giustina, A., & Gazzaruso, C. (2018). Microbiota and metabolic diseases. *Endocrine, 61*(3), 357–371. https://doi.org/10.1007/s12020-018-1605-5 (accessed on 28th June 2025).

Reed, S., Neuman, H., Moscovich, S., Glahn, R. P., Koren, O., & Tako, E. (2015). Chronic zinc deficiency alters chick gut microbiota composition and function. *Nutrients, 7*(12), 9768–9784. https://doi.org/10.3390/nu7125497 (accessed on 28th June 2025).

Reichardt, N., Duncan, S. H., Young, P., Belenguer, A., McWilliam Leitch, C., Scott, K. P., Flint, H. J., & Louis, P. (2014). Phylogenetic distribution of three pathways for propionate production within the human gut microbiota. *ISME Journal, 8*(6), 1323–1335. https://doi.org/10.1038/ismej.2014.14 (accessed on 28th June 2025).

Reilly, S. M., & Saltiel, A. R. (2017). Adapting to obesity with adipose tissue inflammation. *Nature Reviews Endocrinology, 13*(11), 633–643. https://doi.org/10.1038/nrendo.2017.90 (accessed on 28th June 2025).

Ríos-Covián, D., Ruas-Madiedo, P., Margolles, A., Gueimonde, M., De los Reyes-Gavilán, C. G., & Salazar, N. (2016). Intestinal short chain fatty acids and their link with diet and human health. *Frontiers in Microbiology, 7*, 185. https://doi.org/10.3389/fmicb.2016.00185 (accessed on 28th June 2025).

Schroeder, B. O., & Bäckhed, F. (2016). Signals from the gut microbiota to distant organs in physiology and disease. *Nature Medicine, 22*(10), 1079–1089. https://doi.org/10.1038/nm.4185 (accessed on 28th June 2025).

Schroeder, B. O., Birchenough, G. M. H., Ståhlman, M., Arike, L., Johansson, M. E. V., Hansson, G. C., & Bäckhed, F. (2018). *Bifidobacteria* or fiber protects against diet-induced microbiota-mediated colonic mucus deterioration. *Cell Host & Microbe, 23*(1), 27–40.e7. https://doi.org/10.1016/j.chom.2017.11.004 (accessed on 28th June 2025).

Shao, Y., Lei, Z., Yuan, J., Yang, Y., Guo, Y., & Zhang, B. (2014). Effect of zinc on growth performance, gut morphometry, and cecal microbial community in broilers challenged with *Salmonella enterica* serovar *typhimurium*. *Journal of Microbiology, 52*(12), 1002–1011. https://doi.org/10.1007/s12275-014-4347-y (accessed on 28th June 2025).

Sharma, V. K., & Singh, T. G. (2020). Chronic stress and diabetes mellitus: Interwoven pathologies. *Current Diabetes Reviews, 16*(6), 546–556. https://doi.org/10.2174/1573399815666191111152248 (accessed on 28th June 2025).

Simpson, H. L., & Campbell, B. J. (2015). Review article: Dietary fibre–microbiota interactions. *Alimentary Pharmacology & Therapeutics, 42*(2), 158–179. https://doi.org/10.1111/apt.13248 (accessed on 28th June 2025).

Singh, A. K., Cabral, C., Kumar, R., Ganguly, R., Rana, H. K., Gupta, A., Lauro, M. R., Carbone, C., Reis, F., & Pandey, A. K. (2019). Beneficial effects of dietary polyphenols on gut microbiota and strategies to improve delivery efficiency. *Nutrients, 11*(9), 2216. https://doi.org/10.3390/nu11092216 (accessed on 28th June 2025).

Singh, R., Farooq, S. A., Mannan, A., Singh, T. G., Najda, A., Grażyna, Z., Albadrani, G. M., Sayed, A. A., & Abdel-Daim, M. M. (2022). Animal models of diabetic microvascular complications: Relevance to clinical features. *Biomedicine & Pharmacotherapy, 145*, 112305. https://doi.org/10.1016/j.biopha.2021.112305 (accessed on 28th June 2025).

Singh, R., Rao, H. K., & Singh, T. G. (2020). Neuropathic pain in diabetes mellitus: Challenges and future trends. *Obesity Medicine, 18*, 100215. https://doi.org/10.1016/j.obmed.2020.100215 (accessed on 28th June 2025).

Sivamaruthi, B. S., Kesika, P., Suganthy, N., & Chaiyasut, C. (2019). A review on role of microbiome in obesity and antiobesity properties of probiotic supplements. *BioMed Research International, 2019*, 3291367. https://doi.org/10.1155/2019/3291367 (accessed on 28th June 2025).

Soiza, R. L., Donaldson, A. I. C., & Myint, P. K. (2018). Vaccine against arteriosclerosis: An update. *Therapeutic Advances in Vaccines, 9*(6), 259–261. https://doi.org/10.1177/https (accessed on 28th June 2025).

Thursby, E., & Juge, N. (2017). Introduction to the human gut microbiota. *Biochemical Journal, 474*(11), 1823–1836. https://doi.org/10.1042/BCJ20160510 (accessed on 28th June 2025).

Turnbaugh, P. J., Ley, R. E., Mahowald, M. A., Magrini, V., Mardis, E. R., & Gordon, J. I. (2006). An obesity-associated gut microbiome with increased capacity for energy harvest. *Nature, 444*(7122), 1027–1031. https://doi.org/10.1038/nature05414 (accessed on 28th June 2025).

Turnbaugh, P., Bäckhed, F., Fulton, L., & Gordon, J. (2008). Marked alterations in the distal gut microbiome linked to diet-induced obesity. *Cell Host & Microbe, 3*(4), 213–223. https://doi.org/10.1016/j.chom.2008.02.015 (accessed on 28th June 2025).

Vernocchi, P., Del Chierico, F., & Putignani, L. (2016). Gut microbiota profiling: Metabolomics based approach to unravel compounds affecting human health. *Frontiers in Microbiology, 7*, 1144. https://doi.org/10.3389/fmicb.2016.01144 (accessed on 28th June 2025).

Wan, Y., Wang, F., Yuan, J., Li, J., Jiang, D., Zhang, J., Li, H., Wang, R., Tang, J., Huang, T., Zheng, J., Sinclair, A. J., Mann, J., & Li, D. (2019). Effects of dietary fat on gut microbiota and faecal metabolites, and their relationship with cardiometabolic risk factors: A 6-month randomised controlled-feeding trial. *Gut, 68*(8), 1417–1429. https://doi.org/10.1136/gutjnl-2018-317609 (accessed on 28th June 2025).

Wang, B., Jiang, X., Cao, M., Ge, J., Bao, Q., Tang, L., Chen, Y., & Li, L. (2016). Altered fecal microbiota correlates with liver biochemistry in nonobese patients with non-alcoholic fatty liver disease. *Scientific Reports, 6*, 32002. https://doi.org/10.1038/srep32002 (accessed on 28th June 2025).

Wang, Z. Bin, Xin, S. S., Ding, L. N., Ding, W. Y., Hou, Y. L., Liu, C. Q., & Zhang, X. D. (2019). The potential role of probiotics in controlling overweight/obesity and associated metabolic parameters in adults: A systematic review and meta-analysis. *Evidence-Based Complementary and Alternative Medicine, 2019*, 3862971. https://doi.org/10.1155/2019/3862971 (accessed on 28th June 2025).

Wang, Z., Chen, J., Zhu, L., Jiao, S., Chen, Y., & Sun, Y. (2023). Metabolic disorders and risk of cardiovascular diseases: A two-sample Mendelian randomization study. *BMC Cardiovascular Disorders, 23*(1), 1–8. https://doi.org/10.1186/s12872-023-03567-3 (accessed on 28th June 2025).

Ward, Z. J., Bleich, S. N., Cradock, A. L., Barrett, J. L., Giles, C. M., Flax, C., Long, M. W., & Gortmaker, S. L. (2019). Projected U.S. state-level prevalence of adult obesity and severe obesity. *New England Journal of Medicine, 381*(25), 2440–2450. https://doi.org/10.1056/nejmsa1909301 (accessed on 28th June 2025).

Wiese, M., Bashmakov, Y., Chalyk, N., Nielsen, D. S., Krych, Ł., Kot, W., Klochkov, V., Pristensky, D., Bandaletova, T., Chernyshova, M., Kyle, N., & Petyaev, I. (2019). Prebiotic effect of lycopene and dark chocolate on gut microbiome with systemic changes in liver metabolism, skeletal muscles and skin in moderately obese persons. *BioMed Research International, 2019*, 4625279. https://doi.org/10.1155/2019/4625279 (accessed on 28th June 2025).

Wolters, M., Ahrens, J., Romaní-Pérez, M., Watkins, C., Sanz, Y., Benítez-Páez, A., Stanton, C., & Günther, K. (2019). Dietary fat, the gut microbiota, and metabolic health – A systematic review conducted within the MyNewGut project. *Clinical Nutrition, 38*(6), 2504–2520. https://doi.org/10.1016/j.clnu.2018.12.024 (accessed on 28th June 2025).

Wu, G. D., Chen, J., Hoffmann, C., Bittinger, K., Chen, Y.-Y., Keilbaugh, S. A., Bewtra, M., Knights, D., Walters, W. A., Knight, R., Sinha, R., Gilroy, E., Gupta, K., Baldassano, R., … Lewis, J. D. (2011). Linking long-term dietary patterns with gut microbial enterotypes. *Science, 334*(6052), 105–109. https://doi.org/10.1126/science.1208344 (accessed on 28th June 2025).

Wu, J., Wang, K., Wang, X., Pang, Y., & Jiang, C. (2021). The role of the gut microbiome and its metabolites in metabolic diseases. *Protein & Cell, 12*(5), 360–373. https://doi.org/10.1007/s13238-020-00814-7 (accessed on 28th June 2025).

Xiong, R. G., Zhou, D. D., Wu, S. X., Huang, S. Y., Saimaiti, A., Yang, Z. J., Shang, A., Zhao, C. N., Gan, R. Y., & Li, H. Bin. (2022). Health benefits and side effects of short-chain fatty acids. *Foods, 11*(18), 2863. https://doi.org/10.3390/foods11182863 (accessed on 28th June 2025).

Yang, M., Liu, S., & Zhang, C. (2022). The related metabolic diseases and treatments of obesity. *Healthcare (Switzerland), 10*(9), 1916. https://doi.org/10.3390/healthcare10091616 (accessed on 28th June 2025).

Yang, Q., Liang, Q., Balakrishnan, B., Belobrajdic, D. P., Feng, Q. J., & Zhang, W. (2020). Role of dietary nutrients in the modulation of gut microbiota: A narrative review. *Nutrients, 12*(2), 381. https://doi.org/10.3390/nu12020381 (accessed on 28th June 2025).

Zhang, Y. J., Li, S., Gan, R. Y., Zhou, T., Xu, D. P., & Li, H. Bin. (2015). Impacts of gut bacteria on human health and diseases. *International Journal of Molecular Sciences, 16*(4), 7493–7519. https://doi.org/10.3390/ijms16047493 (accessed on 28th June 2025).

Zheng, Y., Ley, S. H., & Hu, F. B. (2018). Global aetiology and epidemiology of type 2 diabetes mellitus and its complications. *Nature Reviews Endocrinology, 14*(2), 88–98. https://doi.org/10.1038/nrendo.2017.151 (accessed on 28th June 2025).

CHAPTER 9

Dietary Influence on Gut Microbiota and Epigenetic Factors in Metabolic Disorders: Exploring Mechanisms and Therapeutic Strategies

GURPREET KAUR,[1,2] AJAY SINGH KUSHWAH,[1,*] and SRINIVAS NAMMI[3]

[1]*Department of Pharmacology, Amar Shaheed Baba Ajit Singh Jujhar Singh Memorial College of Pharmacy, Bela, Ropar, Punjab, India*

[2]*I. K. Gujral Punjab Technical University, Kapurthala, Jalandhar, Punjab, India*

[3]*School of Science, Western Sydney University, Penrith, New South Wales, Australia*

*Corresponding author

ABSTRACT

Metabolic disorders, with their far-reaching impact on public health, stand as prominent global concerns. Recent studies indicate that the intricate connection between the elements in our diet, the composition of the gut microbiome, and epigenetic factors play a vital function in the initiation and advancement of chronic complications. A vast population of 100 trillion beneficial bacteria are present in the gastrointestinal canal of humans, causing disturbances in the intestinal microbiota and dysbiosis, which is further responsible for various health conditions. The gut microbiome has been increasingly recognized for its potential influence on epigenetic modifications. A fundamental pathway combining multiple elements in

Precision Nutrition and Endocrine Health: Synthesis, Characterization, and Applications.
Thakur Gurjeet Singh and Sanjana Mehta (Eds.)

DOI: 10.1201/9781998511877-9

modifying genetics involves metabolic production, a crucial factor and allosteric controller influencing epigenetic phenomena. Epigenetic factors, including DNA methylation, histone modifications, and non-coding RNAs, can significantly impact gene expression related to metabolic pathways. These alterations play an important factor in overall well-being and susceptibility to diseases. The chapter delves into the intricate mechanisms through which dietary choices impact the gut microbiota, microbial metabolism, and the subsequent effects on host epigenetic regulation. It highlights the key players in this complex web of influence, including the immune system and signaling molecules. In conclusion, this chapter underscores the pivotal contribution of dietary intake in forming the intestinal microflora and epigenetic landscape, thereby impacting the development and progression of metabolic disorders. Understanding these complex relationships opens the door to novel therapeutic strategies and preventive approaches considering genetic and environmental influences.

9.1 INTRODUCTION

Lifestyle originates from various health-related complications, primarily poor dietary choices, lack of physical activity, improper body posture, and a disruption in the biological clock. All of these factors alter health conditions. A collaborative report from the World Economic Forum and World Health Organization (WHO) indicates that India is projected to face a cumulative economic downturn of approximately $230–250 billion due to poor dietary lifestyles. The report highlights that in recent years, 60% of global deaths (35 million) were attributed to non-communicable diseases, representing 44% of premature fatalities. Moreover, metabolic disorder (MetD) covers a significant portion of this value (Sharma and Majumdar, 2009). MetD is associated with various health complications that lead to disturbance in normal metabolism that further affects the ability of the body to convert food into energy, leading to various health problems (Park et al., 2006; Sharma and Singh, 2020). A distinct correlation exists among the gut microbiota, dietary patterns, and metabolic results. Evidence indicates that a high-fiber diet is associated with reduced inflammation, enhanced insulin sensitivity, and decreased dyslipidemias. Conversely, a food with high fatty and sugar content is linked to lipid and insulin metabolism conditions. The latest reports prove a substantial involvement of human intestinal microflora in either the onset or resolution of metabolic syndrome (MetS) and related conditions (Thomas et al., 2022). These disruptions can have widespread effects on various physiological processes, often leading to abnormalities and imbalances in essential substances like carbohydrates, proteins, and fats (Thomas et al., 2018). This imbalance further increases the unhealthy condition of the body. It increases the risk of its associated complications, almost doubles the Type 2 Diabetes Mellitus (T2DM) conditions and elevates risk factors by five times related to heart (Bhargava et al., 2022a, b; Seuring et al., 2015; Sharma et al., 2021; Singh et al., 2022; Thomas et al., 2018). Additionally, it raises the susceptibility to various chronic conditions, including fatty liver diseases, systematic disorders, neurodegenerative diseases, cancer, reproductive issues, and lipid and atherosclerosis. Genetic predisposition also plays a significant role in these conditions, but the interconnection of environment and genetic makeup has not been fully proven. Various experimental studies have reported and proved the Epigenetic connection in MetD (Mehta et al., 2022). Epigenetic markers serve as distinctive features of different disorders and states of illness, rendering them promising targets for novel drug therapies. The primary epigenetic mechanisms include DNA methylation, alterations in chromatin structure (posttranslational modifications of histones), and RNA-related processes like microRNAs (miRNAs) and long non-coding RNAs (LncRNAs) (Wilson, 2008). In addition to epigenetics, the human gut and its microbial community are a substantial factor in modifying the body's physiology; it is also strongly linked to MetD (Wu et al., 2023). The human gut contains around 120 trillion microorganisms, more than 10 times that of human cells. In recent decades, comprehension of intestinal microflora's significant involvement in well-being and disease states has expanded considerably (Sawicki et al., 2021). The management and treatment of these conditions often require extensive resources, including medications, regular monitoring, and lifestyle interventions. The economic impact on healthcare systems and societies can be substantial. Addressing these modifiable risk factors is crucial in preventing and managing these conditions. The management of metabolic disorders often involves a multidisciplinary approach, including medical professionals, dietitians, and other healthcare providers (Singh et al., 2020; Vieira et al., 2013). Collaborative efforts are necessary to address the diverse aspects of these conditions, including medical treatment, dietary changes, and lifestyle modifications. In conclusion, the importance of metabolic disorders lies in their widespread impact on health, their chronic nature, and the associated burden on healthcare systems. Prevention, early detection, and comprehensive management strategies are essential to mitigate the effects of these disorders and improve overall health outcomes.

9.2 THE ROLE OF DIET IN METABOLIC DISORDERS

A nutritional dietary intake consists of an appropriate mix of micronutrients (vitamins and minerals) and macronutrients (carbohydrates, proteins, and fats). Their balance is essential for body functioning and has specific effects on energy. Nutrient needs may depend on age, gender, physical work, and well-being. In several cases, micronutrient supplementation may be recommended, but per the doctor's advice for preventing excessive intake, it can have adverse effects (Vieira et al., 2013). Additionally, consultation with a dietitian is mandatory to determine individual dietary requirements. A sole emphasis on individual nutrients in dietary interventions has various constraints, and recommendations should priorities the comprehensive dietary pattern in treating MetD (Thomas et al., 2022). Recent findings advocate adopting dietary interventions centered on foods rather than restrictive approaches targeting calories or isolated nutrients. Table 9.1 summarizes the health advantages related to MetD, explicitly focusing on dietary macronutrient patterns and diverse dietary strategies.

TABLE 9.1 Represent the Dietary Pattern, Nutritional Distribution, and Beneficial Effects of MetS Management

Sr. No.	Dietary Pattern	Nutritional Distribution	Improvements in MetS Criteria
1.	Nordic diet	• High-fiber and whole-grain-rich products. • Low animal-based and processed products.	• Decline in systolic and diastolic BP. • Enhanced HDL-c levels.
2.	Mediterranean diet	• 30–50% kcal/d from total fat (mainly MUFA 1, EVOO and nuts being the resource). • 37–46% kcal/d from CH. • 17–20% kcal/d from protein.	• Decrease in the occurrence and consequences of cardiovascular disease (CVD). • Reduction in systolic and diastolic Blood Pressure. • Opposite relationship with mortality. • Enhancements in hyperlipidemia. • Reduced occurrence of T2DM.

TABLE 9.1 *(Continued)*

Sr. No.	Dietary Pattern	Nutritional Distribution	Improvements in MetS Criteria
3.	Plant-based diets	• Restriction of animal-based diet. • Increased intake of plant-derived diet. • Lipid profile rich in UFAs.	• Decline in systolic and diastolic BP. • Controlled weight and obesity risk factors. • Decreased CVD risk. • Reduced T2DM risk.
4.	DASH diet	• Total fats 25–30% kcal/d. • Saturated fats 5–7% kcal/d. • Food derived Cholesterol. • CH 52–55% kcal/d. • Proteins 15–20% kcal/d.	• Decline in systolic and diastolic BP. • Decreased BMI. • Cardio metabolic profile improvement. • Recover T2DM occurrence.
5.	Low CH diets and deficient CH diets (ketogenic diets)	• Less than 45–50% kcal/d from carbohydrates and less than 7–10% kcal/d. • From CH in ketogenic diets. • High protein (25–28% kcal/d). • Rich fatty component intake (35–75% kcal/d).	• Reduced weight and maintenance of weight. • Decreased DBP. • Management of LDL-c and triglycerides levels. • Elevation of HDL-c levels. • Better insulin resistance. • Decline in HbA1c levels.
6.	High protein diet	• High protein 25–35% kcal/d) Alternatively, 1.35–1.55 g/Kg body weight/d from protein. • Low CH (45–55% kcal/d).	• Decline in triglyceride levels.
7.	Intermittent fasting	• Long period fasting.	• Losing weight. • Better insulin resistance. • Enhancements in hyperlipidemia. • Decline in systolic and diastolic BP. • Decline in risk of T2DM and CVD.
8.	Low-fat diet	• Less than 25–30% kcal/d from total fat (less than 7–10% saturated fat). • 20% kcal/d from protein. • 60% kcal/d from CH.	• Decline in systolic and diastolic BP. • Enhancement of cholesterol profile for the short term. • Weight loss for the short term.

MUFA: Monounsaturated fatty acids; EVOO: extra virgin olive oil; CH: carbohydrates; CVD: cardiovascular disease; BP: blood pressure; T2DM: type 2 diabetes mellitus; DASH: Dietary Approaches to Stop Hypertension; UFAs: unsaturated fatty acids; BMI: body mass index; DBP: diastolic blood pressure; LDL-c: low-density lipoprotein cholesterol; HDL-c: high-density lipoprotein cholesterol; HbA1c: glycated hemoglobin; MUFA: monounsaturated fatty acids.

9.2.1 DIETARY COMPONENTS AND THEIR IMPACT ON GUT MICROBIOTA

The gut microbiome is a dynamic environment impacted by age, genetic makeup, surroundings, personal habits, and, predominantly, dietary choices (Yatsunenko et al., 2012). Dietary adjustments can lead to shifts in intestinal microflora, but the alterations are not permanent. The possibility of causing permanent changes in the gut microbiota through prolonged dietary modifications is unknown because of a lack of extensive studies on the human diet or extended short-term nutritional observations. It is suggested that regular dietary intake might significantly impact the gut microbiome more than immediate diet-related strategies (Gupta et al., 2021; Leeming et al., 2019). Due to geographical variations in dietary practices, the diversity in microbiota across different populations becomes evident. For instance, a comparison between pediatric groups following a Western diet and children in Burkina Faso, who adhere to a low-lipid, vegetable-rich diet with minimal animal proteins, revealed notable differences. The African population exhibited increased levels of *Prevotella* and xylanibacter, whereas the representation of shigella and Escherichia was notably lower. Changes in dietary intake can be noted without considering the age of the population. Additionally, one more study conducted for comparison of microbiome content on dietary intake with fiber-rich, less fat component and animal-extracted protein-rich diet displayed a change of microflora to bile-tolerant metabolism species, such as alistipes, biophilia and Bacteroides, and a reduction in firmicutes, especially roseburiain animal extracted diet consumers. Moreover, a diet with rich fiber leads to an increase in the *Bifidobacterium* genus.

9.2.2 DIETARY FIBERS, PROBIOTICS, PREBIOTICS AND METABOLIC DISORDERS

Dietary fiber supports the development of a healthy gut environment, enabling the flourishing of beneficial bacteria (eubiosis). This, in turn, reduces plasma, cholesterol and glucose levels (Riccardi and Rivellese, 1991). Following the consumption of dietary fiber, there was a notable increase in the abundance of various producers of short-chain fatty acid (SCFA), such as *Bifidobacterium, lachnospira, lactobacillus, echinococcus, akkermansia, faecal bacterium, Rosebery, Dorea and clostridium* (Mann and Cummings, 2009). Probiotics are a form of active microbes, prevailing as a food component and have beneficial impacts in regulating the body's microbial balance (Yoo and Kim, 2016). Prebiotics are unabsorbable dietary components, including oligosaccharides such as fructose, galactose and lactulose, and indigestible carbohydrates combined with probiotics, known as synbiotics. Research has shown that incorporating probiotics Visbiome® into the diet decreases fasting blood glucose levels and modifies the ratio of firmicutes/bacteroidetes in the intestinal microflora. This, in turn, plays a role in facilitating severe obesity in adolescents (Verma et al., 2021). Probiotics, particularly supplements like Biogen®, have been demonstrated to enhance metabolic disorders in individuals at risk of diabetes by modifying the microbiome. A randomised controlled trial shows that individuals with prediabetes experienced a reduction in HbA1C levels after receiving probiotics and synbiotics (Kassaian et al., 2018).

9.2.3 METABOLIC DISORDERS AND COMPOSITION OF GUT MICROBIOTA

Intestinal microflora help produce energy and control local or systemic immunity (Hur and Lee, 2015). Microbes are present almost everywhere in the body, but most microorganisms are in the gut microbiome. Moreover, the combined heritable material of the gut microflora, known as the microbiome, harbors 100 to 150 times more genes than our genome (Ashique et al., 2022; Qiao et al., 2013; Qin et al., 2010). The growth of microbes is initiated by birth in the gastrointestinal tract. The microbiota affects health by controlling nutritional metabolism and acting as a protective barrier against pathogens. (Bäumler and Sperandio, 2016), and signaling immune cells to modify immunity (Gensollen et al., 2016). The microbial makeup and variety vary significantly throughout the gastrointestinal tract. Substantial evidence indicates that firmicutes and Bacteroidetes significantly influence the microbiota composition within the human gastrointestinal system, with actinobacteria and proteobacteria contributing to a lesser extent. (David et al., 2014). Available research suggests that the intestinal microbiome directly leads to metabolic-associated diseases such as diabetes and obesity. Experimental mice(germ-free) showed protection against a diet with high-fat content (HFD)-causing obesity and imbalance of metabolism, owing to the reduction of fasting-induced adipose factor (Fiaf), a suppressant of lipoprotein lipase (LPL) (Bäckhed et al., 2007). Moreover, introducing intestinal microflora to germ-free mice from conventionally raised obese donors resulted in a notable elevation in fat content levels of the body and resistance to insulin in the recipient mice (Turnbaugh et al., 2008). Most human and murine gut bacteria are classified within the Bacteroides and Firmicutes phyla. Ob/ob mice deficient in leptin exhibited a simultaneous increase in firmicutes and reduction in Bacteroides compared to lean mice (Ley et al., 2005; Utzschneider et al., 2016). Gaining insight into the imbalances in gut microbiota associated with metabolic syndrome enhances our understanding of specific clinical situations. It presents promising new avenues for potential therapeutic targets that merit additional investigation. Figure 9.1 depicts the overall MetDs development.

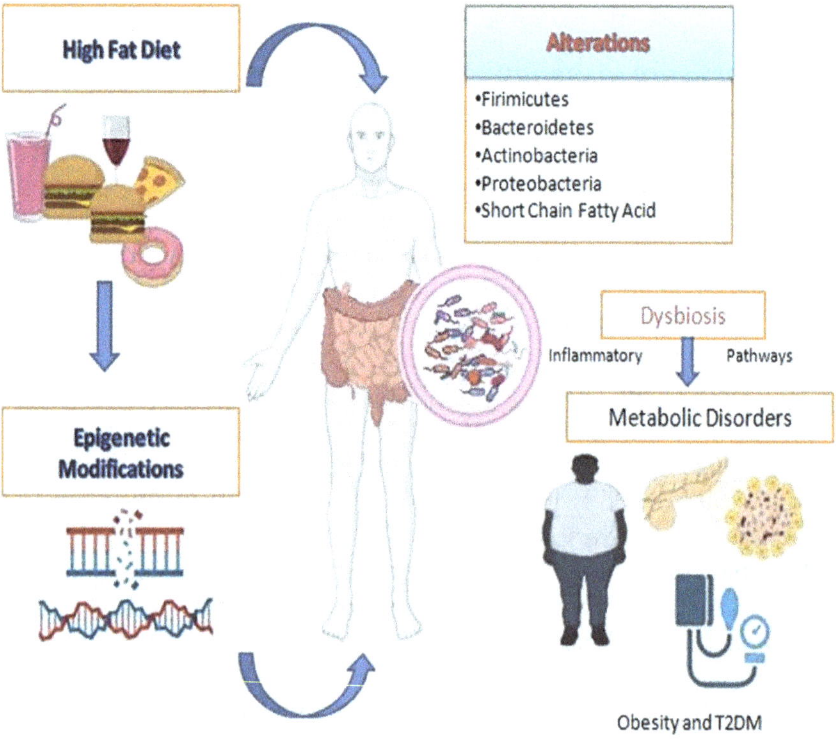

FIGURE 9.1 Depicts the overall MetDs development.

9.3 EPIGENETIC MECHANISMS IN METABOLIC DISORDERS

In addition to diet, the intestinal microflora framework is affected by external variables like lifestyle and medication, as well as internal factors like the immune system, metabolic regulations, and host genetics. Generally, external variables exert a more significant influence, with diet being the most extensively researched (Kaur et al., 2023; Rothschild et al., 2018). Genetics has a confined function in regulating the microbiome; according to a 2016 data analysis of 1120–30 twins, the level was 8.8% (Goodrich et al., 2016). Consequently, the specific arrangement of gut microbiota is personalized to each individual and develops throughout one's lifetime, starting from birth with a distinctive composition of bacterial taxa. (Maier and Typas, 2017). Evaluating genetic capabilities is essential to comprehend intestinal microorganisms' influence on well-being. A research project utilized metagenomic mapping based on Illumina assembly, analyzing 3.3 million unique microbial genes. The genes were extracted from 570–580 gigabases of sequence data obtained from 124 European fecal samples. This vast genetic configuration, approximately 150 times greater than genetic makeup, includes the most prevalent microbial genes in the group. It likely encompasses many prevalent genes found in the human intestinal microbiome. (Suau et al., 1999). The genes are extensively common across individuals in the group, with more than 99% originating from bacteria. This indicates that the entire cohort harbors a range of 1,000 to 1,150 prevailing species of bacteria, and each individual contains a minimum of 160 such species common in each person.

9.3.1 GUT MICROBIOTA AND EPIGENETICS AS EMERGING AREAS OF RESEARCH

Metabolic diseases pose a significant global threat, and exploring the intricate connections between dietary intake, intestinal microflora, and genetic profile holds promise for innovative approaches to treat these conditions. The interplay between dietary patterns, specific microbial species, and epigenetic factors influences the structure of the microbiome; furthermore, environmental variables shape dietary intake and epigenetics, an important role played by the gut microbiota. Microbiota-generated metabolites, particularly SCFAs, serve as epigenetic substrates, modifying chromatin structure. They impact the augmentation of metabolism-associated genes, reprogramming the host's transcriptome. The molecular intricacies of epigenetics encompass various processes, including DNA methylation, histone protein posttranslational modification, the inactivation of one of the X chromosomes in females, and genomic imprinting. Additionally, within the broader scope of epigenetics, non-coding RNAs, such as long non-coding RNA, small interfering RNA and microRNA, play significant roles (Paul et al., 2015).

9.3.2 DNA METHYLATION AND GUT-MICROBIOME

DNA methylation adds a methyl moiety to the fifth-position carbon on the cytosine pyrimidine ring. This modification primarily occurs in CpG islands, regions rich in cytosine guanine dinucleotides situated in the five 'ends of the regulatory position of most base pairs. Biocatalysts responsible for this process are termed DNA methyltransferases (DNMTs). Bacterial toxins induce metabolic alterations, including butyrate, folate, and acetate metabolites, further impacting epigenetic activity. For instance, folate, produced by bifidobacterium spp., provides essential for generating S-adenosylmethionine (SAM), a substrate that donates methyl groups to DNA methyltransferases (Mehta et al., 2022). The existence of 5hmC (5-hydroxymethylcytosine) at bivalent loci and DNase more sensitive regions suggests a dynamic process involving both the removal and renewed deposition of 5mC (5-methylcytosine) by DNMTs. Hence, DNA methylation is a continuous process; positional alterations in DNA methylation have been linked to several cancers. Changes in the chemical contributors for DNA alterations to histones rely on the microbiota's metabolic and nutrition functions (Paul et al., 2015).

9.3.3 NCRNAS AND GUT-MICROBIOME

Non-coding RNAs (ncRNAs) include ncRNAs, microRNAs (miRNAs), and small nucleolar RNAs. MiRNAs are tiny indigenous ncRNAs that play diverse physiological roles by supporting mRNA bases. They regulate genetic modulation after transcription, leading to mRNA deterioration inhibition. Ileal epithelial cells (IECs) in the ileum primarily secrete most miRNAs, eventually found in excretion. MiRNAs interact with the microbiome to regulate host gene expression post-transcriptionally. The modulation of gene expression, either upregulation or downregulation, occurs through the interaction between miRNAs and targeted mRNA within specific regions. Correspondently, the miRNAs and gut microflora regulate microbial cell gene transcripts through complementary nucleic acid sites targeted by miRNAs (Xu et al., 2014). Research has demonstrated that betaine influences the generation of metabolites, like SCFAs, by gut microbes, including akkermansiamuciniphila. Additionally, acetate and butyrate, a key aspect in mitigating metabolic-associated diseases, regulate the methylation level of the host's miR-378A/YY1 facilitator. Fecal microRNA distinctly impacts *Fusobacterium* nucleatum and *Escherichia coli* genetic transcription upon entry. Conversely, mice lacking IEC-miRNA (Dicer1ΔIEC) exhibit significant alterations in gut microbiota (Liu et al., 2016).

9.3.4 HISTONE ACETYLATION AND GUT-MICROBIOME

Acetylation is mainly linked to the activation of gene transcription; most acetylation sites are situated in the tail of histones on the N-terminal position. Lysine acetyltransferases (LATs), enzymes responsible for histone acetylation, facilitate the exchange of acetyl moiety from acetyl coenzyme A (acetyl-CoA) to lysine residues (Nε), simultaneously producing CoA. It increases the availability of nucleosomal DNA to transcription factors, thereby facilitating the process of transcription. The gut microbiome forms SCFAs for ATP production through the TCA cycle. Metabolites like butyrate and propionate, produced by the gut microbiome, can also inhibit histone deacetylases (HDACs). In the cytoplasm and nucleus, ATP citrate lyase (ACL) employs citrate from mitochondria to generate acetyl-CoA. In the cell nucleus, histone acetyltransferases (HATs) support the movement of acetyl groups to specific lysine residues from acetyl-CoA on histone proteins. On a global scale, various metabolites and cofactors, including short-chain fatty acids (SCFAs), SAM, Fe2+/Fe3+, Acetyl-CoA, alpha-ketoglutarate, and ATP, play a role in either inhibiting or promoting histone modifications (Mehta et al., 2022).

9.4 THERAPEUTIC APPROACHES

The interconnection between well-being, microbiome and nutritional intake is a highly promising and complex research topic. The microbiome is a continuously changing ecosystem that undergoes alterations throughout an individual's lifetime, influenced by their dietary habits. Tailored nutrition prescriptions require further investigation and the development of relevant standard guidelines (De Toro-Martín et al., 2017). It possesses substantial metabolic potential and can influence pharmacological targets and bioactive compounds. Despite the recognition that epigenetic modifications triggered by diverse dietary patterns act as a crucial component in regulating the communication within the host cells and microflora, there is still a limited understanding of the molecular and signaling pathways that underlie this interaction. Intrinsic microflora is a crucial factor that affects the body's epigenetic processes directly or indirectly. The low molecular weight molecules created by the intestine microbiome are involved in several pathogenic molecular signaling reactions and the causation of several diseases. While compared with regulatory dietary intake with low-fat, the clinical reports suggest the usage of the MedDiet interference and therapeutic strategy to prevent MetS (De Toro-Martín et al., 2017). However, randomized controlled trials (RCTs) investigating the impacts of a less-carbohydrate Mediterranean diet, which encourages the consumption of grains and protein extracted from plants in individuals with MetS, are necessary to establish the effectiveness of this dietary approach. Table 9.2 details the ongoing randomized clinical trials aiming for diseases and syndromes related to metabolism (Wu et al., 2023).

TABLE 9.2 Ongoing Clinical Trials Targeting Metabolic Diseases and Syndromes (Wu et al., 2023)

Disease	Drug	Status	NCT Number
DNMTi/ T2D	Hydralazine	Phase 3	NCT00000620
Obesity	Valproic acid	Phase 4	NCT00298857
Diabetes	sodium phenylbutyrate	Phase 4	NCT00533559
Diabetes, obesity	Sodium phenylbutyrate	-	NCT00771901
T2D	Curcumin	Phase 4	NCT01052597
T2D, obeisty	Curcumin	-	NCT03542240
Obesity, NAFLD	Curcumin	-	NCT03864783
T2D	Resveratrol	Phase 2	NCT02549924
NAFLD	Resveratrol	Phase 2/3	NCT02030977
Antisense oligonucleotide			
Diabetes	ISIS-GCGRRx	Phase 4	NCT02824003
T2D	ISIS-GCGRRx	Phase 2	NCT02583919
T2D, NAFLD	ISIS 703802	Phase 2	NCT03371355

9.5 CURRENT LIMITATIONS IN THE FIELD

The consensus is widespread that intestinal microflora affects metabolic well-being, and there has been a substantial rise in research specifically examining the relationship between the microbiome and metabolic diseases. The medical application of epigenetics holds significant promise, with the detection of numerous epigenetic prognostic markers and the advancement of certain drugs. Additionally, the potential for treating metabolic diseases is substantial through epigenetic editing. The application of bioinformatics facilitates rapid progress in the study of epigenetics, the availability of extensive publicly accessible datasets, and progress in technologies, including gene editing and high-throughput sequencing. Despite the numerous studies on epigenomic and metabolism disorders, several challenges remain unexplored. While chromatin remodeling is a significant aspect of epigenetic regulation, there is a limited focus on its role in metabolic diseases (Thakore et al., 2016). Drugs targeting DNA methylation and histone acetylation have been developed, but their application in clinical medicine is not widespread. Despite multiple studies on non-coding RNAs and other histone modifications, their clinical implementation remains limited. Notably, none of the epigenetic drugs developed so far have received approval for treating metabolic diseases. Additionally, there is a concern about potential adverse effects, as these drugs may inadvertently impact off-target genes (Altucci and Rots, 2016). While these approaches hold promise, their potential is currently constrained by gaps in the literature. There is a need for further exploration to establish formal connections between the gut community and diseases at the molecular level. Additionally, the safety of these approaches remains uncertain, as they could have both positive and negative effects depending on the clinical context and individual variations.

9.6 POTENTIAL FUTURE RESEARCH DIRECTIONS

A comprehensive analysis of epigenetic mechanisms in MetD is essential for generating innovative approaches and initiatives to prevent, diagnose, and treat such conditions. Given the difference in MetD, even minor individual changes can significantly affect the result. There is an urgent need to develop more epigenetic medications and related technologies designed explicitly for addressing metabolic diseases, requiring extensive cooperation. While this area shows significant promise, numerous challenges still need further exploration.

9.7 THE NEED FOR PERSONALIZED APPROACHES

Recent evidence supports the close interaction between metabolism and epigenetics, which is crucial in advancing metabolism-associated diseases. This two-way relationship could be the foundation for more intricate connections within organisms. Therefore, more fine-tuned research must be performed to reveal the epigenetic players affecting metabolism and vice versa. Identifying molecular pathways engaged in enzyme regulation of epigenetics will help to assist novel therapeutic practices for several metabolism-related disorders. Additionally, discoveries related to the epigenetic regulation of metabolism will unveil the unrealized potential for altering pathological disease conditions.

9.8 CONCLUSION

This chapter underscores that intestinal microflora undergoes continuous dynamic alterations. The formation of intestinal microflora is affected by dietary patterns and specific microbial species. The limited availability of medications that substantially impact long-term outcomes complicates choosing an appropriate therapy. In this scenario, exploring nutraceuticals, which are readily accessible and have minimal side effects, holds potential as a promising avenue for advancing innovative therapies. In addition to offering a comprehensive overview of the human gut microbiome on a global scale, the extensive gene catalogue we have compiled opens the door to future investigations into the correlation between microbial genes and human traits. Furthermore, this catalogue allows for broader examinations of human lifestyles, considering environmental factors such as diet from infancy to old age. The positive impact of balanced dietary intake on MetS appears to result from the cumulative effect of minor diet modifications instead of restricting specific nutrients. Hence, it is crucial to delve deeper into the investigation of the impact of epigenetic drugs on metabolic diseases. Furthermore, the diverse nature of histone modifications across various tissues necessitates additional research exploration. Additionally, there is a need for further studies to understand the interplay between the gut microbiome and the functioning of epigenetic modifications so that they play a beneficial role in the prevention of disease development.

KEYWORDS

- **diet**
- **DNA modification**
- **epigenetics**
- **gut Microbiota**
- **lifestyle**
- **metabolic disorders**
- **metabolic syndrome**

REFERENCES

Altucci, L., & Rots, M. G. (2016). Epigenetic drugs: From chemistry via biology to medicine and back. In *Clinical Epigenetics, 8*, 56. https://doi.org/10.1186/s13148-016-0222-5 (accessed on 28th June 2025).

Ashique, S., De Rubis, G., Sirohi, E., Mishra, N., Rihan, M., Garg, A., Reyes, R.-J., Manandhar, B., Bhatt, S., Jha, N. K., Singh, T. G., Gupta, G., Singh, S. K., Chellappan, D. K., Paudel, K. R., Hansbro, P. M., Oliver, B. G., & Dua, K. (2022). Short chain fatty acids: Fundamental mediators of the gut-lung axis and their involvement in pulmonary diseases. *Chemico-Biological Interactions, 368*, 110231. https://doi.org/10.1016/j.cbi.2022.110231 (accessed on 28th June 2025).

Bäckhed, F., Manchester, J. K., Semenkovich, C. F., & Gordon, J. I. (2007). Mechanisms underlying the resistance to diet-induced obesity in germ-free mice. *Proceedings of the National Academy of Sciences of the United States of America, 104*(3), 979–984. https://doi.org/10.1073/pnas.0605374104 (accessed on 28th June 2025).

Bäumler, A. J., & Sperandio, V. (2016). Interactions between the microbiota and pathogenic bacteria in the gut. *Nature, 535*(7610), 85–93. https://doi.org/10.1038/nature18849 (accessed on 28th June 2025).

Bhargava, S. K., Singh, T. G., Mannan, A., Singh, S., & Gupta, S. (2022). Pharmacological evaluation of *Thuja occidentalis* for the attenuation of nephropathy in streptozotocin-induced diabetes rats. *Obesity Medicine, 31*, 100391. https://doi.org/10.1016/j.obmed.2022.100391 (accessed on 28th June 2025).

Bhargava, S. K., Singh, T. G., Mannan, A., Singh, S., Singh, M., & Gupta, S. (2022). Pharmacological evaluation of *Thuja occidentalis* for the attenuation of neuropathy via AGEs and TNF-α inhibition in diabetic neuropathic rats. *Environmental Science and Pollution Research International, 29*(40), 60542–60557. https://doi.org/10.1007/s11356-022-20106-3 (accessed on 28th June 2025).

David, L. A., Maurice, C. F., Carmody, R. N., Gootenberg, D. B., Button, J. E., Wolfe, B. E., Ling, A. V., Devlin, A. S., Varma, Y., Fischbach, M. A., Biddinger, S. B., Dutton, R. J., & Turnbaugh, P. J. (2014). Diet rapidly and reproducibly alters the human gut microbiome. *Nature, 505*(7484), 559–563. https://doi.org/10.1038/nature12820 (accessed on 28th June 2025).

De Toro-Martín, J., Arsenault, B. J., Després, J.-P., & Vohl, M.-C. (2017). Precision nutrition: A review of personalized nutritional approaches for the prevention and management of metabolic syndrome. *Nutrients, 9*(8). https://doi.org/10.3390/nu9080913 (accessed on 28th June 2025).

Gensollen, T., Iyer, S. S., Kasper, D. L., & Blumberg, R. S. (2016). How colonization by microbiota in early life shapes the immune system. *Science (New York, N.Y.), 352*(6285), 539–544. https://doi.org/10.1126/science.aad9378 (accessed on 28th June 2025).

Goodrich, J. K., Davenport, E. R., Beaumont, M., Jackson, M. A., Knight, R., Ober, C., Spector, T. D., Bell, J. T., Clark, A. G., & Ley, R. E. (2016). Genetic determinants of the gut microbiome in UK twins. *Cell Host & Microbe, 19*(5), 731–743. https://doi.org/10.1016/j.chom.2016.04.017 (accessed on 28th June 2025).

Gupta, M., Krishan, P., Kaur, A., Arora, S., Trehanpati, N., Singh, T. G., & Bedi, O. (2021). Mechanistic and physiological approaches of fecal microbiota transplantation in the management of NAFLD. *Inflammation Research, 70*(7), 765–776. https://doi.org/10.1007/s00011-021-01480-z (accessed on 28th June 2025).

Hur, K. Y., & Lee, M.-S. (2015). Gut microbiota and metabolic disorders. *Diabetes & Metabolism Journal, 39*(3), 198–203. https://doi.org/10.4093/dmj.2015.39.3.198 (accessed on 28th June 2025).

Kassaian, N., Feizi, A., Aminorroaya, A., Jafari, P., Ebrahimi, M. T., & Amini, M. (2018). The effects of probiotics and synbiotic supplementation on glucose and insulin metabolism in adults with prediabetes: A double-blind randomized clinical trial. *Acta Diabetologica, 55*(10), 1019–1028. https://doi.org/10.1007/s00592-018-1175-2 (accessed on 28th June 2025).

Kaur, N., Kishore, L., Farooq, S. A., Kajal, A., Singh, R., Agrawal, R., Mannan, A., & Singh, T. G. (2023). *Cucurbita pepo* seeds improve peripheral neuropathy in diabetic rats by modulating the inflammation and oxidative stress in rats. *Environmental Science and Pollution Research International.* https://doi.org/10.1007/s11356-023-28339-6 (accessed on 28th June 2025).

Leeming, E. R., Johnson, A. J., Spector, T. D., & Le Roy, C. I. (2019). Effect of diet on the gut microbiota: Rethinking intervention duration. *Nutrients, 11*(12). https://doi.org/10.3390/nu11122862 (accessed on 28th June 2025).

Ley, R. E., Bäckhed, F., Turnbaugh, P., Lozupone, C. A., Knight, R. D., & Gordon, J. I. (2005). Obesity alters gut microbial ecology. *Proceedings of the National Academy of Sciences of the United States of America, 102*(31), 11070–11075. https://doi.org/10.1073/pnas.0504978102 (accessed on 28th June 2025).

Liu, S., da Cunha, A. P., Rezende, R. M., Cialic, R., Wei, Z., Bry, L., Comstock, L. E., Gandhi, R., & Weiner, H. L. (2016). The host shapes the gut microbiota via fecal microRNA. *Cell Host & Microbe, 19*(1), 32–43. https://doi.org/10.1016/j.chom.2015.12.005 (accessed on 28th June 2025).

Maier, L., & Typas, A. (2017). Systematically investigating the impact of medication on the gut microbiome. *Current Opinion in Microbiology, 39*, 128–135. https://doi.org/10.1016/j.mib.2017.11.001 (accessed on 28th June 2025).

Mann, J. I., & Cummings, J. H. (2009). Possible implications for health of the different definitions of dietary fibre. *Nutrition, Metabolism, and Cardiovascular Diseases, 19*(3), 226–229. https://doi.org/10.1016/j.numecd.2009.02.002 (accessed on 28th June 2025).

Mehta, V., Nagu, P., Inbaraj, B. S., Sharma, M., Parashar, A., & Sridhar, K. (2022). Epigenetics and gut microbiota crosstalk: A potential factor in pathogenesis of cardiovascular disorders. *[Manuscript]*, 1–21. https://doi.org/10.1038/s41392-023-01333-7 (accessed on 28th June 2025).

Park, J. H., Yoon, S. J., Lee, H., Jo, H. S., Lee, S. I., Kim, Y., Kim, Y. I., & Shin, Y. (2006). Burden of disease attributable to obesity and overweight in Korea. *International Journal of Obesity, 30*(11), 1661–1669. https://doi.org/10.1038/sj.ijo.0803321 (accessed on 28th June 2025).

Paul, B., Barnes, S., Demark-Wahnefried, W., Morrow, C., & Salvador, C. (2015). Influences of diet and the gut microbiome on epigenetic modulation in cancer and other diseases. *Clinical Epigenetics*, 1–11. https://doi.org/10.1186/s13148-015-0144-7 (accessed on 28th June 2025).

Qiao, Y., Sun, J., Ding, Y., Le, G., & Shi, Y. (2013). Alterations of the gut microbiota in high-fat diet mice is strongly linked to oxidative stress. *Applied Microbiology and Biotechnology, 97*(4), 1689–1697. https://doi.org/10.1007/S00253-012-4323-6 (accessed on 28th June 2025).

Qin, J., Li, R., Raes, J., Arumugam, M., Burgdorf, K. S., Manichanh, C., Nielsen, T., Pons, N., Levenez, F., Yamada, T., Mende, D. R., Li, J., Xu, J., Li, S., Li, D., Cao, J., Wang, B., Liang, H., Zheng, H., … Wang, J. (2010). A human gut microbial gene catalogue established by metagenomic sequencing. *Nature, 464*(7285), 59–65. https://doi.org/10.1038/nature08821 (accessed on 28th June 2025).

Riccardi, G., & Rivellese, A. A. (1991). Effects of dietary fiber and carbohydrate on glucose and lipoprotein metabolism in diabetic patients. *Diabetes Care, 14*(12), 1115–1125. https://doi.org/10.2337/diacare.14.12.1115 (accessed on 28th June 2025).

Rothschild, D., Weissbrod, O., Barkan, E., Kurilshikov, A., Korem, T., Zeevi, D., Costea, P. I., Godneva, A., Kalka, I. N., Bar, N., Shilo, S., Lador, D., Vila, A. V., Zmora, N., Pevsner-Fischer, M., Israeli, D., Kosower, N., Malka, G., Wolf, B. C., … Segal, E. (2018). Environment dominates over host genetics in shaping human gut microbiota. *Nature, 555*(7695), 210–215. https://doi.org/10.1038/nature25973 (accessed on 28th June 2025).

Sawicki, T., Ruszkowska, M., & Danielewicz, A. (2021). Factors, development, symptoms and diagnosis. *[Unspecified Source]*, 1–23. (accessed on 28th June 2025).

Seuring, T., Archangelidi, O., & Suhrcke, M. (2015). The economic costs of type 2 diabetes: A global systematic review. *PharmacoEconomics, 33*(8), 811–831. https://doi.org/10.1007/s40273-015-0268-9 (accessed on 28th June 2025).

Sharma, M., & Majumdar, P. K. (2009). Occupational lifestyle diseases: An emerging issue. *Indian Journal of Occupational and Environmental Medicine, 13*(3), 109–112. https://doi.org/10.4103/0019-5278.58912 (accessed on 28th June 2025).

Sharma, T., Kaur, D., Grewal, A. K., & Singh, T. G. (2021). Therapies modulating insulin resistance in Parkinson's disease: A cross talk. *Neuroscience Letters, 749*, 135754. https://doi.org/10.1016/j.neulet.2021.135754 (accessed on 28th June 2025).

Sharma, V. K., & Singh, T. G. (2020). Chronic stress and diabetes mellitus: Interwoven pathologies. *Current Diabetes Reviews, 16*(6), 546–556. https://doi.org/10.2174/1573399815666191111152248 (accessed on 28th June 2025).

Singh, R., Farooq, S. A., Mannan, A., Singh, T. G., Najda, A., Grażyna, Z., Albadrani, G. M., Sayed, A. A., & Abdel-Daim, M. M. (2022). Animal models of diabetic microvascular complications: Relevance to clinical features. *Biomedicine & Pharmacotherapy = Biomedecine & Pharmacotherapie, 145*, 112305. https://doi.org/10.1016/j.biopha.2021.112305 (accessed on 28th June 2025).

Singh, R., Rao, H. K., & Singh, T. G. (2020). Neuropathic pain in diabetes mellitus: Challenges and future trends. *Obesity Medicine, 18*, 100215. https://doi.org/10.1016/j.obmed.2020.100215 (accessed on 28th June 2025).

Suau, A., Bonnet, R., Sutren, M., Godon, J. J., Gibson, G. R., Collins, M. D., & Doré, J. (1999). Direct analysis of genes encoding 16S rRNA from complex communities reveals many novel molecular species within the human gut. *Applied and Environmental Microbiology, 65*(11), 4799–4807. https://doi.org/10.1128/AEM.65.11.4799-4807.1999 (accessed on 28th June 2025).

Thakore, P. I., Black, J. B., Hilton, I. B., & Gersbach, C. A. (2016). Editing the epigenome: Technologies for programmable transcription and epigenetic modulation. *Nature Methods, 13*(2), 127–137. https://doi.org/10.1038/nmeth.3733 (accessed on 28th June 2025).

Thomas, H., Diamond, J., Vieco, A., Chaudhuri, S., Shinnar, E., Cromer, S., Perel, P., Mensah, G. A., Narula, J., Johnson, C. O., Roth, G. A., & Moran, A. E. (2018). Global atlas of cardiovascular disease 2000–2016. *Global Heart*. https://doi.org/10.1016/j.gheart.2018.09.511 (accessed on 28th June 2025).

Thomas, M. S., Blesso, C. N., Calle, M. C., Chun, O. K., Puglisi, M., Fernandez, M. L., & Al, T. E. T. (2022). Dietary influences on gut microbiota with a focus on metabolic syndrome. *Metabolic Syndrome and Related Disorders, 20*(8), 429–439. https://doi.org/10.1089/met.2021.0131 (accessed on 28th June 2025).

Turnbaugh, P. J., Bäckhed, F., Fulton, L., & Gordon, J. I. (2008). Diet-induced obesity is linked to marked but reversible alterations in the mouse distal gut microbiome. *Cell Host & Microbe, 3*(4), 213–223. https://doi.org/10.1016/j.chom.2008.02.015 (accessed on 28th June 2025).

Utzschneider, K. M., Kratz, M., Damman, C. J., & Hullar, M. (2016). Mechanisms linking the gut microbiome and glucose metabolism. *The Journal of Clinical Endocrinology and Metabolism, 101*(4), 1445–1454. https://doi.org/10.1210/jc.2015-4251 (accessed on 28th June 2025).

Verma, A., Nelson, M. T., DePaolo, W. R., Hampe, C., & Roth, C. L. (2021). A randomized double-blind placebo-controlled pilot study of probiotics in adolescents with severe obesity. *Journal of Diabetes & Metabolic Disorders, 20*(2), 1289–1300. https://doi.org/10.1007/s40200-021-00855-7 (accessed on 28th June 2025).

Vieira, A. T., Teixeira, M. M., & Martins, F. S. (2013). The role of probiotics and prebiotics in inducing gut immunity. *Frontiers in Immunology, 4*(December), 1–12. https://doi.org/10.3389/fimmu.2013.00445 (accessed on 28th June 2025).

Wilson, A. G. (2008). Epigenetic regulation of gene expression in the inflammatory response and relevance to common diseases. *Journal of Periodontology, 79*(8 Suppl), 1514–1519. https://doi.org/10.1902/jop.2008.080172 (accessed on 28th June 2025).

Wu, Y., Lin, Z., Li, C., Lin, X., Shan, S., & Guo, B. (2023). Epigenetic regulation in metabolic diseases: Mechanisms and advances in clinical study. *[Manuscript]*, January. https://doi.org/10.1038/s41392-023-01333-7 (accessed on 28th June 2025).

Xu, W., San Lucas, A., Wang, Z., & Liu, Y. (2014). Identifying microRNA targets in different gene regions. *BMC Bioinformatics, 15*(7), S4. https://doi.org/10.1186/1471-2105-15-S7-S4 (accessed on 28th June 2025).

Yatsunenko, T., Rey, F. E., Manary, M. J., Trehan, I., Dominguez-Bello, M. G., Contreras, M., Magris, M., Hidalgo, G., Baldassano, R. N., Anokhin, A. P., Heath, A. C., Warner, B., Reeder, J., Kuczynski, J., Caporaso, J. G., Lozupone, C. A., Lauber, C., Clemente, J. C., Knights, D., … Gordon, J. I. (2012). Human gut microbiome viewed across age and geography. *Nature, 486*(7402), 222–227. https://doi.org/10.1038/nature11053 (accessed on 28th June 2025).

Yoo, J. Y., & Kim, S. S. (2016). Probiotics and prebiotics: Present status and future perspectives on metabolic disorders. *Nutrients, 8*(3). https://doi.org/10.3390/nu8030173 (accessed on 28th June 2025).

CHAPTER 10

Unveiling Phytoconstituents as Anti-Obesity Agents

AKHIL SHARMA,[1] SUSHMA DEVI,[1,*] THAKUR GURJEET SINGH,[1] SIMA SINGH,[2] and SANJANA MEHTA[1]

[1]*Chitkara College of Pharmacy, Chitkara University, Punjab, India*

[2]*Department of Pharmacy, University of Naples Federico II, Naples, Italy*

*Corresponding author

ABSTRACT

The abstract explores the emerging role of phytochemicals as novel anti-obesity agents, shedding light on their intricate mechanisms of action and potential therapeutic applications. Several essential phytochemicals have been identified as promising contributors to obesity management. Resveratrol, known for its presence in red grapes, exhibits anti-obesity effects by modulating adipogenesis and enhancing mitochondrial function. Curcumin, derived from turmeric, displays anti-inflammatory and antioxidant properties, impacting adipose tissue biology and lipid metabolism (Rohilla et al., 2023). Green tea catechins, particularly epigallocatechin gallate (EGCG), demonstrate thermogenic and fat-burning capabilities, influencing energy expenditure and lipid oxidation. Additionally, the abstract delves into the role of berberine in several medicinal plants in regulating adipokine secretion and insulin sensitivity, contributing to its anti-obesity potential. The synergistic effects of quercetin in various fruits and vegetables with adiponectin modulation and lipid metabolism regulation further highlight the multi-faceted nature of phytochemical interventions. The insights

Precision Nutrition and Endocrine Health: Synthesis, Characterization, and Applications.
Thakur Gurjeet Singh and Sanjana Mehta (Eds.)

DOI: 10.1201/9781998511877-10

presented provide a comprehensive understanding of the molecular mechanisms through which phytochemicals exert their anti-obesity effects, encompassing pathways such as adipogenesis, inflammation, and mitochondrial function. This knowledge forms the foundation for potential therapeutic strategies in obesity management. The abstract concludes by emphasizing the therapeutic promise of these phytochemicals, offering a nuanced approach to combatting obesity and its associated health risks.

10.1 INTRODUCTION

Obesity has become a significant global health issue in recent decades, presenting substantial challenges to public health systems around the world. This medical disorder is distinguished by an atypical accumulation of adipose tissue, which arises from a disparity between energy use and expenditure (Gupta et al., 2021; Lin and Li et al., 2021). As per the 2016 statistics provided by the WHO, about 1.6 billion people were categorized as overweight, and 650 million were identified as obese. The likelihood of developing diabetes, gallstones, hypertension, heart disease and stroke escalate with higher levels of overweight and obesity, mainly when the BMI is 35.0 or above. Even individuals in the upper range of healthy weight (BMI 22.0–24.9) demonstrated a dose-response connection with chronic diseases, highlighting the necessity of keeping a BMI between 18.5 and 21.9 (Garg et al., 2021; Sood et al., 2023).

The malfunction of adipose tissue plays a pivotal role in the development of obesity (Khan et al., 2024; Makkar et al., 2020). Adipose tissue is generally classified into two types: brown adipose tissue (BAT), which is found in particular regions of the adult human body, such as the mediastinal, supraclavicular, axillary, cervical, and upper abdominal regions, and white adipose tissue (WAT), which is found throughout the human body (Maurer et al., 2021; Mehta et al., 2021). Numerous mediators secreted by adipocytes play a significant role in controlling several physiological processes. For instance, TNF-α, IL-6, and IL-1β are linked to local inflammation connected to obesity, whereas leptin and adiponectin are implicated in the regulation of body weight (Bhargava et al., 2022; Foudah et al., 2022; Gómez-Hernández et al., 2016). WAT affects the metabolic activity in peripheral tissues and the brain by secreting adipocytokines like leptin and adiponectin (Kershaw and Flier et al., 2004). As a result, establishing a new regulatory capability for WAT seems to be a suitable strategy for combating obesity.

10.1.1 SIGNIFICANCE OF PHYTOCHEMICALS IN OBESITY MANAGEMENT

Although widely used medications for obesity have shown a certain degree of effectiveness in promoting weight loss, sustaining the therapeutic benefits over an extended period remains a pressing challenge in the management of obesity. After that, there have been accounts of unfavorable side effects, possibly stemming from the unfamiliar mechanisms of action and safety profiles of the diverse compounds in anti-obesity medications (Jakab et al., 2021; Kaur et al., 2023; Singh et al., 2022). Connecting metabolic disorders, an expanding array of herbal ingredients with enduring and diverse anti-obesity effects have been recognized. Anthocyanins sourced from blueberries, epigallocatechin gallate derived from green tea, nobiletin found in citrus peel, and curcumin extracted from turmeric are examples of dietary phytochemicals obtained from vegetables, fruits, and edible plants (Maniglia et al., 2021). In general, these natural compounds decrease the formation of lipids by impending adipocyte differentiation and adipogenesis. Additionally, they reduce triacylglycerol levels by either augmenting lipolysis or lowering lipogenesis pathways (Jakab et al., 2021).

Phytochemicals can combat obesity through diverse mechanisms, such as inhibiting the activity of digestive enzymes like pancreatic lipase and amylase, regulating appetite, restricting WAT development, and promoting WAT browning (Fu et al., 2016). Furthermore, the phytoconstituents present in plants have demonstrated various additional mechanisms of action against obesity, such as elevating PPAR-α and PPAR-γ expression, reducing ghrelin levels, and altering plasma lipid profile (Alkholifi et al., 2023; Mannan et al., 2021; Raoof and Kareem, 2020). Specific beneficial substances derived from fruits, vegetables, and edible plants, like curcumin from turmeric (Lee et al., 2009), have been studied. Blueberry anthocyanins, green tea epigallocatechin gallate, and citrus peel nobiletin have all been reported to be beneficial in treating metabolic illnesses (Chan et al., 2021). In general, these natural compounds usually inhibit the discrimination and adipogenesis of adipocytes and reduce triacylglycerol levels by either enhancing lipolysis or suppressing lipogenesis pathways (Sun et al., 2016). The chapter discusses different natural agents that affect the primary molecular pathways involved in WAT browning and the mechanisms of action associated with the antiobesity effect.

10.2 PHYTOCONSTITUENTS AS METABOLIC AND THERMOGENIC STIMULANTS

Phytoconstituents like caffeine, capsaicin, ephedrine and green tea have been tested as a possible aid in managing obesity. This is because they can boost energy expenditure and neutralize the drop-in metabolic rate often accompanying weight loss (Figure 10.1). Although belonging to the same group, the synergistic effect of caffeine and ephedrine aids in long-term weight loss. This is probably because two substances inhibit various enzymes that may have a synergistic effect. The first substance inhibits cAMP degradation caused by phosphodiesterase, while the second enhances catecholamine release in the sympathetic nervous system, thereby thrilling metabolism (Diepvens et al., 2007).

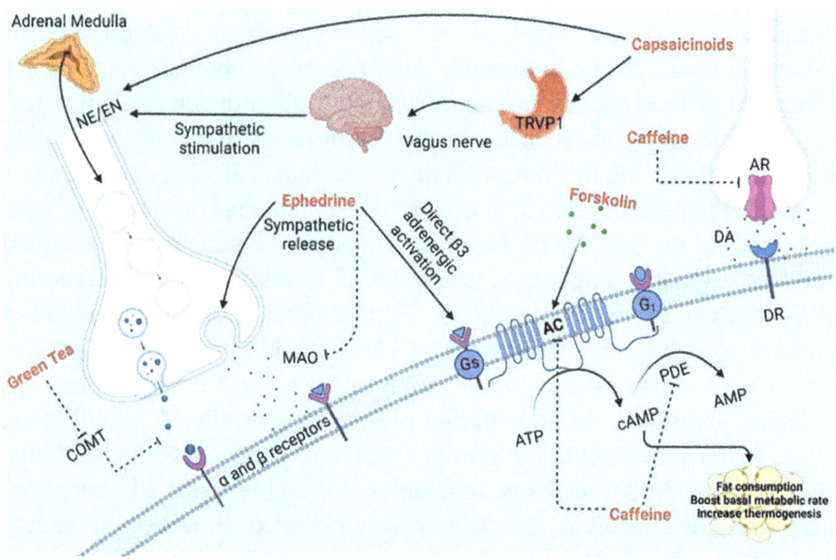

FIGURE 10.1 The impacts of phytoconstituents on metabolic and thermogenic stimulation physiological pathways. AC: adenylyl cyclase; AR: adenosine receptor; DA: dopamine; COMT: catechol-O-methyltransferase; EN: epinephrine; DR: dopamine receptors; MAO: monoamine oxidase; PDE: phosphodiesterase; TAPV1: transient receptor potential vanilloid-1; NE: norepinephrine.

10.2.1 *CAFFEINE*

Caffeine is the most used stimulant globally owing to its diverse effects and mechanism of action (Ferreira et al., 2019). The two most often utilized coffee beans within the Coffea genus are *Coffea arabica L.* and *Coffea canephora Pierre*. Studies have investigated the potential of caffeine as a thermogenic agent for reducing body weight. It is believed that caffeine may affect thermogenesis by inhibiting the breakdown of intracellular cAMP caused by phosphodiesterase (Diepvens et al., 2007). CYP1A2, an enzyme identified as a member of the cytochrome P450 oxidase family, catalyzes the hepatic conversion of caffeine into its three principal metabolites: theobromine (12%), paraxanthine (84%), and theophylline (4%) (Schwarzschild et al., 2003). Caffeine primarily acts by blocking adenosine receptors and modulating the purinergic system, owing to its structural similarities (Van Dam et al., 2020).

10.2.2 EPHEDRINE

Ephedrine is a constituent of *Ephedra sinica*, a plant native to China and Mongolia, and it exists as one of its four isomers. Constituting a sympathomimetic agent and phenylpropanolamine proto alkaloid, it functions as both a stimulant and a thermogenic agent (Stohs and Badmaev, 2016). According to many clinical researches, Ephedrine modulates energy expenditure and facilitates weight reduction. Ephedrine primarily causes thermogenesis by enhancing the release of norepinephrine and epinephrine from sympathetic neurons (Dulloo, 1993). Ephedrine's interaction with β-3 adrenergic receptors is connected to the stimulation of thermogenesis, which facilitates the breakdown of lipids and the regulation of glucose metabolism (Carey et al., 2015).

10.2.3 CAPSAICINOIDS

The hot red peppers of the *Capsicum annuum* L. species, also known as Capsicum frutescens, contain a compilation of solid compounds called capsaicinoids, with capsaicin being the most pungent compound (Barceloux et al., 2009). Research has indicated that capsaicin increases the adrenal medulla's synthesis of catecholamines, particularly norepinephrine and adrenaline. This then interacts with adrenergic receptors to stimulate thermogenesis (Ludy et al., 2012). Capsaicinoids, however, also can alter metabolism through the activation of TRVP1 (transient receptor potential) receptors. Encouraging catabolic processes in adipose tissues may improve energy expenditure and reduce body fat (Yoneshiro and Saito, 2013). Several studies on mice have shown that capsaicin and capsinoids promote thermogenesis via sympathetic activation in brown adipose tissue (BAT), which leads to decreased body fat (Saito et al., 2015). Research has shown that administering a single dose of capsaicin or capsinoids intraperitoneally can enhance body energy expenditure. Research conducted by Yoshioka et al. (1995) revealed that red pepper meals led to higher energy expenditure than control meals. Moreover, studies suggest capsaicin-induced thermogenesis likely depends on the activation of β-adrenergic receptors. The injection of capsaicin results in a rise in the mobilization of lipids and a decrease in the adipose tissue volume (Kawada et al., 1986).

10.2.4 FORSKOLIN

Forskolin is a labdane diterpene that is derived from the roots of the *Coleus forskohlii Briq* plant, which belongs to the Labiatae family (Lamiaceae) (Astell et al., 2013). Forskolin targets the adenylate cyclase enzyme, increasing cAMP levels and promoting lipolysis, breaking down fat in adipose tissues (Litosch et al., 1982). The release of fatty acids from the adipose tissue depot also regulates thermogenesis and promotes an amplification in lean tissue. In general, forskolin has the potential to cause a decrease in body fat while preserving muscle mass (Godard et al., 2005).

10.2.5 GREEN TEA EXTRACTS

Green tea, derived from the plant *Camellia sinensis* L. of the Theaceae family, is a drink mainly consumed in Southeast Asia (Thitimuta et al., 2017). Several studies have demonstrated that green tea and extracts can enhance thermogenesis and fat oxidation (Türközü and Tek, 2017). The thermogenic effect of green tea extract is attributed to the presence of catechins, including epicatechin, epicatechin gallate, epigallocatechin, and epigallocatechin gallate (EGCG). EGCG is the most abundant catechin, comprising 50% to 80% of the total catechins (Stohs and Badmaev, 2016). There is a hypothesis that catechins, particularly EGCG, have a direct inhibitory effect on catechol-O-methyltransferase, an enzyme responsible for the breakdown of norepinephrine. This inhibition is believed to increase the process of fat oxidation (Foudah et al., 2022). The temporary increase in activity of the sympathetic nervous system leads to higher levels of catecholamines, potentially boosting the mobilization and oxidation of fatty acids (Figure 10.1) (Behl et al., 2022; Devi et al., 2023). However, green tea can control the PPAR/FGF21/AMPK/UCP1 pathway, which improves the activation of thermogenic cells by modifying the first stage of adipocyte development (Bolin et al., 2020).

10.3 PHYTOCONSTITUENTS AS APPETITE REGULATORS

Food consumption is affected by the sensations of hunger and fullness, as well as the physiological processes that regulate eating about internal energy reserves and maintaining a consistent body weight (Sayan and Soumya, 2017). By selectively acting on the hypothalamus, a critical satiety region in the central nervous system, anorexic medications efficiently suppress appetite and promote weight loss. These medications alter critical pathways within the neuroendocrine System and the brain-gut axis. Several phytochemicals inhibit hunger, and specific appetite suppressants also facilitate white adipose tissue (WAT) browning, augmenting their efficacy in weight loss while mitigating the adverse effects frequently linked to pharmaceutical therapies.

10.3.1 KHAT EXTRACTS

Khat, produced from the leaves of the *Catha edulis* plant, is a natural stimulant found in East Africa and the Arabian Peninsula. It has effects similar to amphetamines. There is limited knowledge of the natural equivalent of "khat." The primary bioactive constituents of *C. edulis* are cathine (D-nor-pseudoephedrine) and cathinone (1-aminopropiophenone) (Tucci et al., 2010). A recent study has provided evidence that dopamine receptors influence the reduction of food intake caused by D-nor-pseudoephedrine (Fernandes et al., 2020). D-nor-pseudoephedrine has been proposed to possess comparable appetite-suppressing properties to other phenethylamine derivatives such as diethylpropion, phentermine, bupropion, and cathinone. Unsurprisingly, these medications are all structurally related to amphetamines and are expected to have similar effects through similar routes (Khan et al., 2012).

10.3.2 HOODIA GORDONII

An essential characteristic is that *Hoodia gordonii*, alternatively known as Kalahari cactus or Bushman's hat, is a prevalent dietary supplement comprising appetite suppressants derived from natural sources (Jain and Singh, 2013). Significant amounts of pregnane, oxypregnane, and steroidal glycosides are present in *H. gordonii* (Shukla et al., 2009). *Hoodigogenin A* is postulated to be the chemical responsible for augmenting adenosine triphosphate (ATP) levels in hypothalamus neurons that govern food intake while actively inhibiting appetite (Geoffroy et al., 2011; MacLean and Luo, 2004). While the ingestion of *H. gordonii* powder supplements, energy bars, and tea appears to induce appetite suppression and aid in weight reduction, this effect might be attributed in part to the notable adverse effects that accompany the administration of therapeutically relevant high doses (Smith and Krygsman, 2014).

10.3.3 CARALLUMA FIMBRIATA

Caralluma adscendens var. Fimbriata, also called *Caralluma fimbriata,* is widely distributed in the arid parts of Asia (Dutt et al., 2012). It is widely recognized as a food source during famine and a natural appetite reducer and thirst reliever (Kuriyan et al., 2007). The primary phytochemical components of C. fimbriata include pregnane glycosides, flavone glycosides, megastigmane glycosides, bitter principles, saponins, and several other flavonoids, as shown by research. Pregnane glycosides were identified by Bader et al. (2003). These chemicals are plentiful in plants and contribute to Caralluma's ability to reduce appetite (Schneider et al., 1993). The decrease in ghrelin synthesis in the stomach and neuropeptide Y in the hypothalamus is linked to the appetite-suppressing effects of C. fimbriata extract.

10.4 PHYTOCONSTITUENTS AS PANCREATIC LIPASE AND AMYLASE INHIBITORS

There is a widespread acknowledgement that prior use of pancreatic lipase is necessary to enzymatically degrade dietary fat in order for it to be subsequently absorbed from the gut (Rani et al., 2012). Given these facts, inhibiting certain digestive enzymes can be beneficial for addressing obesity, as depicted in Figure 10.2. Several digestive enzyme inhibitors found in plants have been documented in scientific literature. These include crude saponins from *Platycodi radix*, tea saponin, licochalcone A from *Glycyrrhiza uralensis* roots, dioscin from *Dioscorea nipponica*, and phenolic components from the leaves of *Nelumbo nucifera.*

10.4.1 STELLARIA MEDIA

Stellaria media (Linn.) Vill. (*Caryophylaceae*), Also well-known as "Chickweed," it is a popular salad herb that grows in the Himalayas (Sharma, 2003). This species is both edible and medicinal, and it contains significant amounts of β-carotenes, γ-linolenic acid, phenols, vitamins, and minerals. This species has an inhibitory impact on pancreatic α-amylase and lipase that varies depending on the dosage. As reported, *Stellaria media* had a more significant inhibitory effect on lipase than α-amylase (Rani et al., 2012).

10.4.2 ACHYRANTHES ASPERA

Achyranthes aspera Linn (*Amaranthaceae*), often referred to as apamarga, is a prolifically growing plant found in India and traditionally been utilised for its medicinal properties, including its antileprotic, purgative, emmenagogue, oestrogenic, diuretic, antispasmodic, antiarthritic, antimalarial, cardiotonic, antibacterial, and antiviral effects (Goyal et al., 2007). A study showed the impact of phenols, flavonoids, and saponins derived from A. aspera in weight reduction by blocking the enzymes lipases and amylases (Rani et al., 2012). The *in vitro* investigations conducted with extracts of Achyranthes aspera revealed a reduction in lipase and α-amylase activity dependent on the dosage. An additional high-fat diet (HFD) investigation It was observed that the extract significantly reduced the atherogenic index, hepatic total cholesterol, triglyceride, very low-density lipoproteins, and triglyceride levels, in addition to visceral organ weight indices and food efficiency ratio. The antidiabetic effects of A. aspera are primarily attributable to the saponins' antioxidant capabilities (Rani et al., 2012).

10.4.3 NELUMBO NUCIFERA

Nelumbo nucifera Gaertn., popularly known as lotus, remarkably, every component of the plant, such as its leaves, fruits, rhizomes, and seeds, may be consumed and has been used for several objectives, including the control of obesity (Mukherjee et al., 2009). A wide range of phytochemical groups, including alkaloids, flavonoids, megastigmanes, vitamins, and elemanolide sesquiterpenes, were extracted from *N. nucifera*. The use of *N. nucifera* leaves inhibited two primary actions: a) the activity of pancreatic lipases and b) the differentiation of T3-L1 preadipocytes. Benzylisoquinoline alkaloids, namely trans-N-coumaroyltyramine and trans-N-feruloyltyramine, appear responsible for inhibiting pancreatic lipases. However, the compounds 5,6-epoxy-3-hydroxy-7-megastigmen-9-one and annuionone D effectively inhibited the differentiation of adipocytes. This suggests that an epoxy moiety in their structures is essential for the antiadipogenic activity of megastigmanes, as stated by Ahn et al. (2013).

10.4.4 DIOSCOREA NIPPONICA MAKINO

Dioscorea nipponica makino is a perennial herbaceous plant from the Dioscoreaceae family, primarily distributed in northeastern, northern, eastern, and central regions of China. The compounds dioscin and diosgenin, saponins in the form of glycine and aglycone, were extracted from *D. nipponica*. Both compounds exhibited a time-dependent suppression of the elevation in blood triacylglycerol levels when administered orally with maize oil to mice, indicating their ability to block fat absorption. In an 8-week research, rats were given an HFD consisting of 40% beef tallow and 5% *D. nipponica*. Makino exhibited significantly lower body weight and fatty tissue accumulation than the control animals (Kwon et al., 2003).

10.4.5 PLATYCODI RADIX

The root of *Platycodon grandiflorum* known as *Platycodi Radix* is a highly abundant source of saponins, specifically platycosides, with intense biological activity. The *Platycodi Radix* extracts have been utilized in traditional oriental medicine and are associated with several biological advantages (Han et al., 2002b). Lee and Jeong (2002) utilized saponins derived from *Platycodi Radix* to prevent the occurrence of hypercholesterolemia and hyperlipidemia. In their study, (Han et al., 2002) examined the impact of crude saponins derived from *Platycodi Radix* on fat accumulation in mice fed HFD. Supplementing an HFD with either 10 or 30 g/kg of crude saponins resulted in decreased accumulation of fat in adipose tissue and reduced liver fat deposits. This effect is achieved by reducing the levels of blood triacylglycerol, which is likely caused by the blockage of the absorption of dietary fat in the intestines through the action of platycodin D. As reported research identified and isolated 10 triterpenoid saponins from Platycodi Radix, including platycodin A, C, D, and deapioplatycodin D. These compounds were found to reduce the absorption of dietary lipids in the intestines by inhibiting pancreatic lipase (Xu et al., 2005).

10.4.6 LICOCHALCONE A

Glycyrrhiza uralensis (Fisher) is a member of the Leguminosae family and is highly valued for its medicinal properties, including its antiviral and anti-tumor effects. The primary cause of these effects is usually attributed to glycyrrhizin, the primary bioactive component. Licochalcone Isolated from Glycyrrhiza uralensis, a substance that inhibits the action of pancreatic lipase in a reversible and non-competitive manner (Won-Licochalcone et al., 2007). Additionally, the research revealed that inhibition of pancreatic lipase led to the production of oleic acid from triolein, a natural substrate, and an artificial substrate known as 2,4-dinitrophenyl butyrate. Licochalcone A, obtained from *G. uralensis*, increased the expression of UCP-1 in 3T3-L1 adipocytes and induced the browning of inguinal white adipose tissue in obese mice (Lee et al., 2018). Some plant species contain phytochemicals or groups that can inhibit lipases and amylases, as shown in Figure 10.2.

10.5 PHYTOCONSTITUENTS IMPROVE INSULIN SENSITIVITY AND INDUCE HYPOGLYCEMIA

Multiple studies have shown that natural products can effectively improve insulin sensitivity and reduce insulin resistance, aiding in treating diabetes and other metabolic disorders. This can be accomplished by implementing calorie restriction and engaging in physical exercise. In addition, pharmaceutical drugs and natural substances that sensitize cells ultimately impede ATP synthesis in mitochondria (Alharthy et al., 2023; Sharma and Singh, 2020). These drugs enhance the sensitivity of cells to insulin by primarily

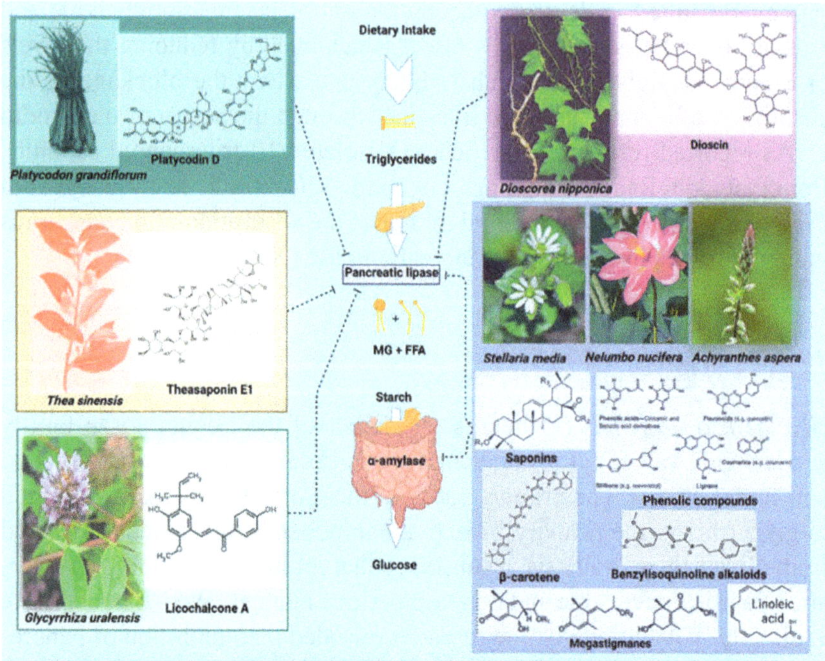

FIGURE 10.2 Some plant species contain phytochemicals or groups that can inhibit lipases and amylases. MG stands for mono glycerol, while FFA refers to free fatty acids.

targeting PPARγ, a regulator of several genes involved in the metabolism of glucose and lipids (Tan et al., 2022).

10.5.1 TRIGONELLA FOENUM-GRAECUM

Fenugreek *(Trigonella foenum-graecum)* originates in India and North America. It consists of steroidal sapogenins, including alkaloids, diosgenin, and furostanol glycosides such as trigonelline, trigocoumarin, trimethyl coumarin, and nicotinic acid (Wani and Kumar, 2018). Fenugreek extract has decreased insulin resistance and enhanced blood glucose control in individuals with diabetes (Gupta et al., 2001). The anti-hyperglycemic effects of this substance have been associated with enhancing the release of insulin and increasing insulin sensitivity (Puri et al., 2002), as well as inhibiting the digestion and absorption of carbohydrates in the intestines (Hannan et al., 2007). The fenugreek seeds are believed to provide anti-hyperglycemic characteristics due to the presence of steroids, saponins, alkaloids, and fiber (Snehlata and Payal, 2012). A clinical investigation conducted on a sample of 18 persons found that soaking fenugreek seeds in hot water resulted in a substantial reduction in fasting blood glucose, triglycerides, and very low-density lipoprotein cholesterol (VLDL-C) levels (Kassaian et al., 2009). In addition, trigonelline has shown significant promise in the treatment of obesity due to its involvement in the process of browning 3T3-L1 white adipocytes. Trigonelline injection significantly increased the expression of BAT hallmark proteins, such as PGC-1α, PRDM16, and UCP1, as well as the corresponding genes (*PPARGC1A*, *PRDM16*, and *UCP1*) in 3T3-L1 white adipocytes (Choi et al., 2021).

10.5.2 ALLIUM SATIVUM

Garlic (*Allium sativum*) is a multifaceted plant that comprises sulphur compounds, amino acids, vitamins, and minerals, among others. Several sulfuric compounds, including diallyl sulphide, diallyl disulphide, and diallyl trisulfide, rapidly decompose into other sulphur compounds, including allicin, which is among the sulphur-containing molecules present in garlic (Zhang et al., 2020). The potential therapeutic effects of S-allyl cysteine and diallyl disulphide on blood glucose, lipid profile, and insulin levels are unknown (Behera et al., 2023). The efficacy of garlic in treating hyperglycemia has been examined through various studies. In a study, it was observed that garlic led to a reduction in serum fructosamine, triglycerides, and fasting blood glucose levels. Garlic is believed to enhance hyperglycemia by promoting insulin production and improving insulin sensitivity (Liu et al., 2005). In 3T3-L1 cells, the garlic extracts reduced the expression of several genes involved in lipid metabolism at the molecular and genetic levels. These genes included PPAR-γ, CCAAT/enhancer-binding proteins a and b, acetyl-CoA carboxylase, fatty acid synthase, sterol regulatory element binding protein 1c, diacylglycerol acyltransferase 1, and perilipin-1. Furthermore, when garlic scape extract was administered during cellular growth, higher levels of carnitine palmitoyl transferase-1α and hormone-sensitive lipase were seen together with the activation of AMPK and its subsequent proteins (Balogun and Kang, 2022). It has been observed that the active component (1R,3S)-1-methyl-1,2,3,4-tetrahydro-β-carboline-3-carboxylic acid, which was extracted from garlic, inhibits the differentiation of adipocytes in 3T3-L1 preadipocytes. This is accomplished by inhibiting cytoskeleton remodeling, an essential process for adipogenesis (Baek et al., 2019).

10.5.3 *ZINGIBER OFFICINALE*

Zingiber officinale Roscoe, is a member of the Zingiberaceae family and main active components are phenolic and terpene chemicals, specifically gingerols, which are changed to shogaols by heat and lengthy storage (Khandouzi et al., 2015; Stoner, 2013). The administration of gingerol in mice resulted in an augmentation of adipocyte differentiation, leading to better insulin sensitivity and glucose absorption. Consequently, gingerol is expected to have potential benefits in managing diabetes (Sekiya et al., 2004). In a research study, 2% ginger showed significantly elevated insulin levels in their blood and improved ability to tolerate glucose (Islam and Choi, 2008) in HFD rats. In addition, ginger nanoparticles can prevent insulin resistance by restoring the homeostasis of the transcription factor Foxa2 in the gut epithelia (Kumar et al., 2022). In addition, when compared to gingerols and 6-shogaol, gingerenone A exhibited a more potent inhibitory impact on adipogenesis and lipid accumulation in 3T3-L1 preadipocyte cells. Moreover, gingerenone A has the potential to modify the metabolism of fatty acids in living organisms by activating AMPK, which can reduce the occurrence of obesity caused by food 6-shogaol and 6-gingerol elevated the expression of the peroxisome proliferator-activated receptor δ (PPAR-δ)-dependent genes in cultured skeletal muscle myotubes, leading to an enhancement in cellular fatty acid catabolism (Mao et al., 2019).

10.5.4 *CROCUS SATIVUS*

The plant species is known as *Crocus sativus*. Linn belongs to the Iridaceae family, and its desiccated stigmas have historically been utilized as a spice or culinary component (Kang et al., 2012). Saffron has a rich historical background as a medical substance, and its extracts contain powerful carotenoids such as crocin and its aglycone crocetin, as well as the monoterpene glycoside picrocrocin and safranal. These compounds have pharmacological effects on many disorders (Rios et al., 1996). In a clinical trial involving type II diabetes patients, saffron significantly reduced fasting blood glucose and TNF-α serum levels. Additionally, there was a downregulation of TNF-α and IL-6 mRNA expression. (Mobasseri et al., 2020a). The study found that eight-week daily saffron supplementation substantially reduced fasting blood glucose levels (Milajerdi et al., 2018). In placebo-controlled randomized clinical research showed that 15 mg of oral crocin daily resulted in a substantial reduction in HbA1C levels in diabetic patients compared to the control placebo groups (Sepahi et al., 2018). Saffron is thought to improve the treatment of diabetes by enhancing insulin sensitivity, stimulating insulin signaling pathways, improving β-cell activities, promoting the expression of glucose transporter type 4 (GLUT-4), regulating oxidative stress, and repressing inflammatory pathways (Mobasseri et al., 2020b).

10.5.5 GINSENG

Ginseng comes under the genus Panax; Ginsenosides are the main constituents of ginseng that show a variety of pharmacological actions (Attele et al., 1999). Research studies have indicated that ginseng can be an alternative therapy for T2DM due to its ability to decrease insulin resistance and fasting blood glucose levels significantly. Ginseng may lower blood glucose levels by enhancing insulin production, protecting pancreatic islets, improving insulin sensitivity, and promoting glucose absorption (Xie et al., 2011). Specifically, ginseng and ginsenosides reduce energy consumption and enhance energy expenditure by stimulating the AMPK pathway. Furthermore, a study discovered that black ginseng substantially increased brown adipocyte markers (*UCP1*, *PRDM16*, and *PGC-1*) levels in 3T3-L1 cells and primary white adipocytes. The study found that treating ginsenoside Rb1 increased the expression of brown adipocyte markers in 3T3-L1 cells and primary white adipocytes in a dose-dependent manner (Park et al., 2019). Enhancing insulin sensitivity and inducing browning of WAT through the chemical elements found in ginseng can effectively enhance weight reduction and prevent obesity.

10.5.6 ESSENTIAL OILS FROM THE GENUS CINNAMOMUM

Cinnamon, a spice, is obtained from the bark of Cinnamomum plants, which are classified under the Lauraceae family. Such species as Cinnamomum zeylanicum and Cinnamomum cassia are included. Cinnamon's principal components consist of volatile oils extracted from the stems, leaves, and roots of Cinnamon zeylanicum and Cinnamon cassia (Alkholifi et al., 2023). The leaf oil contains eugenol, whereas the root-bark oil is predominantly camphoric. Additionally, the bark oil comprises cinnamaldehyde. The dehydrated stem bark of C. cassia was utilized to extract four distinct oils: coumarin, cinnamaldehyde, cinnamic acid, and cinnamyl alcohol (Devi et al., 2023). Cinnamon possesses both traditional and culinary applications and exhibits antioxidant, anti-inflammatory, antibacterial, and anticancer effects (Cao et al., 2008; Hariri and Ghiasvand, 2016). Cinnamon enhances the body's insulin sensitivity and positively impacts metabolism (Couturier et al., 2010). Compared to conventional therapy alone, cinnamon decreased haemoglobin A1c (*HbA1C*) levels by 0.83%, according to a randomized, controlled clinical study. HbA1C levels in individuals with type 2 diabetes mellitus (*T2DM*) were reduced by 0.37% when conventional medication was used in isolation (Crawford et al., 2009). Furthermore, Kwan et al. observed that the treatment of cinnamon extract induced browning in subcutaneous adipocytes derived from obese mouse models, as elaborated in their study. An increase in the levels of UCP1 and other brown adipocyte-specific markers on subcutaneous and 3T3-L1 adipocytes distinguished the WAT browning process. Moreover, introducing cinnamon extract into the body increases the synthesis of proteins within the mitochondria (Kwan et al., 2017).

10.5.7 CAPSAICIN

Capsaicin, the primary compound in chilli peppers, is commonly used as a spice. It activates transient receptor potential vanilloid channel 1 (TRPV1) (Saito et al., 2015). The receptor has a crucial function in regulating metabolic syndrome, which is characterized by the presence of insulin resistance and obesity and is linked with an elevated risk of developing cardiovascular disease, T2DM, and non-alcoholic fatty liver disease (Panchal et al., 2018). Activating the TRPV1 protein receptor by capsaicin can control the process of adipocyte thermogenesis. This activation also influences the functioning of metabolic modulators such as AMPK, PPARα, UCP1, and GLP-1 (Panchal et al., 2018). Capsaicin improves insulin sensitivity, promotes fat oxidation, and decreases body fat, all of which positively affect liver and heart health. According to Aryaeian et al.

(2017), it was shown to help treat diabetic neuropathy and possesses qualities that reduce inflammation and diabetes. The study conducted by Hsu and Yen in 2007 discovered that capsaicin reduces the buildup of lipids in 3T3-L1 adipocytes by lowering the expression of PPARγ, C/EBPα, and leptin proteins. However, it also increases the production of adiponectin.

10.5.8 URSOLIC ACID

The pentacyclic triterpene ursolic acid (3β-hydroxy-12-urs-12-en-28-oic acid) is extensively recognized in conventional Chinese medicine. The primary sources of ursolic acid include malus pumila, Ocimum basilicum, Vaccinium macrocarpon, Olea europaea, Origanum vulgare, Thymus vulgaris, etc. (Ikeda et al., 2008). Ursolic acid (0.05% w/w) affected blood glucose levels and improved insulin sensitivity and glucose intolerance in rats with diabetes, according to the study. An alternative strategy has been proposed to preserve pancreatic β-cells and elevate insulin levels (Jang et al., 2009). The activity of protein tyrosine phosphatase 1B (PTP1B), an enzyme implicated in inhibiting the insulin receptor, is impeded by sulfuric acid. This inhibition results in a proliferation of insulin receptors and an augmentation in the number of operational receptors in response to hypoglycemia stimuli (Jung et al., 2007).

10.5.9 CINNAMIC ACID

Cinnamic acid is primarily derived from several sources such as cinnamon, Presl, citrus fruits, *Vitis vinifera, Camellia sinensis, Theobroma cacao, Apium graveolens, Spinacia oleracea, brassica,* etc. (Adisakwattana, 2017; Devi and Singh, 2017). Cinnamic acid and its derivatives exhibit significant efficacy in treating diabetes, its associated problems, and several other biological functions. Cinnamon extract enhances glucose and lipid metabolism control through the activation of PPAR. This can potentially lead to improvements in hyperglycemia and hyperlipidemia, increased insulin sensitivity, and reduced blood and hepatic lipids (Kim and Choung, 2010). Lee et al. (2022) evaluated the influence of cinnamic acid on obesity and its effects on inflammation in peripheral and hypothalamic regions, metabolic profiles, and inflammatory responses associated with macrophages in mice fed an HFD. Cinnamic acid in the diet decreases obesity and its related symptoms, including fat buildup in the epididymis, insulin resistance, glucose intolerance, and abnormal cholesterol levels (Lee et al., 2022). In addition, cinnamic acid decreased the accumulation of fat, TNF-α, and the infiltration of macrophages in the liver and adipose tissue generated by an HFD. In addition, cinnamic acid decreased the levels of Ly6chigh monocytes, M1 adipose tissue macrophages, and hypothalamus microglial activation. The results suggest that cinnamic acid hinders the inflammatory monocyte/macrophage system in the peripheral and hypothalamic regions, improving metabolic issues related to obesity.

10.5.10 RESVERATROL

Resveratrol, a polyphenolic compound known for its anti-inflammatory and antioxidant properties, has been found in various species of plants, including *Polygonum cuspidatum, Arachis hypogaea, Veratrum grandiflorum, V. vinifera*, and *Vaccinium oxycoccos* (Bishayee et al., 2010). Resveratrol shows excellent potential as a beneficial agent for treating diabetes and other serious diseases. It works in different ways, such as improving insulin sensitivity, promoting the movement of GLUT4, reducing oxidative stress, regulating enzymes involved in carbohydrate metabolism, activating critical signaling pathways mediated by SIRT1 and AMPK, and potentially reducing the expression of genes related to fat cell formation (*adipogenic* genes) (Bagul and Banerjee, 2015). Resveratrol regulates blood sugar levels via activating mitochondrial sirtuin proteins. These proteins govern the metabolic processes of carbohydrates and lipids, substantially influencing the body's energy production at different stages. This is accomplished by augmenting the thermogenesis mechanisms, which elevate energy expenditure by incinerating more adipose tissue (Moshawih et al., 2019).

10.5.11 PROCYANIDINS

Procyanidins are the main flavonoids, commonly referred to as flavan-3-ols, within the proanthocyanidins (Aron and Kennedy, 2008). Oligomeric structures are created by polymerization by combining 2 to 10 subunits of the monomeric flavanols catechin and epicatechin. Procyanidins may be found in several legumes, fruits, grains, vegetables, and nuts, including *Malus domestica, Prunus domestica, Prunus salicina, V. vinifera, Prunus amygdalus*, and *Cicer arietinum* (Bahrin et al., 2022; Rue et al., 2018).

Research has examined the impact of various types of procyanidins on GLP-1. Proanthocyanidins raised the levels of active GLP-1 in healthy people, resulting in a significant reduction in blood glucose levels. Furthermore, the Injection of an additional derivative of procyanidins, cinnamtannin A2, enhances the production of insulin and active GLP-1 in fasting healthy mice (Törrönen et al., 2012; Yamashita et al., 2013). Additionally, it promotes the growth of β-cell mass via stimulating cell division, reducing cell death, and enhancing β-cell specialization. Procyanidin has been identified as a probable target for enteroendocrine cells, including L-cells. According to González-Abuín et al. (2015), these substances have decreased the harm the diet produces, improving glycemic status and insulin sensitivity in models of insulin resistance generated by fructose or high-fat consumption.

10.5.12 MANGIFERIN

Mangiferin (MF) is a glucosylxanthone found in the mango tree (*Mangifera indica*) and demonstrated that it possesses antioxidant activities, anti-diabetic, anti-cancer, antiviral and anti-aging (Dar et al., 2005). Research findings demonstrated that MF enhanced the phosphorylation of AMPK in 3T3-L1 cells, pancreatic β-cell mass, and glucose and insulin uptake (Han et al., 2015). In order to clarify the mechanism by which mangiferin reduces insulin resistance, Qiao Zhang and their colleagues promoted the buildup of lipids in HepG2 and C2C12 cell lines by using palmitic acid (Zhang et al., 2019). The results indicated that MF greatly enhanced the absorption of insulin-driven glucose and substantially reduced the amount of glucose in HepG2 and C2C12 cells. This was due to the increased expression of phosphorylated protein kinase B (*AKT*), GLUT2, and GLUT4 proteins. MF also markedly decreased intracellular FFA and lipid accumulations while enhancing FFA uptake. MF enhanced the rate of fatty acid oxidation and raised the activity of the PPAR protein and its downstream proteins, CD36 and CPT1, which are involved in the metabolism of fatty acids in HepG2 and C2C12 cells. In an experimental setting using isolated cells, administering mangiferin orally at a 20 mg/kg dose enhanced insulin responsiveness in diabetic rats. MF changes the body's fat levels, decreases the quantity of adipokine, and mitigates inflammation and the development of metabolic syndrome (Saleh et al., 2014).

10.6 PHYTOCONSTITUENTS INHIBITING ADIPOGENESIS AND INDUCING ADIPOCYTES APOPTOSIS

Adipogenesis refers to converting preadipocytes into adipocytes by halting the growth of preadipocytes, collecting lipid droplets, and generating fully developed adipocytes with specific morphological and biochemical characteristics (Ghaben and Scherer, 2019). C/EBPα and PPARγ are the primary transcriptional regulators of adipogenesis, playing a crucial role in producing many functional proteins in adipocytes. Leptin and TNF-α are the two most notable adipokines that natural compounds can effectively address (Zhang and Huang, 2012). Natural compounds and phytochemicals that influence enzymes or pathways associated with appetite or fullness might indirectly impact adipogenesis and induce apoptosis, ultimately reducing obesity. Various natural compounds, such as EGCG, genistein, berberine, esculetin, resveratrol, capsaicin, baicalein, and procyanidins, have demonstrated the ability to hinder the formation of fat cells, as evidenced by multiple research investigations. The protein expression of PPAR and C/EBP was reduced in adipocytes treated with genistein, berberine, and rhein (Rayalam et al., 2008).

10.6.1 GENISTEIN

Genistein, an isoflavone initially found and extracted from the *Genista tinctoria* plant, has decreased C/EBPβ inhibition and PPARγ activation via the Wnt/β-catenin pathway. Moreover, it controls the transcriptional activity of PPAR by stimulating AMPK during adipogenesis. This suggests that genistein can be a potent agent against obesity (Harmon et al., 200; Mukund et al., 2017).

10.6.2 BERBERINE

Berberine is the main constituent found in Cortidis rhizome and is known for its antibacterial properties, which are employed in traditional Chinese medicine. The mechanism of Berberine demonstrates its ability to inhibit the differentiation, proliferation, and accumulation of lipids in 3T3-L1 adipocytes. These effects can arise from several biological targets and complex pathways, including the suppression of PPARγ and PPARα trans-activation's, as well as the inhibition of mRNA and protein production of early transcription factors C/EBPβ, PPARγ, and PPARα (Huang et al.,

2006). Berberine further triggers the activation of AMPK and promotes the stimulation of PGC-1α, resulting in the induction of UCP1 expression associated with browning (Zhang et al., 2014).

10.6.3 ESCULETIN

In addition, Esculetin is a dihydroxy coumarin obtained from natural sources, with the majority of its extraction occurring from the trunk bark and twig skin of the Chinese plant Fraxinus rhynchophylla Hance (Zhang et al., 2022). By inhibiting the proliferation of cells, esculetin, also known as 6,7-dihydroxy-2H-1-benzopyran-2-one, exerts its effect. This causes programmed cell death in immature and adult fat cells and prevents fat cell formation in 3T3-L1 immature fat cells. According to a study conducted by Yang et al. in 2006, esculetin effectively prevented the formation of fat cells (adipocytes) in 3T3-L1 cells by reducing the buildup of lipids. This effect was seen to be dependent on the dosage of esculetin.

10.6.4 DELPHINIDIN

Delphinidin, an anthocyanin found in colored fruits and vegetables, has been shown to hinder the formation of fat cells by suppressing markers of fat cell formation and fat production, preventing the buildup of lipids, and enhancing the activity of genes involved in fatty acid metabolism. This was demonstrated in laboratory experiments conducted by Park et al. (2019).

10.6.5 BAICALEIN

Moreover, baicalein, an essential flavonoid in *Scutellaria baicalensis* (*Chinese Skullcap*), has been associated with several biological functions. The ability of baicalein to enhance the production of cyclooxygenase-2 (*COX-2*), which is typically suppressed throughout the process of adipogenesis, may elucidate its anti-adipogenic effects (Cha et al., 2006).

10.6.6 RHEIN

Rhein, a naturally occurring anthraquinone, has various advantageous therapeutic uses. The compound is extracted from the rhizomes of medicinal plants such as *Rheum undulatum*, *Rheum palmatum*, and *Cassia reticulata*

(Huang et al., 2021). Rhein was observed to significantly decrease PPARγ and C/EBPα protein levels and mRNA levels in 3T3-L1 cells treated with differentiation medium (Liu et al., 2011). Recent work by (Huang et al., 2021) found that treating cells with rhein during the mitotic clonal expansion stage resulted in a deceleration of 3T3-L1 differentiation. This was accompanied by a significant reduction in the formation of lipid droplets and the expression of adipocyte genes. Additionally, it was shown that Rhein inhibits the growth of 3T3-L1 adipocytes in a manner dependent on both the dosage and duration of exposure.

10.7 CONCLUSION

Obesity has extended its impact beyond mere physical appearance. It is now acknowledged as a medical problem that needs treatment in order to reduce the likelihood of acquiring additional metabolic disorders such as diabetes. Marketed anti-obesity drugs utilize many techniques to achieve their effects. These include suppressing appetite by boosting norepinephrine, dopamine, and serotonin levels in the spaces between nerve cells, inhibiting pancreatic lipase and amylase enzymes, and slowing down the stomach-emptying process. Phytochemicals obtained from plants appear to be a viable reservoir of anti-obesity medications, as many of them provide advantages through similar processes while causing fewer adverse effects. Remarkably, several natural substances also exhibit other significant characteristics that may be crucial as anti-obesity medications, including the promotion of white adipose tissue browning, stimulation of thermogenesis and induction of adipocyte death, and prevention of adipogenesis.

KEYWORDS

- **adipogenesis inflammation**
- **antioxidants**
- **metabolism**
- **mitochondrial dysfunction**
- **obesity**
- **resveratrol**

REFERENCES

Adisakwattana, S. (2017). Cinnamic acid and its derivatives: Mechanisms for preventing and managing diabetes and its complications. *Nutrients, 9*(2), 163. https://doi.org/10.3390/nu9020163 (accessed on 28th June 2025).

Ahn, J. H., Kim, E. S., Lee, C., Kim, S., Cho, S. H., Hwang, B. Y., et al. (2013). Chemical constituents from *Nelumbo nucifera* leaves and their anti-obesity effects. *Bioorganic & Medicinal Chemistry Letters, 23*(12), 3604–3608. https://doi.org/10.1016/j.bmcl.2013.04.013 (accessed on 28th June 2025).

Alharthy, K. M., Balaha, M. F., Devi, S., Altharawi, A., Yusufoglu, H. S., Aldossari, R. M., ... & Di Giacomo, V. (2023). Ameliorative effects of isoeugenol and eugenol against impaired nerve function and inflammatory and oxidative mediators in diabetic neuropathic rats. *Biomedicines, 11*(4), 1203. https://doi.org/10.3390/biomedicines11041203 (accessed on 28th June 2025).

Alkholifi, F. K., Devi, S., Alam, A., Kamal, M., & Yusufoglu, H. S. (2023). Caraway oil as a multimodal therapy for neuropathic pain: Investigating the mechanisms of action in rats with chronic constriction injury. *Applied Sciences, 13*(5), 2989. https://doi.org/10.3390/app13052989 (accessed on 28th June 2025).

Alkholifi, F. K., Devi, S., Yusufoglu, H. S., & Alam, A. (2023). The cardioprotective effect of corosolic acid in the diabetic rats: A possible mechanism of the PPAR-γ pathway. *Molecules, 28*(3), 929. https://doi.org/10.3390/molecules28030929 (accessed on 28th June 2025).

Aodah, A. H., Devi, S., Alkholifi, F. K., Yusufoglu, H. S., Foudah, A. I., & Alam, A. (2023). Effects of taraxerol on oxidative and inflammatory mediators in isoproterenol-induced cardiotoxicity in an animal model. *Molecules, 28*(10), 4089. https://doi.org/10.3390/molecules28104089 (accessed on 28th June 2025).

Aron, P. M., & Kennedy, J. A. (2008). Flavan-3-ols: Nature, occurrence and biological activity. *Molecular Nutrition & Food Research, 52*(1), 79–104. https://doi.org/10.1002/mnfr.200700137 (accessed on 28th June 2025).

Aryaeian, N., Sedehi, S. K., & Arablou, T. (2017). Polyphenols and their effects on diabetes management: A review. *Medical Journal of the Islamic Republic of Iran, 31*, 134. https://doi.org/10.14196/mjiri.31.134 (accessed on 28th June 2025).

Astell, K. J., Mathai, M. L., & Su, X. Q. (2013). A review of botanical species and chemical compounds with appetite-suppressing properties for body weight control. *Plant Foods for Human Nutrition, 68*(3), 213–221. https://doi.org/10.1007/s11130-013-0361-1 (accessed on 28th June 2025).

Attele, A. S., Wu, J. A., & Yuan, C.-S. (1999). Ginseng pharmacology: Multiple constituents and multiple actions. *Biochemical Pharmacology, 58*(11), 1685–1693. https://doi.org/10.1016/s0006-2952(99)00212-9 (accessed on 28th June 2025).

Bader, A., Braca, A., De Tommasi, N., & Morelli, I. (2003). Further constituents from *Caralluma negevensis*. *Phytochemistry, 62*, 1277–1281. https://doi.org/10.1016/s0031-9422(02)00678-7 (accessed on 28th June 2025).

Baek, S. C., Nam, K. H., Yi, S. A., Jo, M. S., Lee, K. H., Lee, Y. H., et al. (2019). Anti-adipogenic effect of β-carboline alkaloids from garlic (*Allium sativum*). *Foods, 8*(12), 673. https://doi.org/10.3390/foods8120673 (accessed on 28th June 2025).

Bagul, P. K., & Banerjee, S. K. (2015). Application of resveratrol in diabetes: Rationale, strategies and challenges. *Current Molecular Medicine, 15*(4), 312–330. https://doi.org/10.2174/1566524015666150505155702 (accessed on 28th June 2025).

Bahrin, A. A., Moshawih, S., Dhaliwal, J. S., Kanakal, M. M., Khan, A., Lee, K. S., et al. (2022). Cancer protective effects of plums: A systematic review. *Biomedicine & Pharmacotherapy, 146*, 112568. https://doi.org/10.1016/j.biopha.2021.112568 (accessed on 28th June 2025).

Balogun, O., & Kang, H. W. (2022). Garlic scape (*Allium sativum* L) extract decreases adipogenesis by activating AMPK-activated protein kinase during the differentiation in 3T3-L1 adipocytes. *Journal of Medicinal Food, 25*(1), 24–32. https://doi.org/10.1089/jmf.2021.0014 (accessed on 28th June 2025).

Barceloux, D. G. (2009). Pepper and capsaicin (*Capsicum* and *Piper* species). *Disease-a-Month, 55*(6), 380–390. https://doi.org/10.1016/j.disamonth.2009.03.008 (accessed on 28th June 2025).

Behera, P. K., Devi, S., & Mittal, N. (2023). Therapeutic potential of gallic acid in obesity: Considerable shift! *Obesity Medicine, 37*, 100473. https://doi.org/10.1016/j.obmed.2023.100473 (accessed on 28th June 2025).

Behl, T., Makkar, R., Sehgal, A., Sharma, N., Singh, S., Albratty, M., Najmi, A., Meraya, A. M., & Bungau, S. G. (2022). Insights into the explicit protective activity of herbals in the management of neurodegenerative and cerebrovascular disorders. *Molecules, 27*(15), 4970. https://doi.org/10.3390/molecules27154970 (accessed on 28th June 2025).

Bhargava, S. K., Singh, T. G., Mannan, A., Singh, S., Singh, M., & Gupta, S. (2022). Pharmacological evaluation of *Thuja occidentalis* for the attenuation of neuropathy via AGEs and TNF-α inhibition in diabetic neuropathic rats. *Environmental Science and Pollution Research, 29*(40), 60542–60557. https://doi.org/10.1007/s11356-022-20000-5 (accessed on 28th June 2025).

Bishayee, A., Barnes, K. F., Bhatia, D., Darvesh, A. S., & Carroll, R. T. (2010). Resveratrol suppresses oxidative stress and inflammatory response in diethylnitrosamine-initiated rat hepatocarcinogenesis. *Cancer Prevention Research, 3*(6), 753–763. https://doi.org/10.1158/1940-6207.CAPR-09-0171 (accessed on 28th June 2025).

Bolin, A. P., Sousa-Filho, C. P. B., Dos Santos, G. T. N., Ferreira, L. T., de Andrade, P. B. M., Figueira, A. C. M., et al. (2020). Adipogenic commitment induced by green tea polyphenols remodel adipocytes to a thermogenic phenotype. *Journal of Nutritional Biochemistry, 83*, 108429. https://doi.org/10.1016/j.jnutbio.2020.108429 (accessed on 28th June 2025).

Cao, H., Urban, J. F., & Anderson, R. A. (2008). Cinnamon polyphenol extract affects immune responses by regulating anti-, proinflammatory, and glucose transporter gene expression in mouse macrophages. *Journal of Nutrition, 138*(5), 833–840. https://doi.org/10.1093/jn/138.5.833 (accessed on 28th June 2025).

Carey, A., Paitak, R., Formosa, M., Van Every, B., Bertovic, D. A., Anderson, M. J., et al. (2015). Chronic ephedrine administration decreases brown adipose tissue activity in a randomised controlled human trial: Implications for obesity. *Diabetologia & Metabolic Syndrome, 58*, 1045–1054. https://doi.org/10.1007/s00125-015-3543-6 (accessed on 28th June 2025).

Cha, M.-H., Kim, I. C., Lee, B. H., & Yoon, Y. (2006). Baicalein inhibits adipocyte differentiation by enhancing COX-2 expression. *Journal of Medicinal Food, 9*(2), 145–153. https://doi.org/10.1089/jmf.2006.9.145 (accessed on 28th June 2025).

Chan, Y., Ng, S. W., Tan, J. Z. X., Gupta, G., Negi, P., Thangavelu, L., et al. (2021). Natural products in the management of obesity: Fundamental mechanisms and pharmacotherapy. *South African Journal of Botany, 143*, 176–197. https://doi.org/10.1016/j.sajb.2021.07.026 (accessed on 28th June 2025).

Choi, M., Mukherjee, S., & Yun, J. W. (2021). Trigonelline induces browning in 3T3-L1 white adipocytes. *Phytotherapy Research, 35*(2), 1113–1124. https://doi.org/10.1002/ptr.6892 (accessed on 28th June 2025).

Couturier, K., Batandier, C., Awada, M., Hininger-Favier, I., Canini, F., Anderson, R. A., et al. (2010). Cinnamon improves insulin sensitivity and alters the body composition in an animal model of the metabolic syndrome. *Archives of Biochemistry and Biophysics, 501*(1), 158–161. https://doi.org/10.1016/j.abb.2010.05.032 (accessed on 28th June 2025).

Crawford, P. (2009). Effectiveness of cinnamon for lowering hemoglobin A1C in patients with type 2 diabetes: A randomised, controlled trial. *Journal of the American Board of Family Medicine, 22*(5), 507–512. https://doi.org/10.3122/jabfm.2009.05.080093 (accessed on 28th June 2025).

Dar, A., Faizi, S., Naqvi, S., Roome, T., Zikr-ur-Rehman, S., Ali, M., et al. (2005). Analgesic and antioxidant activity of mangiferin and its derivatives: The structure-activity relationship. *Biological & Pharmaceutical Bulletin, 28*(4), 596–600. https://doi.org/10.1248/bpb.28.596 (accessed on 28th June 2025).

Devi, S., & Singh, R. (2017). Evaluation of antioxidant and anti-hypercholesterolemic potential of *Vitis vinifera* leaves. *Food Science and Human Wellness, 6*(3), 131–136. https://doi.org/10.1016/j.fshw.2017.06.002 (accessed on 28th June 2025).

Devi, S., Chauhan, S., Mannan, A., & Singh, T. G. (2023). Targeting cardiovascular risk factors with eugenol: An anti-inflammatory perspective. *Inflammopharmacology*, 1–11. https://doi.org/10.1007/s10787-023-01195-9 (accessed on 28th June 2025).

Devi, S., Kaur, N., Kumar, M., & Kumar, P. (2023). *In vitro* and *in vivo* evaluation of antidiabetic potential and drug-herb interactions of *Euphorbia neriifolia* in streptozotocin-induced diabetes in rats and *in vitro* antioxidant studies. *Food Chemistry Advances*, 100199. https://doi.org/10.1016/j.focha.2023.100199 (accessed on 28th June 2025).

Diepvens, K., Westerterp, K. R., & Westerterp-Plantenga, M. S. (2007). Obesity and thermogenesis related to caffeine, ephedrine, capsaicin, and green tea consumption. *American Journal of Physiology – Regulatory, Integrative and Comparative Physiology, 292*, R77–R85. https://doi.org/10.1152/ajpregu.00832.2005 (accessed on 28th June 2025).

Dulloo, A. (1993). Ephedrine, xanthines and prostaglandin-inhibitors: Actions and interactions in the stimulation of thermogenesis. *International Journal of Obesity and Related Metabolic Disorders, 17*, S35–S40.

Dutt, H. C., Singh, S., Avula, B., Khan, I. A., & Bedi, Y. S. (2012). Pharmacological review of *Caralluma* R.Br. with particular reference to appetite suppression and anti-obesity. *Journal of Medicinal Food, 15*(2), 108–119. https://doi.org/10.1089/jmf.2010.1555 (accessed on 28th June 2025).

Fernandes, A. B., Alves da Silva, J., Almeida, J., Cui, G., Gerfen, C. R., Costa, R. M., et al. (2020). Postingestive modulation of food seeking depends on vagus-mediated dopamine neuron activity. *Neuron, 106*(5), 778–788. https://doi.org/10.1016/j.neuron.2020.03.009 (accessed on 28th June 2025).

Ferreira, T., Shuler, J., Guimarães, R. J., & Farah, A. (2019). Chapter 1: Introduction to the coffee plant and genetics: Production, quality and chemistry. In *Coffee* (pp. 1–39). Royal Society of Chemistry. https://doi.org/10.1039/9781788014927-00001 (accessed on 28th June 2025).

Foudah, A. I., Alqarni, M. H., Devi, S., Singh, A., Alam, A., Alam, P., & Singh, S. (2022). The analgesic action of catechin on chronic constriction injury–induced neuropathic pain in Sprague–Dawley rats. *Frontiers in Pharmacology, 13*, 895079. https://doi.org/10.3389/fphar.2022.895079 (accessed on 28th June 2025).

Foudah, A. I., Devi, S., Alqarni, M. H., Alam, A., Salkini, M. A., Kumar, M., & Almalki, H. S. (2022). Quercetin attenuates nitroglycerin-induced migraine headaches by inhibiting oxidative stress and inflammatory mediators. *Nutrients, 14*(22), 4871. https://doi.org/10.3390/nu14224871 (accessed on 28th June 2025).

Fu, C., Jiang, Y., Guo, J., & Su, Z. (2016). Natural products with anti-obesity effects and different mechanisms of action. *Journal of Agricultural and Food Chemistry, 64*(51), 9571–9585. https://doi.org/10.1021/acs.jafc.6b04468 (accessed on 28th June 2025).

Garg, N., Singh, T. G., Khan, H., Arora, S., Kaur, A., & Mannan, A. (2021). Mechanistic interventions of selected *Ocimum* species in management of diabetes, obesity and liver disorders: Transformative developments from preclinical to clinical approaches. *Biointerface Research in Applied Chemistry, 12*(1), 1304–1323.

Geoffroy, P., Ressault, B., Marchioni, E., & Miesch, M. (2011). Synthesis of hoodigogenin A, the aglycone of natural appetite suppressant glycosteroids extracted from *Hoodia gordonii*. *Steroids, 76*(7), 702–708. https://doi.org/10.1016/j.steroids.2011.03.014 (accessed on 28th June 2025).

Ghaben, A. L., & Scherer, P. E. (2019). Adipogenesis and metabolic health. *Nature Reviews Molecular Cell Biology, 20*(4), 242–258. https://doi.org/10.1038/s41580-018-0093-z (accessed on 28th June 2025).

Godard, M. P., Johnson, B. A., & Richmond, S. R. (2005). Body composition and hormonal adaptations associated with forskolin consumption in overweight and obese men. *Obesity Research, 13*(8), 1335–1343. https://doi.org/10.1038/oby.2005.162 (accessed on 28th June 2025).

Gómez-Hernández, A., Beneit, N., Díaz-Castroverde, S., & Escribano, Ó. (2016). Differential role of adipose tissues in obesity and related metabolic and vascular complications. *International Journal of Endocrinology, 2016*, 1216783. https://doi.org/10.1155/2016/1216783 (accessed on 28th June 2025).

González-Abuín, N., Pinent, M., Casanova-Marti, A., Arola, L., Blay, M., & Ardevol, A. (2015). Procyanidins and their healthy protective effects against type 2 diabetes. *Current Medicinal Chemistry, 22*(1), 39–50. https://doi.org/10.2174/0929867321666140916115519 (accessed on 28th June 2025).

Goyal, B. R., Goyal, R. K., & Mehta, A. A. (2007). *Phcog rev.* Plant review phytopharmacology of *Achyranthes aspera*: A review. *Pharmacognosy Reviews, 1*(1).

Gupta, A., Gupta, R., & Lal, B. (2001). Effect of *Trigonella foenum-graecum* (fenugreek) seeds on glycaemic control and insulin resistance in type 2 diabetes mellitus: A double-blind placebo-controlled study. *Journal of the Association of Physicians of India, 49*, 1057–1061.

Gupta, M., Krishan, P., Kaur, A., Arora, S., Trehanpati, N., Singh, T. G., & Bedi, O. (2021). Mechanistic and physiological approaches of fecal microbiota transplantation in the management of NAFLD. *Inflammation Research, 70*(7), 765–776. https://doi.org/10.1007/s00011-021-01480-z (accessed on 28th June 2025).

Han, J., Yi, J., Liang, F., Jiang, B., Xiao, Y., Gao, S., et al. (2015). X-3, a mangiferin derivative, stimulates AMP-activated protein kinase, reducing hyperglycemia and obesity in db/db mice. *Molecular and Cellular Endocrinology, 405*, 63–73. https://doi.org/10.1016/j.mce.2015.02.008 (accessed on 28th June 2025).

Han, L. K., Zheng, Y. N., Xu, B. J., Okuda, H., & Kimura, Y. (2002). Saponins from *Platycodi radix* ameliorate high-fat diet-induced obesity in mice. *Journal of Nutrition, 132*(8), 2241–2245. https://doi.org/10.1093/jn/132.8.2241 (accessed on 28th June 2025).

Hannan, J. M., Ali, L., Rokeya, B., Khaleque, J., Akhter, M., Flatt, P. R., et al. (2007). The soluble dietary fibre fraction of *Trigonella foenum-graecum* (fenugreek) seed improves glucose homeostasis in animal models of type 1 and type 2 diabetes by delaying carbohydrate digestion and absorption and enhancing insulin action. *British Journal of Nutrition, 97*(3), 514–521. https://doi.org/10.1017/S0007114507657869 (accessed on 28th June 2025).

Hariri, M., & Ghiasvand, R. (2016). Cinnamon and chronic diseases. In *Advances in Experimental Medicine and Biology, 929*, 1–24. https://doi.org/10.1007/978-3-319-41342-6_1 (accessed on 28th June 2025).

Harmon, A. W., Patel, Y. M., & Harp, J. B. (2002). Genistein inhibits CCAAT/enhancer-binding protein beta (C/EBPβ) activity and 3T3-L1 adipogenesis by increasing C/EBP homologous protein expression. *Biochemical Journal, 367*, 203–208. https://doi.org/10.1042/BJ20020300 (accessed on 28th June 2025).

Hsu, C.-L., & Yen, G.-C. (2007). Effects of capsaicin on induction of apoptosis and inhibition of adipogenesis in 3T3-L1 cells. *Journal of Agricultural and Food Chemistry, 55*(5), 1730–1736. https://doi.org/10.1021/jf062912b (accessed on 28th June 2025).

Huang, C., Zhang, Y., Gong, Z., Sheng, X., Li, Z., Zhang, W., et al. (2006). Berberine inhibits 3T3-L1 adipocyte differentiation through the PPARγ pathway. *Biochemical and Biophysical Research Communications, 348*(2), 571–578. https://doi.org/10.1016/j.bbrc.2006.07.095 (accessed on 28th June 2025).

Huang, L., Zhang, J., Zhu, X., Mi, X., Li, Q., Gao, J., et al. (2021). The phytochemical rhein mediates M(6)a-independent suppression of adipocyte differentiation. *Frontiers in Nutrition, 8*, 756803. https://doi.org/10.3389/fnut.2021.756803 (accessed on 28th June 2025).

Ikeda, Y., Murakami, A., & Ohigashi, H. (2008). Ursolic acid: An anti- and pro-inflammatory triterpenoid. *Molecular Nutrition & Food Research, 52*(1), 26–42. https://doi.org/10.1002/mnfr.200700389 (accessed on 28th June 2025).

Islam, M., & Choi, H. K. (2008). Comparative effects of dietary ginger (*Zingiber officinale*) and garlic (*Allium sativum*) investigated in a type 2 diabetes model of rats. *Journal of Medicinal Food, 11*(1), 152–159. https://doi.org/10.1089/jmf.2007.634 (accessed on 28th June 2025).

Jain, S., & Singh, S. N. (2013). Metabolic effect of short-term administration of *Hoodia gordonii*, an herbal appetite suppressant. *South African Journal of Botany, 86*, 51–55. https://doi.org/10.1016/j.sajb.2013.02.002 (accessed on 28th June 2025).

Jakab, J., Miškić, B., Mikšić, Š., Juranić, B., Ćosić, V., Schwarz, D., & Včev, A. (2021). Adipogenesis as a potential anti-obesity target: A review of pharmacological treatment and natural products. *Diabetes, Metabolic Syndrome and Obesity, 2021*(Jan 8), 67–83.

Jang, S.-M., Yee, S. T., Choi, J., Choi, M. S., Do, G. M., Jeon, S. M., et al. (2009). Ursolic acid enhances the cellular immune system and pancreatic β-cell function in streptozotocin-induced diabetic mice fed a high-fat diet. *International Immunopharmacology, 9*, 113–119. https://doi.org/10.1016/j.intimp.2008.10.013 (accessed on 28th June 2025).

Jeukendrup, A. E., & Randell, R. (2011). Fat burners: Nutrition supplements that increase fat metabolism. *Obesity Reviews, 12*(10), 841–851. https://doi.org/10.1111/j.1467-789X.2011.00908.x (accessed on 28th June 2025).

Jung, S., Ha, Y. J., Shim, E. K., Choi, S. Y., Jin, J. L., Yun-Choi, H. S., et al. (2007). Insulin-mimetic and insulin-sensitizing activities of a pentacyclic triterpenoid insulin receptor activator. *Biochemical Journal, 403*, 243–250. https://doi.org/10.1042/BJ20061123 (accessed on 28th June 2025).

Kang, C., Lee, H., Jung, E. S., Seyedian, R., Jo, M., Kim, J., et al. (2012). Saffron (*Crocus sativus* L) increases glucose uptake and insulin sensitivity in muscle cells via multipathway mechanisms. *Food Chemistry, 135*(4), 2350–2358. https://doi.org/10.1016/j.foodchem.2012.06.092 (accessed on 28th June 2025).

Kaur, N., Kishore, L., Farooq, S. A., Kajal, A., Singh, R., Agrawal, R., ... & Singh, T. G. (2023). *Cucurbita pepo* seeds improve peripheral neuropathy in diabetic rats by modulating the inflammation and oxidative stress in rats. *Environmental Science and Pollution Research, 30*(36), 85910–85919.

Kawada, T., Watanabe, T., Takaishi, T., Tanaka, T., & Iwai, K. (1986). Capsaicin-induced beta-adrenergic action on energy metabolism in rats: Influence of capsaicin on oxygen consumption, the respiratory quotient, and substrate utilisation. *Proceedings of the Society for Experimental Biology and Medicine, 183*, 250–256. https://doi.org/10.3181/00379727-183-42414 (accessed on 28th June 2025).

Kershaw, E. E., & Flier, J. S. (2004). Adipose tissue is an endocrine organ. *Journal of Clinical Endocrinology and Metabolism, 89*(6), 2548–2556. https://doi.org/10.1210/jc.2004-0395 (accessed on 28th June 2025).

Khan, H., Tiwari, C., Kalra, P., Vyas, D., Grewal, A. K., & Singh, T. G. (2024). Mechanistic correlation of molecular pathways in obesity-mediated stroke pathogenesis. *Pharmacological Reports*. Advance online publication. https://doi.org/10.1007/s43440-024-00590-9 (accessed on 28th June 2025).

Khan, J. I., Kennedy, T. J., & Christian, D. R. (2012). Phenethylamines. In J. I. Khan, T. J. Kennedy, & D. R. Christian Jr (Eds.), *Basic Principles of Forensic Chemistry* (pp. 157–176). Humana Press.

Khandouzi, N., Shidfar, F., Rajab, A., Rahideh, T., Hosseini, P., & Mir Taheri, M. (2015). The effects of ginger on fasting blood sugar, hemoglobin A1C, apolipoprotein B, apolipoprotein A-I and malondialdehyde in type 2 diabetic patients. *Iranian Journal of Pharmaceutical Research (IJPR), 14*(1), 131–140.

Kim, S. H., & Choung, S. Y. (2010). Antihyperglycemic and antihyperlipidemic action of *Cinnamomum cassia* (cinnamon bark) extract in C57BL/Ks db/db mice. *Archives of Pharmacal Research, 33*(2), 325–333. https://doi.org/10.1007/s12272-010-0219-0 (accessed on 28th June 2025).

Kumar, A., Sundaram, K., Teng, Y., Mu, J., Sriwastva, M. K., Zhang, L., et al. (2022). Ginger nanoparticles mediated induction of Foxa2 prevents high-fat diet-induced insulin resistance. *Theranostics, 12*(3), 1388–1403. https://doi.org/10.7150/thno.62514 (accessed on 28th June 2025).

Kuriyan, R., Raj, T., Srinivas, S. K., Vaz, M., Rajendran, R., & Kurpad, A. V. (2007). Effect of *Caralluma fimbriata* extract on appetite, food intake and anthropometry in adult Indian men and women. *Appetite, 48*(3), 338–344. https://doi.org/10.1016/j.appet.2006.09.013 (accessed on 28th June 2025).

Kwan, H. Y., Wu, J., Su, T., Chao, X. J., Liu, B., Fu, X., et al. (2017). Cinnamon induces browning in subcutaneous adipocytes. *Scientific Reports, 7*(1), 2447. https://doi.org/10.1038/s41598-017-02263-5 (accessed on 28th June 2025).

Kwon, C. S., Sohn, H. Y., Kim, S. H., Kim, J. H., Son, K. H., Lee, J. S., et al. (2003a). Anti-obesity effect of *Dioscorea nipponica* Makino with lipase-inhibitory activity in rodents. *Bioscience, Biotechnology, and Biochemistry, 67*(7), 1451–1456. https://doi.org/10.1271/bbb.67.1451 (accessed on 28th June 2025).

Latha, B. P. (2011). Therapeutic efficacy of *Achyranthes aspera* saponin extract in high-fat diet-induced hyperlipidaemia in male Wistar rats. *African Journal of Biotechnology, 10*(74), 17038–17042.

Lee, A. G., Kang, S., Im, S., & Pak, Y. K. (2022). Cinnamic acid attenuates peripheral and hypothalamic inflammation in high-fat diet-induced obese mice. *Pharmaceutics, 14*(8), 1675. https://doi.org/10.3390/pharmaceutics14081675 (accessed on 28th June 2025).

Lee, H. E., Yang, G., Han, S. H., Lee, J. H., & Jang, J. K. (2018). Anti-obesity potential of *Glycyrrhiza uralensis* and licochalcone A through induction of adipocyte browning. *Biochemical and Biophysical Research Communications, 503*(3), 2117–2123. https://doi.org/10.1016/j.bbrc.2018.07.168 (accessed on 28th June 2025).

Lee, K. J., & Jeong, H. G. (2002). Protective effect of *Platycodi radix* on carbon tetrachloride-induced hepatotoxicity. *Food and Chemical Toxicology, 40*(4), 517–525. https://doi.org/10.1016/s0278-6915(01)00104-1 (accessed on 28th June 2025).

Lefebvre, P., & Staels, B. (2012). Naturally improving insulin resistance with amorfrutins. *Proceedings of the National Academy of Sciences of the United States of America, 109*(19), 7136–7137. https://doi.org/10.1073/pnas.1204455109 (accessed on 28th June 2025).

Lin, J., Della-Fera, M. A., & Baile, C. A. (2005). Green tea polyphenol epigallocatechin gallate inhibits adipogenesis and induces apoptosis in 3T3-L1 adipocytes. *Obesity Research, 13*(6), 982–990. https://doi.org/10.1038/oby.2005.115 (accessed on 28th June 2025).

Lin, X., & Li, H. (2021). Obesity: Epidemiology, pathophysiology, and therapeutics. *Frontiers in Endocrinology (Lausanne), 12*, 706978. https://doi.org/10.3389/fendo.2021.706978 (accessed on 28th June 2025).

Litosch, I., Hudson, T. H., Mills, I., & Fain, J. N. (1982). Forskolin as an activator of cyclic AMP accumulation and lipolysis in rat adipocytes. *Molecular Pharmacology, 22*(1), 109–115.

Liu, Q., Zhang, X. L., Tao, R. Y., Niu, Y. J., Chen, X. G., Tian, J. Y., et al. (2011). Rhein, an inhibitor of adipocyte differentiation and adipogenesis. *Journal of Asian Natural*

Products Research, 13(8), 714–723. https://doi.org/10.1080/10286020.2011.586341 (accessed on 28th June 2025).

Ludy, M.-J., Moore, G. E., & Mattes, R. D. (2012). The effects of capsaicin and capsiate on energy balance: Critical review and meta-analyses of studies in humans. *Chemical Senses, 37*(2), 103–121. https://doi.org/10.1093/chemse/bjr100 (accessed on 28th June 2025).

MacLean, D. B., & Luo, L. G. (2004). Increased ATP content/production in the hypothalamus may signal energy-sensing of satiety: Studies of the anorectic mechanism of a plant steroidal glycoside. *Brain Research, 1020*(1–2), 1–11. https://doi.org/10.1016/j.brainres.2004.04.041 (accessed on 28th June 2025).

Makkar, R., Behl, T., Bungau, S., Zengin, G., Mehta, V., Kumar, A., Uddin, M. S., Ashraf, G. M., Abdel-Daim, M. M., Arora, S., & Oancea, R. (2020). Nutraceuticals in neurological disorders. *International Journal of Molecular Sciences, 21*(12), 4424. https://doi.org/10.3390/ijms21124424 (accessed on 28th June 2025).

Maniglia, B. C., Rebelatto, E. A., Andrade, K. S., Zielinski, A., & de Andrade, C. J. (2021). Polyphenols. In *Food Bioactives and Health* (pp. 1–39).

Mannan, A., Garg, N., Singh, T. G., & Kang, H. K. (2021). Peroxisome proliferator-activated receptor-gamma (PPAR-ɣ): Molecular effects and its importance as a novel therapeutic target for cerebral ischemic injury. *Neurochemical Research, 46*(11), 2800–2831. https://doi.org/10.1007/s11064-021-03402-1 (accessed on 28th June 2025).

Mao, Q. Q., Xu, X. Y., Cao, S. Y., Gan, R. Y., Corke, H., Beta, T., et al. (2019). Bioactive compounds and bioactivities of ginger (*Zingiber officinale* Roscoe). *Foods, 8*(6), 185. https://doi.org/10.3390/foods8060185 (accessed on 28th June 2025).

Maurer, S., Harms, M., & Boucher, J. (2021). The colourful versatility of adipocytes: White-to-brown transdifferentiation and its therapeutic potential in humans. *FEBS Journal, 288*(12), 3628–3646. https://doi.org/10.1111/febs.15470 (accessed on 28th June 2025).

Mehta, S., Nain, P., Agrawal, B. K., Singh, R. P., Kaur, J., Maity, S., Bhattacharjee, A., Peela, J., Nauhria, S., & Nauhria, S. (2021). Effectiveness of empagliflozin with vitamin D supplementation in peripheral neuropathy in type 2 diabetic patients. *Cureus, 13*(12), e20208. https://doi.org/10.7759/cureus.20208 (accessed on 28th June 2025).

Milajerdi, A., Jazayeri, S., Hashemzadeh, N., Shirzadi, E., Derakhshan, Z., Djazayeri, A., et al. (2018). The effect of saffron (*Crocus sativus* L) hydroalcoholic extract on metabolic control in type 2 diabetes mellitus: A triple-blinded randomised clinical trial. *Journal of Research in Medical Sciences, 23*, 16. https://doi.org/10.4103/jrms.JRMS_286_17 (accessed on 28th June 2025).

Mobasseri, M., Ostadrahimi, A., Tajaddini, A., Asghari, S., Barati, M., Akbarzadeh, M., et al. (2020). Effects of saffron supplementation on glycemia and inflammation in patients with type 2 diabetes mellitus: A randomised, double-blind, placebo-controlled clinical trial study. *Diabetes & Metabolic Syndrome: Clinical Research & Reviews, 14*(4), 527–534. https://doi.org/10.1016/j.dsx.2020.04.031 (accessed on 28th June 2025).

Moshawih, S., Mydin, R. B., Kalakotla, S., & Jarrar, Q. B. (2019). Potential application of resveratrol in nanocarriers against cancer: Overview and future trends. *Journal of Drug Delivery Science and Technology, 53*, 101187. https://doi.org/10.1016/j.jddst.2019.101187 (accessed on 28th June 2025).

Mukherjee, P. K., Mukherjee, D., Maji, A. K., Rai, S., & Heinrich, M. (2009). The sacred lotus (*Nelumbo nucifera*)–Phytochemical and therapeutic profile. *Journal of Pharmacy and Pharmacology, 61*(4), 407–422. https://doi.org/10.1211/jpp/61.04.0001 (accessed on 28th June 2025).

Mukund, V., Mukund, D., Sharma, V., Mannarapu, M., & Alam, A. (2017). Genistein: Its role in metabolic diseases and cancer. *Critical Reviews in Oncology/Hematology, 119*, 13–22. https://doi.org/10.1016/j.critrevonc.2017.09.004 (accessed on 28th June 2025).

Panchal, S., Bliss, E., & Brown, L. (2018). Capsaicin in metabolic syndrome. *Nutrients, 10*(5), 630. https://doi.org/10.3390/nu10050630 (accessed on 28th June 2025).

Park, M., Sharma, A., & Hj, L. (2019). Anti-adipogenic effects of delphinidin-3-O-β-glucoside in 3T3-L1 preadipocytes and primary white adipocytes. *Molecules, 24*(10), 1848. https://doi.org/10.3390/molecules24101848 (accessed on 28th June 2025).

Puri, D., Prabhu, K. M., & Murthy, P. S. (2002). Mechanism of action of a hypoglycemic principle isolated from fenugreek seeds. *Indian Journal of Physiology and Pharmacology, 46*(4), 457–462.

Rani, N., Sharma, S. K., & Vasudeva, N. (2012). Assessment of the antiobesity potential of *Achyranthes aspera* Linn. seed. *Evidence-Based Complementary and Alternative Medicine, 2012*, 715912. https://doi.org/10.1155/2012/715912 (accessed on 28th June 2025).

Rani, N., Vasudeva, N., & Sharma, S. K. (2012). Quality assessment and anti-obesity activity of *Stellaria media* (Linn) Vill. *BMC Complementary and Alternative Medicine, 12*, 145. https://doi.org/10.1186/1472-6882-12-145 (accessed on 28th June 2025).

Raoof, G. F. A., & Kareem, A. M. Z. A. E. (2020). The golden role of natural products in obesity. *International Journal of Pharmaceutical Research and Health Sciences, 8*(6), 3248–3255. https://doi.org/10.21276/ijprhs.2020.06.03 (accessed on 28th June 2025).

Rayalam, S., Della-Fera, M. A., & Baile, C. A. (2008). Phytochemicals and regulation of the adipocyte life cycle. *Journal of Nutritional Biochemistry, 19*(11), 717–726. https://doi.org/10.1016/j.jnutbio.2007.12.007 (accessed on 28th June 2025).

Rios, J., Recio, M. C., Giner, R. M., & Máñez, S. (1996). An updated review of saffron and its active constituents. *Phytotherapy Research, 10*, 189–193. https://doi.org/10.1002/(sici)1099-1573(199605)10 (accessed on 28th June 2025).

Rohilla, M., Rishabh, Bansal, S., Garg, A., Dhiman, S., Dhankhar, S., Saini, M., Chauhan, S., Alsubaie, N., Batiha, G. E., Albezrah, N. K. A., & Singh, T. G. (2023). Discussing pathologic mechanisms of diabetic retinopathy & therapeutic potentials of curcumin and β-glucogallin in the management of diabetic retinopathy. *Biomedicine & Pharmacotherapy, 169*, 115881. https://doi.org/10.1016/j.biopha.2023.115881 (accessed on 28th June 2025).

Rue, E. A., Rush, M. D., & van Breemen, R. B. (2018). Procyanidins: A comprehensive review encompassing structure elucidation via mass spectrometry. *Phytochemical Reviews, 17*(1), 1–16. https://doi.org/10.1007/s11101-017-9507-3 (accessed on 28th June 2025).

Saito, M. (2015). Capsaicin and related food ingredients reduce body fat by activating TRP and brown fat thermogenesis. *Advances in Food and Nutrition Research, 76*, 1–28. https://doi.org/10.1016/bs.afnr.2015.07.002 (accessed on 28th June 2025).

Saleh, S., El-Maraghy, N., Reda, E., & Barakat, W. (2014). Modulation of diabetes and dyslipidemia in diabetic insulin-resistant rats by mangiferin: Role of adiponectin and TNF-α. *Anais da Academia Brasileira de Ciências, 86*(4), 1935–1948. https://doi.org/10.1590/0001-3765201420140212 (accessed on 28th June 2025).

Sayan, M., & Soumya, M. (2017). The potential role of phytochemicals in regulating human appetite: A novel approach towards diet management 1. *Botanica, 67*, 34–39.

Schneider, C., Rotscheidt, K., & Breitmaier, E. (1993). Vier neue Pregnanglycoside aus *Gongronema latifolium* (Asclepiadaceae). *Liebigs Annalen der Chemie, 1993*(10), 1057–1062. https://doi.org/10.1002/jlac.1993199301170 (accessed on 28th June 2025).

Schwarzschild, M. A., Xu, K., Oztas, E., Petzer, J. P., Castagnoli, K., Castagnoli, N., et al. (2003). Neuroprotection by caffeine and, more specifically, A2A receptor antagonists in animal models of Parkinson's disease. *Neurology, 61*(11), S55–S61. https://doi.org/10.1212/01.wnl.0000095214.53646.72 (accessed on 28th June 2025).

Sekiya, K., Ohtani, A., & Kusano, S. (2004). Enhancement of insulin sensitivity in adipocytes by ginger. *BioFactors, 22*(1–4), 153–156. https://doi.org/10.1002/biof.5520220130 (accessed on 28th June 2025).

Sepahi, S., Mohajeri, S. A., Hosseini, S. M., Khodaverdi, E., Shoeibi, N., Namdari, M., et al. (2018). Effects of crocin on diabetic maculopathy: A placebo-controlled randomised clinical trial. *American Journal of Ophthalmology, 190*, 89–98. https://doi.org/10.1016/j.ajo.2018.03.007 (accessed on 28th June 2025).

Sharma, R. (2003). *Medicinal plants of India: An encyclopaedia.* Daryaganj: Daya Publishing House.

Sharma, V. K., & Singh, T. G. (2020). Insulin resistance and bioenergetic manifestations: Targets and approaches in Alzheimer's disease. *Life Sciences, 262*, 118401. https://doi.org/10.1016/j.lfs.2020.118401 (accessed on 28th June 2025).

Shukla, Y. J., Pawar, R. S., Ding, Y., Li, X. C., Ferreira, D., & Khan, I. A. (2009). Pregnane glycosides from *Hoodia gordonii. Phytochemistry, 70*(5), 675–683. https://doi.org/10.1016/j.phytochem.2009.02.006 (accessed on 28th June 2025).

Singh, R., Farooq, S. A., Mannan, A., Singh, T. G., Najda, A., Grażyna, Z., ... & Abdel-Daim, M. M. (2022). Animal models of diabetic microvascular complications: Relevance to clinical features. *Biomedicine & Pharmacotherapy, 145*, 112305. https://doi.org/10.1016/j.biopha.2021.112305 (accessed on 28th June 2025).

Smith, C., & Krygsman, A. (2014). *Hoodia gordonii*: To eat, or not to eat. *Journal of Ethnopharmacology, 155*(2), 987–991. https://doi.org/10.1016/j.jep.2014.06.033 (accessed on 28th June 2025).

Snehlata, H. S., & Payal, D. R. (2012). Fenugreek (*Trigonella foenum-graecum* L): An overview. *International Journal of Current Pharmaceutical Review and Research, 2*(4), 169–187.

Sood, S., Devi, S., Singh, T. G., & Mittal, N. (2023). Pathogenesis of obesity-associated cardiovascular diseases: Critical role of biomolecules. *Health Sciences Review*, 100098.

Stohs, S. J., & Badmaev, V. (2016). A review of natural stimulant and non-stimulant thermogenic agents. *Phytotherapy Research, 30*(5), 732–740. https://doi.org/10.1002/ptr.5583 (accessed on 28th June 2025).

Stoner, G. D. (2013). Ginger: Is it ready for prime time? *Cancer Prevention Research, 6*(4), 257–262. https://doi.org/10.1158/1940-6207.CAPR-13-0055 (accessed on 28th June 2025).

Sun, N. N., Wu, T. Y., & Chau, C. F. (2016). Natural dietary and herbal products in anti-obesity treatment. *Molecules, 21*(10), 1351. https://doi.org/10.3390/molecules21101351 (accessed on 28th June 2025).

Tan, J., Kumar, M., Devi, S., & Kumar, M. (2022). Neuroprotective effects of arbutin against oxygen and glucose deprivation-induced oxidative stress and neuroinflammation in rat cortical neurons. *Acta Pharmaceutica, 72*(1), 123–134.

Tasić-Kostov, M., Arsić, I., Pavlović, D., Stojanović, S., Najman, S., Naumović, S., et al. (2019). Towards a modern approach to traditional use: In vitro and in vivo evaluation of *Alchemilla vulgaris* L. gel wound healing potential. *Journal of Ethnopharmacology, 83*, 111789. https://doi.org/10.1016/j.jep.2019.03.016 (accessed on 28th June 2025).

Thitimuta, S., Pithayanukul, P., Nithitanakool, S., Bavovada, R., Leanpolchareanchai, J., & Saparpakorn, P. (2017). *Camellia sinensis* L. extract and its potential beneficial effects in antioxidant, anti-inflammatory, anti-hepatotoxic, and anti-tyrosinase activities. *Molecules, 22*(3), 401. https://doi.org/10.3390/molecules22030401 (accessed on 28th June 2025).

Törrönen, R., Sarkkinen, E., Niskanen, T., Tapola, N., Kilpi, K., & Niskanen, L. (2012). In healthy subjects, postprandial glucose, insulin and glucagon-like peptide one responds to sucrose ingested with berries. *British Journal of Nutrition, 107*(10), 1445–1451. https://doi.org/10.1017/S0007114511004557 (accessed on 28th June 2025).

Tucci, S. A. (2010). Phytochemicals in the control of human appetite and body weight. *Pharmaceuticals (Basel), 3*(3), 748–763. https://doi.org/10.3390/ph3030748 (accessed on 28th June 2025).

Türközü, D., & Tek, N. A. (2017). A minireview of effects of green tea on energy expenditure. *Critical Reviews in Food Science and Nutrition, 57*(2), 254–258. https://doi.org/10.1080/10408398.2014.986672 (accessed on 28th June 2025).

Van Dam, R. M., Hu, F. B., & Willett, W. C. (2020). Coffee, caffeine, and health. *The New England Journal of Medicine, 383*, 369–378. https://doi.org/10.1056/NEJMra1816604 (accessed on 28th June 2025).

Wani, S. A., & Kumar, P. (2018). Fenugreek: A review of its nutraceutical properties and utilisation in various food products. *Journal of the Saudi Society of Agricultural Sciences, 17*(2), 97–106. https://doi.org/10.1016/j.jssas.2016.01.007 (accessed on 28th June 2025).

Won, S.-R., Kim, Y. M., Lee, P. H., Ryu, J. H., & Kim, J. W. (2007). Licochalcone A: A lipase inhibitor from the roots of *Glycyrrhiza uralensis*. *Food Research International, 40*, 1046–1050. https://doi.org/10.1016/j.foodres.2007.05.005 (accessed on 28th June 2025).

Xie, W., Zhao, Y., & Zhang, Y. (2011). Traditional Chinese medicines in the treatment of patients with type 2 diabetes mellitus. *Evidence-Based Complementary and Alternative Medicine, 2011*, 726723. https://doi.org/10.1155/2011/726723 (accessed on 28th June 2025).

Xu, B. J., Han, L. K., Zheng, Y. N., Lee, J. H., & Sung, C. K. (2005). In vitro inhibitory effect of triterpenoidal saponins from *Platycodi Radix* on pancreatic lipase. *Archives of Pharmacal Research, 28*(2), 180–185. https://doi.org/10.1007/BF02977712 (accessed on 28th June 2025).

Yamashita, Y., Okabe, M., Natsume, M., & Ashida, H. (2013). Cinnamtannin A2, a tetrameric procyanidin, increases GLP-1 and insulin secretion in mice. *Bioscience, Biotechnology, and Biochemistry, 77*(4), 888–891. https://doi.org/10.1271/bbb.130095 (accessed on 28th June 2025).

Yang, J. Y., Della-Fera, M. A., Hartzell, D. L., Nelson-Dooley, C., Hausman, D. B., & Baile, C. A. (2006). Esculetin induces apoptosis and inhibits adipogenesis in 3T3-L1 cells. *Obesity (Silver Spring), 14*(10), 1691–1699. https://doi.org/10.1038/oby.2006.194 (accessed on 28th June 2025).

Yoneshiro, T., & Saito, M. (2013). Transient receptor potential activated Brown fat thermogenesis as a target of food ingredients for obesity management. *Current Opinion in Clinical Nutrition and Metabolic Care, 16*, 625–631. https://doi.org/10.1097/MCO.0b013e3283653ee1 (accessed on 28th June 2025).

Yoshioka, M., Lim, K., Kikuzato, S., Kiyonaga, A., Tanaka, H., Shindo, M., et al. (1995). Effects of red-pepper diet on the energy metabolism in men. *Journal of Nutritional Science and Vitaminology (Tokyo), 41*, 647–656. https://doi.org/10.3177/jnsv.41.647 (accessed on 28th June 2025).

Zhang, L., Xie, Q., & Li, X. (2022). Esculetin: A review of its pharmacology and pharmacokinetics. *Phytotherapy Research, 36*(1), 279–298. https://doi.org/10.1002/ptr.7311 (accessed on 28th June 2025).

Zhang, Q., Huang, Y., Li, X., Liu, H., He, B., Wang, B., et al. (2019). Mangiferin improved palmitate-induced insulin resistance by promoting free fatty acid metabolism in HepG2 and C2C12 cells via PPARα: Mangiferin improved insulin resistance. *Journal of Diabetes Research, 2019*, 7403978. https://doi.org/10.1155/2019/7403978 (accessed on 28th June 2025).

Zhang, Y., & Huang, C. (2012). Targeting adipocyte apoptosis: A novel strategy for obesity therapy. *Biochemical and Biophysical Research Communications, 417*(1), 1–4. https://doi.org/10.1016/j.bbrc.2011.11.158 (accessed on 28th June 2025).

Zhang, Y., Liu, X., Ruan, J., Zhuang, X., Zhang, X., & Li, Z. (2020). Phytochemicals of garlic: Promising candidates for cancer therapy. *Biomedicine & Pharmacotherapy, 123*, 109730. https://doi.org/10.1016/j.biopha.2019.109730 (accessed on 28th June 2025).

Zhang, Z., Zhang, H., Li, B. E. A., Meng, X., Wang, J., Zhang, Y., et al. (2014). Berberine activates thermogenesis in white and Brown adipose tissue. *Nature Communications, 5*, 5493. https://doi.org/10.1038/ncomms6493 (accessed on 28th June 2025).

CHAPTER 11

Natural Phytochemicals in Diabetic Mellitus (Mechanistic Approach)

MADHUKAR GARG,[1,*] PARUL SOOD,[2] RAJAN SWAMI,[1] LOVELEEN KAUR,[1] ATHRV ARORA,[1] LAVISH VAID,[1] BIKASH MANANDHAR,[3,4] THAKUR GURJEET SINGH,[1] and SANJANA MEHTA[1]

[1]*Chitkara College of Pharmacy, Chitkara University, Punjab, India*

[2]*School of Pharmacy, Chitkara University, Solan, Himachal Pradesh, India*

[3]*Discipline of Pharmacy, Graduate School of Health, University of Technology Sydney, Sydney, New South Wales, Australia*

[4]*Faculty of Health, Australian Research Center in Complementary and Integrative Medicine, University of Technology Sydney, Ultimo, New South Wales, Australia*

*Corresponding author

ABSTRACT

Diabetes mellitus, diagnosed as a complex metabolic disorder, has impacted adversely all age groups, posing constraints worldwide for its management. Insulin and synthetic orals have consistently fallen short and render it more difficult with times compelling the exploration and development of innovative drugs seeking desperate diversion for alternatives, mainly natural phytochemicals such as NCEs and bioactive compounds derived from natural sources. The stated ones ameliorated the Pathophysiological mechanisms while minimizing the side effects compared to

Precision Nutrition and Endocrine Health: Synthesis, Characterization, and Applications.
Thakur Gurjeet Singh and Sanjana Mehta (Eds.)

DOI: 10.1201/9781998511877-11

established ones. The chapter offers the mechanistic approach working behind mentioned entities including polyphenols, alkaloids, terpenoids, plant extracts etc. containing bioactive principles such as Angeline, berberine, curcumin, resveratrol, turmerone and many others in mitigation as evidenced by preclinical and clinical trials too. The content aims to bridge the gap between traditional and modern approaches, offering novel perspectives on the holistic treatment of pervasive and challenging issues.

11.1 INTRODUCTION

The treatment of diseases by using herbal medicines and the phytochemicals obtained has been an integral approach in different systems of medicine. Several putative active compounds isolated, identified and purified showed significant effects in reducing the severity of ailments (Kaur et al., 2023; Singh et al., 2020). Various compounds obtained from plant sources have been able to exert their action either through an increase in insulin secretion to control glucose concentrations in blood or inhibited α-glucosidase, DPP IV, and so forth (Kaur et al., 2017; Sharma and Singh, 2020). Despite significant progress in understanding and managing diabetes, the rising prevalence and the associated complications persist. Recent insights into the disease's pathophysiology have unveiled new avenues for innovative therapies, including exploring phytochemicals from traditional medicinal plants (Bhargava et al., 2022; Garg et al., 2021; Hunter et al., 1998; Mehta et al., 2021). Since ancient times, plants have been widely acknowledged as dependable sources of therapeutic agents, with many synthetic drugs originating directly or indirectly from them as they were believed to be cost-effective and safe (Arora et al., 2021; Garg et al., 2023). The book chapter will provide a concise overview of the pathophysiology of diabetes mellitus and explore the multimodal therapeutic effects of phytochemicals derived from medicinal plants, preceded by the discussion revolving around the status and prospects of these treatments.

11.2 PHYTOCHEMICALS: MECHANISM OF ACTION (EVIDENCE FROM PRE-CLINICAL AND CLINICAL STUDIES)

Chemicals extracted from the plants are known as Phyto-chemicals. With the increase in the side effects of synthetic medicines, there has been a constant search for natural management of diseases with minimal side effects. Evidence from pre-clinical and clinical studies on ongoing research on phytochemicals in diabetes management showed extraordinary results. Some of them and their mechanism of action are given below, claiming positive results for managing diabetes (Alam et al., 2022).

11.2.1 BERBERINE

Berberis aristata DC has been found in the Northern Himalayan part, and the Phyto-constituent berberine extracted showed meaningful results in managing diabetes (Gupta et al., 2021; Rehman et al., 2017). It was found to act by different mechanisms such as by enhancement of GLP-1 (Glucagon-like peptide 1) excretion and regulation, insulin mimetic activity, initiation of 5′ adenosine monophosphate-engaged protein kinase, aldose reductase inhibition, reducing inflammation and fighting oxidative stress (Potdar et al., 2012). Researchers have conducted pre-clinical trials to determine the efficacy of berberine, and the very first report showed the effect in mice against T2DM. Action relationship assays, in silico molecular docking, and cell-based assays were performed to uncover the effect within the cell. Clinical studies (Yin et al., 2008) exhibited that administering 0.5g of it thrice a day to people diagnosed with type 2 diabetes revealed effectiveness comparable to metformin monotherapy improved fasting blood glucose level and HbA1c (Sarker et al., 2020). Further studies showed that it could be helpful when administered alongside the ongoing synthetic medicine in treating type 2 diabetic patients. Berberine became the most valuable alternative treatment for diabetes and was found to be one of the best natural treatments (Guarino et al., 2017).

11.2.2 VINDOLINE, VINDOLILININE, VINDOLICINE, VINDOLIDINE

Catharanthus roseus (L.) G. Don is a natural herbals originated from Madagascar but are distributed worldwide due to their high survival rate (Tiong et al., 2013). Pre-clinical trials confirmed the dose-dependent action in lowering blood glucose levels in both the control and diabetic rat groups upon administering the extracts of leaves of this plant. Tolbutamide is an anti-diabetic drug used to treat diabetes; an equivalent performance was performed by the extract of this plant in lowering the blood sugar level in animal models (Chattopadhyay et al., 1999). Compared to animals without any disease, the biochemical action of glycogen synthase, succinate dehydrogenase, malate dehydrogenase and glucose 6-phosphate- dehydrogenase were observed to decline in diabetic animals in the liver. When the leaves of *C. roseus* were extracted, dichloromethane–methanol and twigs were given to diabetic animals at 500mg/kg for seven days, and the enzymatic activity was gradually increased. Alkaloids like indoline, vindoline, indoline and vinylidene compounds of *C. roseus* are very effective in diabetes management as these compounds help improve glucose uptake in myoblast C2 and C12 or pancreatic β-TC6 cells. Extracted compounds substantially inhibited the protein tyrosine phosphatase–1B required for managing type 2 diabetes. Prohibiting the protein improved blood glucose levels, whereas the extracts showed enhanced glucose metabolism and insulin-related activities (Singh et al., 2001).

11.2.3 CHLOROGENIC ACID AND CHICORY

Cichorium intybus L., known as Chicory, was founded in Asia, Europe, Africa and Southern America (Street et al., 2013). Plant ethanolic extract has been found to reduce hepatic 6 phosphatase performance, suggesting a decline in hepatic gluconeogenesis (Nishimura et al., 2015). Chlorogenic acid and chicoric, an anti-diabetic compound, enhance glucose uptake in L6 muscular cells. They also stimulate insulin excretion from the INS-1Einsuline secretory cell line and rat's pancreatic islets. Preclinical studies show that when diabetic rats are treated with CIE, the hepatic Glc-6-Pase activity drops (Pushparaj et al., 2007). Moreover, this enzyme is responsible for glucose production in the liver. Moreover, when its activity decreases, glucose production in the lives decreases, resulting in a decrease in blood glucose levels. A random clinical trial was conducted on 100 individuals diagnosed with type 2 diabetes, and the result we got was that the HbA1c level reduced from 8.6% to 7.42% after 12 weeks of supplementation (Chandra et al., 2020).

This shows its tremendous effect of medicinal efficacy in type 2 diabetes. All pre-clinical and clinical studies suggested that it is proven to be an excellent alternative to synthetic drugs against diabetes.

11.2.4 CHAMAEMELOSIDE

Chamaemelum nobile is commonly known as Roman chamomile. It has been found in Southeastern Morocco (Eddoukset al., 2005). It has been found to follow an insulin-independent pathway, as liquid extracts displayed a decline in blood glucose levels when performed in a diabetic rat model without altering plasma insulin level, suggesting an insulin secretion-independent pathway. Several studies also found that it may exert a hypoglycemic effect on the digestive system, decelerating carbohydrate incorporation's digestion rate. This whole regulation suggested its multifaceted mechanism. Chamaemeloside, a significant compound in it, showed hypoglycemic property activity in the Swiss-Webster mice model, which helped in improved pre-meal glucose level, enhanced glycemic tolerance, and reduced plasma glucose concentration (König et al., 1998). Chamaemeloside, containing flavonoid glucoside, is a significant component that helps improve pre-meal glucose levels and enhance glycemic tolerance. An eight-week clinical study demonstrated that 26 pre-diabetic volunteers were given mixed herbal extracts. The extract was combined with hot water retrieve of roman chamomile and Vitis vinifera at an intake of 1200 mg, and it has been found that there is a reduction in abnormal glucose values, suggesting it contains potential in diabetes management (Yonei et al., 2010)

11.2.5 MASOPROCOL

Larrea tridentata, commonly known as Coville. It is commonly found in North American warm deserts and Mexico (Arteaga et al., 2005). Studies have illustrated that Masoprocol components contain antihyperglycemic effects, which act as lipoxygenase inhibitors. In preclinical studies, type 2 diabetic models were taken, and it was revealed that they can decline the plasma glucose level without modifying the concentration of plasma insulin (Luo et al., 1998). it has also been found that it helps to enhance oral glucose tolerance and augments insulin performance.

11.2.6 B-GLUCANS

Hordeum vulgare L., known as Barley, has been founded in Fertile Crescent, including Israel, Jordan, and Syria (Von Bothmer et al., 1985). It contains the β-glucans dietary fiber that is highly therapeutic in diabetes management. When orally given to mice with type 2 diabetes and those on a high-level fat diet, it has resulted in a cutback in the blood glucose level (Cao et al., 2017). There is a suppression of a protein called intestinal glucose transporter. It has been found that it encourages glycogen synthesis and prevents fat build-up in the liver. Decreasing glucose creation and promoting glucose uptake in the body regulates glucose. Various clinical studies showed that β-glucans also help to optimize glucose regulation for diabetic patients (Ying Sun et al., 2023). Various antidiabetic herbal sources have been shown in Figure 11.1.

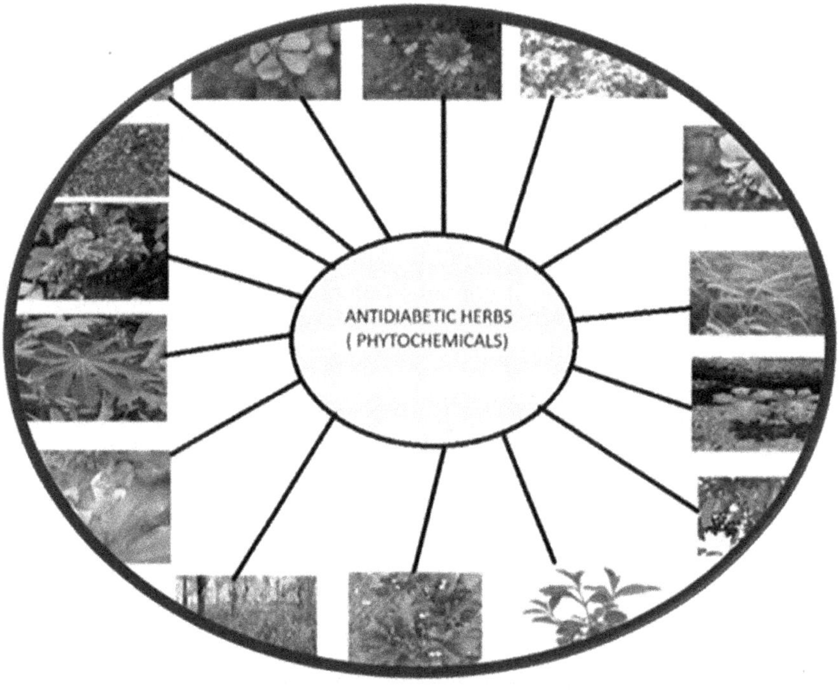

FIGURE 11.1 Pictorial depiction of antidiabetic herbal sources.

11.2.7 PELTALOSA

Psacalium peltatum (Kunth) Cass. is commonly known as 'Matarique' and has been found in Mexico. Peltalosa, isolated from the roots and rhizomes of the mentioned plant, contained hypoglycemic activity results inferred when given to mice with mild diabetes (Contreras et al., 2005). Studies demonstrated that it promotes excretion of insulin from the pancreatic islets.

11.2.8 MYCAMINOSE

Syzygium cumini (L.) Skeels, commonly known as Jamun, was founded in India. *S. cumin* seeds contain remarkable therapeutic effects in diabetic management as it lowers blood glucose levels by stimulating insulin release (Kumar et al., 2013). Mycaminose, a major component extracted from it, helps reduce blood sugar levels, as suggested by various studies and research (Karthic et al., 2008). In a clinical trial involving 99 individuals with type 2 diabetes, 10 g of its enrichment was daily, decreasing pre-meal blood glucose by 30% and meal blood sugar by 22% (Sidana et al., 2017).

11.2.9 STEVIOSIDE

Stevia rebounding Bertoni was founded in the Amambay region northeast of Paraguay. Stevioside, a chemical compound obtained from it, holds the property to control diabetes. Studies have shown that it plays a significant role in anti-hyperglycemic, insulinotropic, and glucagon static (Li et al., 2013). Trials have been done to know its efficacy. A 60-day trial was conducted; 1g of powder was given to 20 individuals diagnosed with type 2 diabetes, resulting in a decline in pre and post-meal sugar levels (Anton et al., 2010). A 45-day clinical trial was also conducted where 0.5 g and 1 g of powdered leaves of S. rebaudiana with tea were given to 15 diabetic patients thrice a day, resulting in the decline of FBG and PPBG.

11.2.10 D-PINITOL

Bougainvillea spectabilis Willd. Natural herbal plants originated in Brazil and hold good therapeutic efficacy in diabetes management. D-pinitol compound extracted from it was found to help elevate the performance of glucose-6-phosphate dehydrogenase (Holt et al., 2004). To examine its efficacy, a randomized controlled clinical study was executed on 66 individuals with type 2 diabetes; 1.2g of it was given to them, which led to a reduction in pre-meal blood sugar levels and HbA1c, HOMA-IR (Jawla et al., 2013).

11.2.11 4-HYDROXYBENZOIC ACID

Pandanus amaryllifolius Roxb Herbal plant, also known as *Pandanu Diodorus*,isfoundinThailand(Chiabchalardetal.,2015).4-Hydroxybenzoic acid phytoconstituent extracted from it contained hypoglycemic occurrences. Studies on mice models have shown that it declines the blood sugar level in streptozotocin. By restraining α-glucosidase enzyme and regulating blood production, it showed antihyperglycemic activity. A clinical trial implemented involving 30 healthy individuals (15 males and 15 females) determined that tea consisting of approximately 30 g helps in the downturn of post-meal production of glucose levels and suggested it is relevant in managing blood sugar levels in a real-world setting (Chiabchalard et al., 2015).

11.2.12 B-AMYRIN AND METHYL TETRACOSANATE

Costus pictus D. Don, a medicinal herbal widely known as the 'Insulin plant' known for its anti-diabetic properties, originated in Southern and Central America. β-amyrin and methyl tetracosanate are found to be the significant phytochemicals that perform enhanced glucose uptake (Shilpa et al., 2009). Impedes α-amylase and glucosidase activity, due to which it controls blood sugar levels (Tranetal et al., 2020). When studying its functionality in model mice, it was concluded that there was an increase in plasma insulin level and a decrease in blood sugar level. It helps to augment glucose utilization by advancing peripheral glucose utilization and elevating hepatic glycogen synthesis while diminishing glycogenolysis; it decreases the glycemic index of carbohydrates, further regulating glucose homeostasis (Jayasri et al., 2007). Clinical trials were carried out on diabetic patients when administered to them, resulting in a diminution in their fasting and post-meal blood glucose levels (Shetty et al., 2010). Mechanisms of different phytochemicals to manage diabetes can be seen in Figure 11.2.

11.2.13 ISOORIENTIN AND CHLOROGENIC ACID

Cecropia obtusifolia Bertol. is an herbal plant found in Mexico and Ecuador. Isoorientin and Chlorogenic acid are its major components,

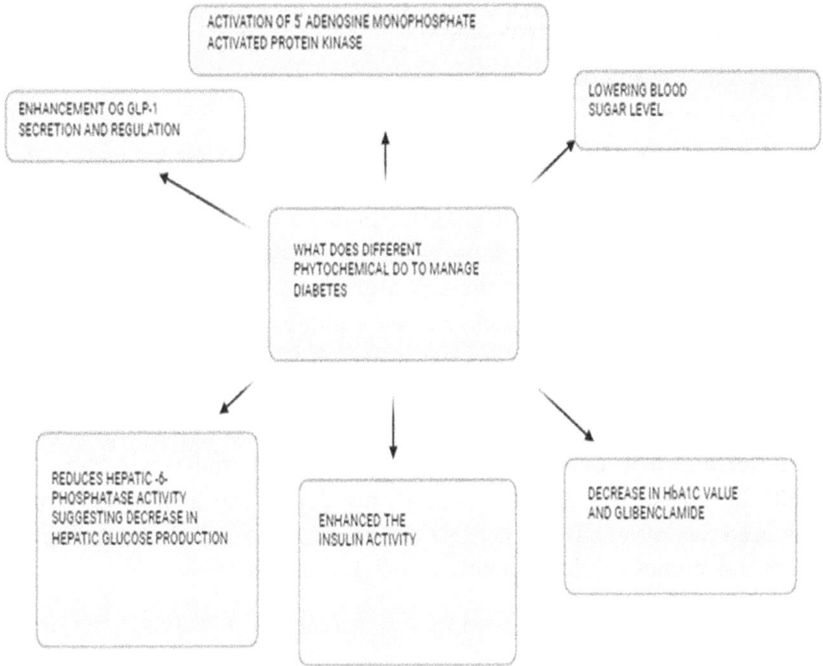

FIGURE 11.2 Mechanism of different phytochemicals to manage diabetes.

which are believed to have beneficial antidiabetic properties as they help decrease Hba1c and blood glucose levels (Yang et al., 2020). A 21-day clinical trial in which dry leaf infusions were dispensed to 43 individuals with type 2 diabetes brought about a 15.25% decline in pre-meal blood sugar levels (Revilla et al., 2007).

11.2.14 COROSOLIC ACID

Lagerstroemia speciosa (L.) Pers. is an herbal plant commonly found in tropical southern areas. Corosolic acid is the main constituent of it, which is found to facilitate glucose transport, stimulating activity back in blood glucose levels and stimulating glucose uptake in 3T3-L1(Miao et al., 2018). Researchers conducted a two-week randomized clinical trial of almost 48 g of a daily dose of it gels with 1% corosolic acid administered to 10 individuals having type 2 diabetes, which resulted in approximately

30% and 20% decline in blood glucose levels for respective soft and hard gel formulation (Judy et al., 2003). The above studies confirmed its anti-diabetic activity and performance.

11.2.15 SALACINOL AND KOTALANOL

Salacia reticulates Wight, originating in Sri Lanka, contains Salacinol and Kotalanol, their major component in diabetic management. They have been found to suppress the alpha-glucosidase enzyme (Trpkovic et al., 2015). To know its efficaciousness, a clinical trial was implemented a six-month clinical trial conducted in which 51 individuals with type 2 diabetes were given mixed herbal preparations, which yielded a decrease in HbA1C value and glibenclamide (Jayawardena et al., 2005). Another crossover and 6-week endured placebo-controlled trial was operated in which 20 individuals with type 2, 240 mg daily dose of it were given a decreased fasting glucose level (Nakamura et al., 2010). An easy illustration of the studies of phytochemicals can be seen in Table 11.1.

11.3 CHALLENGES

Recently, many individuals have been shifting towards herbal medicines for several reasons. As they suggested, herbal medicines contain less toxicity than synthetic treatments. Unsatisfied pharmaceutical results, higher costs and side effects of synthetic drugs have drawn attention towards the shift. Rather than scientific information, some choose them because of their personal experiences. However, sometimes, caution is needed as the lack of safety study is a concern. To know these specific points should be kept in mind (Tan et al., 2014).

1. Herbal products should pass quality certification, including standardization and stability checks. Using herbal products without valid authorization is unsafe.
2. Not always herbal medicines are safe, so safety assessment should be conducted
3. It should not be administered Without pre-clinical and clinical trial results.
4. After checking all the above challenges, herbal medicines should only be administered.

TABLE 11.1 Different Phytochemicals Used in Preclinical and Clinical Studies to Manage Diabetes

S. No.	Plant Name	Phytochemical	Origin	Preclinical and Clinical Studies	References
1.	*Berberis aristata* DC	Berberine	Northern Himalayan	Effect in mice against T2DM. of 0.5 g of it thrice a day to people diagnosed with type 2 diabetes revealed effectiveness in improving fasting blood glucose level	Yin et al. (2008)
2.	*Catharanthus roseus* (L.) G. Don	Vindoline, Vindolilinine, Vindolicine, Vindolidine	Madagascar	Dose-dependent action in lowering the blood glucose levels in both the control and diabetic rat group, dichloromethane–methanol and twigs were given to diabetic animals 500mg/kg for seven days, gradually increasing the enzymatic activity	Tiong et al. (2013)
3.	*Cichorium intybus* L	Chlorogenic acid and chicory	Asia, Europe, Africa and Southern America	Diabetic rat treated with CIE, the hepatic Glc-6-Pase activity drops; a clinical trial conducted on 100 individuals diagnosed with type 2 diabetes results see HbA1c level gets reduced from8.6% to 7.42% after12 weeks of it supplementation	Chandra et al. (2020); Street et al. (2013)
4.	*Chamaemelum nobile*	Chamaemeloside	South eastern Morocco	Hypo glycemic property activity in Swiss-Webster mice model, which helps in improved fasting glucose level and enhanced glucose tolerance	Eddouksetal. (2005); König et al. (1998)
5.	*Larrea tridentata* (Sess)	Masoprocol	North American warm deserts and Mexico	Type 2 diabetic models were taken, and it showed that it contains the ability to reduce the plasma glucose level without altering the concentration of plasma insulin	Arteaga et al. (2005); Luo et al. (1998)
6.	*Hordeum vulgare* L.	β-glucans	Israel	Orally given to mice with type 2 diabetes and those on a level-fat diet, it has resulted in a reduction in the blood glucose level	Cao et al. (2017); Von Bothmer et al. (1985)
7.	*Psacalium peltatum* (Kunth) Cass	Peltalosa	Mexico	Contained anti-glycemic activity results concluded when given to mice with mild diabetes	Contreras et al. (2005)
8.	*Syzygium cumini* (L.)	Mycaminose	India and Malaya	The clinical trial involves 99 individuals Diagnosed type 2 diabetes, a 10 g quantity of *Syzygium cumini* supplementation was given daily, resulting in a decrease in fasting blood glucose level	Sidana et al. (2017)

TABLE 11.1 *(Continued)*

S. No.	Plant Name	Phytochemical	Origin	Preclinical and Clinical Studies	References
9.	*Stevia rebaundiana Bertoni*	Stevioside	Amambay	The 60-day long trial has been conducted,1g S. powder was given to 20 individuals diagnosed with type 2 diabetes, resulting in a decline in pre and post-meal glucose level	Anton et al. (2010)
10.	*Bougainvillea spectabilis Willd.*	D-pinitol	Brazil	The randomized controlled clinical study was executed on 66 individuals with type 2 diabetes; 1.2g of it was given to them, which led to a reduction in fasting blood glucose level and HbA1c, HOMA-IR	Jawla et al. (2013)
11.	*Pandanus amaryllifolius Roxb.*	4-Hydroxybenzoic acid	Thailand	A clinical trial involving 30 healthy individuals (15 males and 15 females) was implemented, and it was determined that tea, consisting of approximately 30 g, helps in the downturn of post-meal production of glucose level.	Chiabchalar et al. (2015)
12.	*Costus pictures* D. Don	β-amyrin and methyl tetracosanate	Southern and Central America	When studying its functionality in model mice, it concluded increase in plasma insulin level and decrease blood sugar level. Clinical trials were carried out on diabetic patients, when it was administered to them, resulted in a diminution in their pre and post-meal blood sugar levels	Shetty et al. (2010)
13.	*Cecropia obtusifolia Bertol.*	Isoorientin and Chlorogenic acid	Mexico and Ecuador	A 21-day clinical trial was performed in which dry leaf infusions were dispensed to 43 individuals having type 2 diabetic patients, brought about 15.25% decline in pre-meal blood sugar level	Revilla- Monsalve et al. (2007)
14.	*Lagerstroemia speciosa* (L.) Pers.	Corosolicacid	Tropical southern area	A two-week clinical trial conducted 48 g of a daily dose of it gels with 1% corosolic acid administered to 10 individuals having type 2 diabetic patients resulted in approximately 30% and 20% decline in blood glucose levels for respective soft, hard gel formulation	Judy et al. (2003)
15.	*Salacia reticulate Wight*	Salacinoland Kotalanol	Srilanka	Week endured placebo-controlled trials were operated in which 20 individuals having type 2 diabetes, 240 mg daily dose of it were given the concluded decline in pre-meal glucose level	Jayawarden et al. (2005); Nakamura et al. (2010)

11.4 FUTURE DIRECTIONS

Advancements in the research field open new avenues for exploring innovative ideas and drug discoveries, aiming to focus on the action of phytochemicals in managing diabetes.

11.4.1 NANO-FORMULATIONS

Advancements in nano-science and nanotechnology bring various applications in medical and health science. It has proven to be a game changer in drug delivery systems and has proven to be better than conventional approaches (Bhattacharya et al., 2022; Dhiman and Singh, 2011). Improving biopharmaceutical attributes, target specificity, and pharmacokinetic profile of therapeutic agents' nano formulations enhances their clinical efficacy. Extensive studies and development of medical science came up with the conclusion that nano-carrier-assembled drug nano-particles like polymeric nanoparticles, dendrimers, liposomes, etc., were found to be more successful than the conventional drug delivery system in terms of stability, drug release, bioavailability, and effectiveness. It has also been found that if nano-carriers are attached to ligands, their target specificity gradually increases, protecting against drug degradation (Dewanjee et al., 2020).

Traditional local remedies, learnings, and treatment styles have resulted in the discovery of herbal medicines we use recently. Scientists have found valuable treatments against diseases by observing natural home remedies and have started working on them to find their best efficacy. As per the reports, 70% of modern medicines in India are derived from natural sources. In the future, plant-based medicines will play a significant role as there will be an increase in the side effects of synthetic drugs. The medicinal plant contributes dually to both economic and healthcare solutions

11.5 CONCLUSION

This article evaluates the properties of plants that can help to manage diabetes. Natural compounds in these plants can lower blood sugar levels without causing significant side effects. Moreover, plants are generally considered safe and have good therapeutic efficacy. More research on plant properties can give plants more useful therapeutic efficacy, which can be helpful to humans.

KEYWORDS

- **alkaloids**
- **bioactive compounds**
- **clinical validation**
- **diabetes mellitus**
- **phytochemicals**
- **polyphenols**

REFERENCES

Alam, S., Sarker, M. M. R., Sultana, T. N., Chowdhury, M. N. R., Rashid, M. A., Chaity, N. I., Zhao, C., Xiao, J., Hafez, E. E., Khan, S. A., & Mohamed, I. N. (2022). Antidiabetic phytochemicals from medicinal plants: Prospective candidates for new drug discovery and development. *Frontiers in Endocrinology, 13*, 800714. https://doi.org/10.3389/fendo.2022.800714 (accessed on 28th June 2025).

Anton, S. D., Martin, C. K., Han, H., Coulon, S., Cefalu, W. T., Geiselman, P., & Williamson, D. A. (2010). Effects of stevia, aspartame, and sucrose on food intake, satiety, and postprandial glucose and insulin levels. *Appetite, 55*(1), 37–43. https://doi.org/10.1016/j.appet.2010.03.009 (accessed on 28th June 2025).

Arora, A., Behl, T., Sehgal, A., Singh, S., Sharma, N., Bhatia, S., Sobarzo-Sanchez, E., & Bungau, S. (2021). Unravelling the involvement of gut microbiota in type 2 diabetes mellitus. *Life Sciences, 273*, 119311. https://doi.org/10.1016/j.lfs.2021.119311 (accessed on 28th June 2025).

Arteaga, S., Andrade-Cetto, A., & Cárdenas, R. (2005). *Larrea tridentata* (Creosote Bush), an abundant plant of Mexican and US-American deserts and its metabolite nordihydroguaiaretic acid. *Journal of Ethnopharmacology, 98*(3), 231–239. https://doi.org/10.1016/j.jep.2005.02.002 (accessed on 28th June 2025).

Bhargava, S. K., Singh, T. G., Mannan, A., Singh, S., Singh, M., & Gupta, S. (2022). Pharmacological evaluation of *Thuja occidentalis* for the attenuation of neuropathy via AGEs and TNF-α inhibition in diabetic neuropathic rats. *Environmental Science and Pollution Research International, 29*(40), 60542–60557. https://doi.org/10.1007/s11356-022-20106-3 (accessed on 28th June 2025).

Bhattacharya, T., Soares, G. A. B. E., Chopra, H., Rahman, M. M., Hasan, Z., Swain, S. S., & Cavalu, S. (2022). Applications of phyto-nanotechnology for the treatment of neurodegenerative disorders. *Materials (Basel, Switzerland), 15*(3), 804. https://doi.org/10.3390/ma15030804 (accessed on 28th June 2025).

Cao, Y., Sun, Y., Zou, S., Li, M., & Xu, X. (2017). Orally administered baker's yeast β-glucan promotes glucose and lipid homeostasis in the livers of obesity and diabetes model mice. *Journal of Agricultural and Food Chemistry, 65*, 9665–9674. https://pubs.acs.org/doi/10.1021/acs.jafc.7b03782 (accessed on 28th June 2025).

Chandra, K., Jain, V., Jabin, A., Dwivedi, S., Joshi, S., Ahmad, S., et al. (2020). Effect of *Cichorium intybus* seeds supplementation on the markers of glycemic control, oxidative stress, inflammation, and lipid profile in type 2 diabetes mellitus: A randomized, double-blind placebo study. *Phytotherapy Research, 34*, 1609–1618. https://doi.org/10.1002/ptr.6624 (accessed on 28th June 2025).

Chattopadhyay, R. R. (1999). A comparative evaluation of some blood sugar lowering agents of plant origin. *Journal of Ethnopharmacology, 67*, 367–372. https://doi.org/10.1016/S0378-8741(99)00095-1 (accessed on 28th June 2025).

Chiabchalard, A., & Nooron, N. (2015). Antihyperglycemic effects of *Pandanus amaryllifolius* Roxb. leaf extract. *Pharmacognosy Magazine, 11*, 117–122. https://www.ncbi.nlm.nih.gov/pmc/articles/PMC4329610/ (accessed on 28th June 2025).

Contreras, C., Román, R., Pérez, C., Alarcón, F., Zavala, M., & Pérez, S. (2005). Hypoglycemic activity of a new carbohydrate isolated from the roots of *Psacalium peltatum*. *Chemical & Pharmaceutical Bulletin (Tokyo), 53*, 1408–1410. https://doi.org/10.1248/cpb.53.1408 (accessed on 28th June 2025).

Dewanjee, S., Chakraborty, P., Mukherjee, B., & De Feo, V. (2020). Plant-based antidiabetic nanoformulations: The emerging paradigm for effective therapy. *International Journal of Molecular Sciences, 21*(6), 2217. https://doi.org/10.3390/ijms21062217 (accessed on 28th June 2025).

Dhiman, S., & Thakur, G. S. (2011). Nanosuspension: A recent approach for nano drug delivery system. *International Journal of Current Pharmaceutical Research, 3*(4), 96–101. https://doi.org/10.1016/j.appet.2010.03.009 (accessed on 28th June 2025).

Eddouks, M., Lemhadri, A., Zeggwagh, N. A., & Michel, J.-B. (2005). Potent hypoglycaemic activity of the aqueous extract of *Chamaemelum nobile* in normal and streptozotocin-induced diabetic rats. *Diabetes Research and Clinical Practice, 67*, 189–195. https://doi.org/10.1016/j.diabres.2004.07.015 (accessed on 28th June 2025).

Garg, M., Sharma, A., Bansal, S., Grover, R., Sharma, T., Kumari, S., Goyal, A., Bhatia, S., Vaid, L., Deswal, G., & Grewal, A. S. (2023). Role of medicinal plants in the management of inflammatory disorders: An overview. *Recent Advances in Inflammation & Allergy Drug Discovery, 17*(1), 20–30. https://doi.org/10.2174/27722708176662302271406 59 (accessed on 28th June 2025).

Garg, N., Singh, T. G., Khan, H., Arora, S., Kaur, A., & Mannan, A. (2021). Mechanistic interventions of selected *Ocimum* species in management of diabetes, obesity and liver disorders: Transformative developments from preclinical to clinical approaches. *Biointerface Research in Applied Chemistry, 12*(1), 1304–1323.

Guarino, G., Strollo, F., Carbone, L., Della Corte, T., Letizia, M., Marino, G., et al. (2017). Bioimpedance analysis, metabolic effects and safety of the association *Berberis aristata/Silybum marianum*: A 52-week double-blind, placebo-controlled study in obese patients with type 2 diabetes. *Journal of Biological Regulators and Homeostatic Agents, 31*, 495–502.

Gupta, S., Khan, A., Vishwas, S., Gulati, M., Singh, T. G., Dua, K., Singh, S. K., Najda, A., Sayed, A. A., Almeer, R., & Abdel-Daim, M. M. (2021). Demethyleneberberine: A possible treatment for Huntington's disease. *Medical Hypotheses, 153*, 110639. https://doi.org/10.1016/j.mehy.2021.110639 (accessed on 28th June 2025).

Holt, R. I. (2004). Diagnosis, epidemiology and pathogenesis of diabetes mellitus: An update for psychiatrists. *The British Journal of Psychiatry. Supplement, 47*, S55–S63. https://doi.org/10.1192/bjp.184.47.s55 (accessed on 28th June 2025).

Hunter, S. J., & Garvey, W. T. (1998). Insulin action and insulin resistance: Diseases involving defects in insulin receptors, signal transduction, and the glucose transport effector system. *The American Journal of Medicine, 105*(4), 331–345. https://doi.org/10.1016/s0002-9343(98)00300-3 (accessed on 28th June 2025).

Jawla, S., Kumar, Y., & Khan, M. S. Y. (2013). Isolation of antidiabetic principle from *Bougainvillea spectabilis* Willd (*Nyctaginaceae*) stem bark. *Tropical Journal of Pharmaceutical Research, 12*(5), 761–765. https://www.ajol.info/index.php/tjpr/article/view/95947 (accessed on 28th June 2025).

Jayasri, M. A., Gunasekaran, S., Radha, A., & Mathew, T. L. (2008). Anti-diabetic effect of *Costus pictus* leaves in normal and streptozotocin-induced diabetic rats. *International Journal of Diabetes and Metabolism, 16*(3), 117–122. https://doi.org/10.1159/000497662 (accessed on 28th June 2025).

Jayawardena, M. H., de Alwis, N. M., Hettigoda, V., & Fernando, D. J. (2005). A double blind randomised placebo controlled cross over study of a herbal preparation containing *Salacia reticulata* in the treatment of type 2 diabetes. *Journal of Ethnopharmacology, 97*(2), 215–218. https://doi.org/10.1016/j.jep.2004.10.026 (accessed on 28th June 2025).

Judy, W. V., Hari, S. P., Stogsdill, W. W., Judy, J. S., Naguib, Y. M. A., & Passwater, R. (2003). Antidiabetic activity of a standardized extract (Glucosol) from *Lagerstroemia speciosa* leaves in type II diabetics: A dose-dependence study. *Journal of Ethnopharmacology, 87*, 115–117. https://doi.org/10.1016/S0378-8741(03)00122-3 (accessed on 28th June 2025).

Karthic, K., Kirthiram, K. S., Sadasivam, S., & Thayumanavan, B. (2008). Identification of alpha amylase inhibitors from *Syzygium cumini* Linn seeds. *Indian Journal of Experimental Biology, 46*(9), 677–680.

Kaur, J., Singla, M., Saini, B., & Bansal, G. (2017). Standardization of some commercial anti-diabetic herbal products containing *Syzygium cumini*. *Journal of Pharmaceutical Technology, Research and Management, 5*(1), 21–30.

Kaur, N., Kishore, L., Farooq, S. A., Kajal, A., Singh, R., Agrawal, R., Mannan, A., & Singh, T. G. (2023). *Cucurbita pepo* seeds improve peripheral neuropathy in diabetic rats by modulating the inflammation and oxidative stress in rats. *Environmental Science and Pollution Research International, 30*(36), 85910–85919. https://doi.org/10.1007/s11356-023-28339-6 (accessed on 28th June 2025).

König, G. M., Wright, A. D., Keller, W. J., Judd, R. L., Bates, S., & Day, C. (1998). Hypoglycaemic activity of an HMG-containing flavonoid glucoside, chamaemeloside, from *Chamaemelum nobile*. *Planta Medica, 64*(7), 612–614. https://doi.org/10.1055/s-2006-957532 (accessed on 28th June 2025).

Kumar, A., Ilavarasan, R., Jayachandran, T., Deecaraman, M., Aravindan, P., Padmanabhan, N., & Krishan, M. R. V. (2008). Anti-diabetic activity of *Syzygium cumini* and its isolated compound against streptozotocin-induced diabetic rats. *Journal of Medicinal Plants Research, 2*(9), 246–249.

Li, G. Q., Kam, A., Wong, K. H., Zhou, X., Omar, E. A., Alqahtani, A., Li, K. M., Razmovski-Naumovski, V., & Chan, K. (2012). Herbal medicines for the management of diabetes. In *Advances in Experimental Medicine and Biology, 771*, 396–413. https://doi.org/10.1007/978-1-4614-5441-0_28 (accessed on 28th June 2025).

Luo, J., Chuang, T., Cheung, J., Quan, J., Tsai, J., Sullivan, C., Hector, R. F., Reed, M. J., Meszaros, K., King, S. R., Carlson, T. J., & Reaven, G. M. (1998). Masoprocol (nordihydroguaiaretic acid): A new antihyperglycemic agent isolated from the creosote bush (*Larrea tridentata*). *European Journal of Pharmacology, 346*(1), 77–79. https://doi.org/10.1016/s0014-2999(98)00139-3 (accessed on 28th June 2025).

Mehta, S., Nain, P., Agrawal, B. K., Singh, R. P., Kaur, J., Maity, S., Bhattacharjee, A., Peela, J., Nauhria, S., & Nauhria, S. (2021). Effectiveness of empagliflozin with vitamin D supplementation in peripheral neuropathy in type 2 diabetic patients. *Cureus, 13*(12), e20208. https://doi.org/10.7759/cureus.20208 (accessed on 28th June 2025).

Miao, C., Zhang, G., Xie, Z., & Chang, J. (2018). MicroRNAs in the pathogenesis of type 2 diabetes: New research progress and future direction. *Canadian Journal of Physiology and Pharmacology, 96*(2), 103–112. https://doi.org/10.1139/cjpp-2017-0452 (accessed on 28th June 2025).

Nakamura, S., Takahira, K., Tanabe, G., Morikawa, T., Sakano, M., Ninomiya, K., Yoshikawa, M., Muraoka, O., & Nakanishi, I. (2010). Docking and SAR studies of salacinol derivatives as alpha-glucosidase inhibitors. *Bioorganic & Medicinal Chemistry Letters, 20*(15), 4420–4423. https://doi.org/10.1016/j.bmcl.2010.06.059 (accessed on 28th June 2025).

Nishimura, M., Ohkawara, T., Kanayama, T., Kitagawa, K., Nishimura, H., & Nishihira, J. (2015). Effects of the extract from roasted chicory (*Cichorium intybus* L.) root containing inulin-type fructans on blood glucose, lipid metabolism, and fecal properties. *Journal of Traditional and Complementary Medicine, 5*(3), 161–167. https://doi.org/10.1016/j.jtcme.2014.11.016 (accessed on 28th June 2025).

Potdar, D., Hirwani, R. R., & Dhulap, S. (2012). Phyto-chemical and pharmacological applications of *Berberis aristata. Fitoterapia, 83*(5), 817–830. https://doi.org/10.1016/j.fitote.2012.04.012 (accessed on 28th June 2025).

Pushparaj, P. N., Low, H. K., Manikandan, J., Tan, B. K., & Tan, C. H. (2007). Anti-diabetic effects of *Cichorium intybus* in streptozotocin-induced diabetic rats. *Journal of Ethnopharmacology, 111*(2), 430–434. https://doi.org/10.1016/j.jep.2006.11.028 (accessed on 28th June 2025).

Rehman, K., & Akash, M. S. H. (2017). Mechanism of generation of oxidative stress and pathophysiology of type 2 diabetes mellitus: How are they interlinked? *Journal of Cellular Biochemistry, 118*(11), 3577–3585. https://doi.org/10.1002/jcb.26097 (accessed on 28th June 2025).

Revilla-Monsalve, M. C., Andrade-Cetto, A., Palomino-Garibay, M. A., Wiedenfeld, H., & Islas-Andrade, S. (2007). Hypoglycemic effect of *Cecropia obtusifolia* Bertol aqueous extracts on type 2 diabetic patients. *Journal of Ethnopharmacology, 111*(3), 636–640. https://doi.org/10.1016/j.jep.2007.01.014 (accessed on 28th June 2025).

Sarker, M. M. R., & Soma, M. A. (2020). Updates on clinical study reports of phytotherapy in the management of type 2 diabetes mellitus. *Phytotherapy in the Management of Diabetes and Hypertension, 4*, 1–60.

Sharma, V. K., & Singh, T. G. (2020). Insulin resistance and bioenergetic manifestations: Targets and approaches in Alzheimer's disease. *Life Sciences, 262*, 118401. https://doi.org/10.1016/j.lfs.2020.118401 (accessed on 28th June 2025).

Shetty, A. J., Choudhury, D., Rejeesh, Nair, V., Kuruvilla, M., & Kotian, S. (2010). Effect of the insulin plant (*Costus igneus*) leaves on dexamethasone-induced hyperglycemia. *International Journal of Ayurveda Research, 1*(2), 100–102. https://doi.org/10.4103/0974-7788.64396 (accessed on 28th June 2025).

Shilpa, K., Sangeetha, K. N., Muthusamy, V. S., Sujatha, S., & Lakshmi, B. S. (2009). Probing key targets in insulin signaling and adipogenesis using a methanolic extract of *Costus pictus* and its bioactive molecule, methyl tetracosanoate. *Biotechnology Letters, 31*(12), 1837–1841. https://doi.org/10.1007/s10529-009-0105-3 (accessed on 28th June 2025).

Sidana, S., Singh, V. B., Meena, B. L., Beniwal, S., Singh, K., Kumar, D., & Singla, R. (2017). Effect of *Syzygium cumini* (jamun) seed powder on glycemic control: A double-blind randomized controlled trial. *Journal of Medical Society, 31*(3), 185–189. https://doi.org/10.4103/jms (accessed on 28th June 2025).

Singh, S. N., Vats, P., Suri, S., Shyam, R., Kumria, M. M., Ranganathan, S., & Sridharan, K. (2001). Effect of an antidiabetic extract of *Catharanthus roseus* on enzymic activities in streptozotocin-induced diabetic rats. *Journal of Ethnopharmacology, 76*(3), 269–277. https://doi.org/10.1016/s0378-8741(01)00254-9 (accessed on 28th June 2025).

Singh, V., & Kumar, A. (2020). Antioxidant potential of *Glycyrrhiza glabra* L. roots: In-vitro evidences. *Journal of Pharmaceutical Technology, Research and Management, 8*(1), 9–13. https://doi.org/10.15415/jptrm.2020.81002 (accessed on 28th June 2025).

Street, R. A., Sidana, J., & Prinsloo, G. (2013). *Cichorium intybus*: Traditional uses, phytochemistry, pharmacology, and toxicology. *Evidence-Based Complementary and Alternative Medicine, 2013*, 579319. https://doi.org/10.1155/2013/579319 (accessed on 28th June 2025).

Sun, Y., Liang, L., Yi, Y., Meng, Y., Peng, K., Jiang, X., & Wang, H. (2023). Synthesis, characterization and anti-inflammatory activity of selenium nanoparticles stabilized by aminated yeast glucan. *International Journal of Biological Macromolecules, 245*, 125187. https://doi.org/10.1016/j.ijbiomac.2023.125187 (accessed on 28th June 2025).

Tan, J., McKenzie, C., Potamitis, M., Thorburn, A. N., Mackay, C. R., & Macia, L. (2014). The role of short-chain fatty acids in health and disease. *Advances in Immunology, 121*, 91–119. https://doi.org/10.1016/B978-0-12-800100-4.00003-9 (accessed on 28th June 2025).

Tiong, S. H., Looi, C. Y., Hazni, H., Arya, A., Paydar, M., Wong, W. F., Cheah, S. C., Mustafa, M. R., & Awang, K. (2013). Antidiabetic and antioxidant properties of alkaloids from *Catharanthus roseus* (L.) G. Don. *Molecules (Basel, Switzerland), 18*(8), 9770–9784. https://doi.org/10.3390/molecules18089770 (accessed on 28th June 2025).

Tran, N., Pham, B., & Le, L. (2020). Bioactive compounds in anti-diabetic plants: From herbal medicine to modern drug discovery. *Biology, 9*(9), 252. https://doi.org/10.3390/biology9090252 (accessed on 28th June 2025).

Trpkovic, A., Resanovic, I., Stanimirovic, J., Radak, D., Mousa, S. A., Cenic-Milosevic, D., Jevremovic, D., & Isenovic, E. R. (2015). Oxidized low-density lipoprotein as a biomarker of cardiovascular diseases. *Critical Reviews in Clinical Laboratory Sciences, 52*(2), 70–85. https://doi.org/10.3109/10408363.2014.992063 (accessed on 28th June 2025).

von Bothmer, R., & Jacobsen, N. (1985). Origin, taxonomy, and related species. In *Barley, 26*, 19–56.

Yang, S., Zhou, R., Zhang, C., He, S., & Su, Z. (2020). Mitochondria-associated endoplasmic reticulum membranes in the pathogenesis of type 2 diabetes mellitus. *Frontiers in Cell and Developmental Biology, 8*, 571554. https://doi.org/10.3389/fcell.2020.571554 (accessed on 28th June 2025).

Yin, J., Xing, H., & Ye, J. (2008). Efficacy of berberine in patients with type 2 diabetes mellitus. *Metabolism: Clinical and Experimental, 57*(5), 712–717. https://doi.org/10.1016/j.metabol.2008.01.013 (accessed on 28th June 2025).

Yoshikazu, Y., Ryo, M., Yoko, T., Hozumi, T., Keitaro, N., Masayuki, Y., … & Nobuyasu, M. (2010). Anti-glycation effect of mixed herbal extract in individuals with pre-diabetes mellitus. *Anti-Aging Medicine, 7*(5), 26–35. https://doi.org/10.3793/jaam.7.26 (accessed on 28th June 2025).

CHAPTER 12

Novel Phyto-Nanotherapeutics Targeting Approaches for Diabetes Mellitus

RAJAN SWAMI,[1,*] KOMAL SALL,[1] MADHUKAR GARG,[1]
PANKAJ POPLI,[1,2] NIDHI RANI,[1] SAMIR MEHNDIRATTA,[3,4]
THAKUR GURJEET SINGH,[1] and SANJANA MEHTA[1]

[1]Chitkara College of Pharmacy, Chitkara University, Punjab, India

[2]Department of Pharmacy, Jagannath University, Bahadurgarh, Haryana, India

[3]Discipline of Pharmacy, Graduate School of Health, University of Technology Sydney, Sydney, New South Wales, Australia

[4]Faculty of Health, Australian Research Center in Complementary and Integrative Medicine, University of Technology Sydney, Ultimo, New South Wales, Australia

*Corresponding author

ABSTRACT

Diabetes mellitus (DM), commonly referred to as diabetes, has become a prevalent health concern in the contemporary world due to our evolving lifestyles. Our bodies continuously process glucose as a primary energy source, but when diabetes occurs, it signifies a disruption in the production and regulation of insulin. This leads to elevated blood glucose levels, placing chronic stress on various organs. Traditional drug treatments have been explored, but the necessity for escalating doses often results in unwanted side effects. However, ancient systems of medicine

Precision Nutrition and Endocrine Health: Synthesis, Characterization, and Applications.
Thakur Gurjeet Singh and Sanjana Mehta (Eds.)

DOI: 10.1201/9781998511877-12

like Ayurveda and Traditional Chinese Medicine have proposed natural remedies that can help maintain blood glucose levels when consistently administered, with minimal adverse effects. These natural remedies face challenges due to their limited bioavailability, primarily due to unfavorable physicochemical properties. Innovative formulation techniques offer a solution by enhancing the overall bioavailability and targeting these remedies to specific sites. The advent of nanotechnology has played a pivotal role in this regard, and the combination of nano-sized natural remedies has ushered in a new era of DM management. This chapter delves into this journey and how nanoparticles assist natural remedies in shaping the future of DM treatment, offering valuable insights to the readers.

12.1 INTRODUCTION

Glucose plays a vital role in energy use. All the major nutrients, that is carbohydrates, proteins, and lipids, are ultimately metabolized into glucose, which serves as mammals' primary energy source. Glycolysis, a process in glucose metabolism, is the primary mechanism responsible for extracting energy from glucose, generating two pyruvic acid molecules. Gluconeogenesis occurs when glucose is synthesized from non-carbohydrate substrates within the mitochondria of hepatic cells (Nakrani et al., 2020; Singh et al., 2022).

DM is marked by the body's reduced ability to regulate and maintain systemic glucose levels due to dysfunction in hormone creation or response (Bhargava et al., 2022a, b). Pancreatic β-cells undergo autoimmune destruction, resulting in inadequate insulin synthesis. Additionally, the body's cells exhibit inherent resistance to insulin (Sharma and Singh, 2020; Sharma et al., 2021). Complications of DM can be divided into two primary types: microvascular complications (Mehta et al., 2021), which affect small blood vessels in different body regions and, hence, cause multiple ailments in the affected regions, such as neuropathy, retinopathy, and nephropathy (Devi et al., 2023; Kaur et al., 2023; Mezil and Abed, 2021). Other macrovascular complications, including microvascular complications and cardiovascular disease, further increase mortality or cause permanent blindness or a general decline in quality of life for patients (Rohilla et al., 2023).

Type 1 diabetes is an autoimmune condition in which T cells destroy pancreatic β-cells, leading to insulin deficiency and hyperglycaemia. Without the insulin hormone, the body cannot control blood sugar levels properly. Type 1 diabetes manifests in childhood and persists into adulthood (Banday et al., 2020).

Type 2 diabetes is primarily characterized by three metabolic abnormalities that work together: increased hepatic production, decreased insulin secretion, and inadequate glucose absorption into peripheral tissues. These factors collectively contribute to the dysfunction of β-cells (Ekta et al., 2020; Garg et al., 2021; Najar et al., 2022; Tesauro and Mazzotta et al., 2020). However, many therapeutic interventions were presented that helped decrease the diabetic burden, as illustrated in Table 12.1. However, many challenges are limiting the effectiveness of diabetic drug delivery. These are as follows:

- Enhancing existing treatments to manage blood glucose, blood pressure, and lipid levels and reduce complications.
- Providing education to patients about how to manage their diabetes independently.
- Enhancing patient compliance with lifestyle changes and drug interventions.
- Reducing barriers to early initiation of insulin therapy.
- Enhancing the provision of health services for individuals with long-term conditions.

Table 12.1 represents the treatment approaches for the management of diabetes condition.

TABLE 12.1 Current Treatments for the Management of Diabetes (Tan et al., 2019)

S. No.	Treatment	Inference
1.	Insulin	Insulin injection is a primary therapeutic intervention for managing DM, especially when all other medicines stop working.
2.	Biguanides	The most common class of drug prescribed for the management of DM (is Metformin).
		It works by modulating the glucose production by activating AMP-activated protein kinase.
3.	Sulfonylureas	Work as insulin sensitizers.
		Stimulate β-cells of the pancreas to release insulin in a potassium-dependent manner.
4.	Thiazolidinediones	Activate peroxisome proliferator-activated receptor γ.
		They act on β-cells to maintain insulin secretion.
5.	Dipeptidyl peptidase-4 (DPP4) inhibitors	DPP4 inhibitors suppress the activity of dipeptidyl peptidase 4, thus inactivating the incretin hormone and reducing glucagon release from pancreatic α-cells, thereby increasing glycaemia control.

12.2 NANOTECHNOLOGY-PHYTOTHERAPEUTICS FUSION

Nanotechnology is the study of material characteristics in between 1–100 nm. This research aims to develop or modify new products. (Dhiman and Thakur, 2011; Sim and Wong, 2021). Their low particle size makes NPs more likely to reach the desired site. Besides, the higher surface helps to regulate the drug release efficiently, hence aiding in controlled drug release. There are multiple NPs available, which have their advantages and disadvantages. Polymeric NPs, Lipidic NPs, elemental NPs, and miscellaneous NPs are used. However, till now, the lipid NPs were only able to commercialize. Other particles are still only at the research level.

Herbal medicines are used primarily to promote health and treat chronic diseases rather than life-threatening ones (Wachtel-Galor and Benzie, 2011). Phytopharmaceuticals require a systematic and scientific strategy to administer their components and enhance patient compliance. Specific nano-formulations can reduce dose by increasing the adequate biological availability of drugs. It can help selectively target the phytoconstituents to selective binding sites to specific receptors. Nano-Phototherapeutics has recently emerged as a promising therapeutic option for managing infectious and non-infectious diseases. The present review focuses on the therapeutic use of diverse nano-phytopharmaceuticals in the field of DM (Lim et al., 2022).

12.3 NANO-PHYTOPHARMACEUTICALS IN THE FIELD OF DIABETES

12.3.1 CURCUMIN (CUR)

Curcuma longa is an herb classified under the Zingiberaceae family. It is a lipophilic polyphenol with a crystalline orange-yellow color and exhibits insolubility in aqueous physiological media, resulting in inadequate distribution and bioavailability. However, it exhibits solubility in polar solvents such as acetone, methanol, DMSO, and ethanol (Rathore et al., 2020).

CUR hampers microorganism growth through antioxidant action. It can hinder bacteria's virulence factors, impede the formation of bacterial biofilms, and thwart bacteria's attachment to host receptors (Zheng et al., 2020).

Its potential anti-diabetic effects may stem from its capacity to inhibit oxidative stress and processes associated with pro-inflammatory cytokines. It also significantly lowers fasting blood sugar levels, glycated hemoglobin, and body mass index (Marton et al., 2021). The notable connection between CUR's anti-diabetic attributes and its influence on inflammation and oxidation is significant, given that inflammation is pivotal in disrupting the structure of β cells (Bozkurt et al., 2022). In diabetes, CUR demonstrates hypocholesterolaemia and hypoglycaemic effects while enhancing insulin sensitivity (Hussain et al., 2022).

However, the clinical applicability of CUR is limited due to the challenges associated with CUR, such as poor oral bioavailability and solubility, so CUR NPs were developed. Unlike CUR, these NPs displayed excellent water dispersibility without needing any surfactant (Bhawana et al., 2011).

Taweel et al. designed CUR-NPs to address reduced tetrahydrobiopterin levels in DM. Results indicated a marked rise in mean malondialdehyde levels in the diabetic group. Nonetheless, CUR-NPs demonstrated effective regulation of glucose and insulin levels, enhancing the bioavailability of nitric oxide in the vascular wall. The outcomes suggested that CUR-NPs exhibited superior efficacy in free CUR in treating DM (Abu-Taweel et al., 2020).

Boarescu et al. formulated CUR-NPs to counter acute myocardial infarction in animal models with DM, showcasing extensive organ protection. The study aimed to assess the hepatoprotective, nephroprotective, and cardioprotective impacts of CUR-NPs. Employing CUR NPs in type 1 DM demonstrated safeguarding beta cells, diminishing serum glucose levels, and yielding improved C-peptide levels in contrast to conventional CUR. Consequently, CUR-NPs helped treat T1DM (Boarescu et al., 2021).

Laddha et al. engineered a novel method to target diabetic retinopathy (DR) using tailored nano synthesis encapsulating CUR in PLGA-NPs. In an *in vivo* study using rats, a dose-dependent decrease in vascular endothelial growth factor (VEGF) concentration in the vitreous fluid was noted. Consequently, it can be inferred that the developed formulation holds promise for the effective treatment of diabetics (Laddha et al., 2022).

Liao et al. developed a bioactive and multifunctional nanofiber membrane by grafting heparin onto aligned PLGA/CUR nanofibers to expedite diabetic wound healing. Initially, CUR-loaded nanofiber membranes were prepared using PLGA. The grafted heparin attracted and stabilized growth factors crucial for wound healing. Additionally, the released CUR mitigated high oxidative stress and inflammation during the diabetic wound healing process (Liao et al., 2021).

12.3.2 BERBERINE (BER)

BER, also known as *Coptis rhizome*, classified as an isoquinoline alkaloid, is a plant metabolite found in the stem, rhizomes, bark, and roots of Chinese herb Coptis chinensis and *Berberis vulgaris* as well as various other plants (Gupta et al., 2021). BER's most widely researched features in several randomized clinical trials include its effects on reducing lipid levels and improving insulin resistance. When given at specific doses, BER exhibits minimal toxicity and provides clinical benefits without significant side effects (Imenshahidi and Hosseinzadeh, 2019; Och et al., 2020). BER shows therapeutic promise in several conditions, including cancer, digestive problems, metabolic disorders, cardiovascular concerns, and neurological disorders (Song et al., 2020).

In addition to the advantageous impacts of BER, its application has been impeded by several barriers, such as its poor solubility in water, minimal absorption, and short oral bioavailability (<1%). Nanotechnology has been identified as a primary approach to address the mentioned constraints. (Mirhadi et al., 2018; Murakami et al., 2023). BER is sparingly soluble in methanol and minimally soluble in water. Consequently, the poor water solubility of BER leads to a significantly decreased dissolution rate and oral bioavailability, thereby imposing limitations on its clinical utility (Singh et al., 2020).

In a study by Zhang et al., a BER nano-colloidal hydrogel (BNH) was developed to improve wound healing in diabetic animal models. It was found from the molecular studies that BNH inhibits the expression of various molecular inflammation markers such as Tumor Necrosis Factor-alpha, NF-κB and IL-6 while concurrently promoting the expression of α-Smooth Muscle Actin, VEGF, adhesion molecules like CD21 through the activation of Sirt1. These molecular alterations positively influence the wound-healing process in diabetic rats (Zhang et al., 2020).

Panda et al. formulated BER-encapsulated lecithin-chitosan NPs as a novel therapeutic agent for wound healing in individuals with DM. By mitigating inflammation, stimulating angiogenesis, and facilitating the migration of fibroblasts, the nanoparticulate system facilitated the deposition of mature collagen fibers. Results indicate that the utilization of lecithin-chitosan NPs containing BER helped in the treatment of DM (Panda et al., 2021).

12.3.3 RESVERATROL (RES)

RES is a BCS class II polyphenolic stilbene and is found in several plant sources such as grapes, mulberries, peanuts and rhubarb (Malaguarnera et al., 2019). The administration of RES demonstrates a mitigating effect on heart oxidative damage, fibrosis, and hypertrophy that DM generates (Wang et al., 2018). RES exhibits a partial capacity to mitigate β-cell dysfunction and enhance β-cell function, subsequently reducing blood glucose levels. Additionally, it aids in preserving beta cells and improves insulin action, thereby serving as a therapeutic intervention to treat DM (Koushki et al., 2018).

RES is limited by its inherent characteristics, including low water solubility, susceptibility to light-induced isomerization, auto-oxidation, and fast metabolism. Hence, nanotechnology has emerged as a promising alternative for enhancing the substance's solubility and stability, thereby permitting its medicinal application using several methodologies (Santos et al., 2019).

Mohseni et al. conducted a study involving the oral administration of solid lipid NPs (SLNs) loaded with RES to enhance insulin resistance in rats with DM. Administration of SLNs containing RES via the oral route prevented weight loss and displayed better hypoglycemic effects than administering RES alone. The findings indicate that SLN-RES is a viable therapeutic strategy for treating DM (Mohseni et al., 2019).

Çiğdem et al. generated nanoliposomal RES as a novel strategy to enhance insulin levels to treat DM. Results indicated that the developed liposomal formulation exhibited a reduction in elevated glucose levels within diabetic cell clusters. The liposomal formulation surpassed the effectiveness of the RES solution and displayed extended antioxidant activity. These results highlighted the potential of the liposomal formulation in treating DM (Yücel et al., 2018).

Rahman et al. formulated cationic solid lipid NPs of RES (RES-SLN) to treat hepatocellular carcinoma associated with DM. The administration of cationic RSV-SLN restored antioxidant enzyme balance and reduced the expression of pro-inflammatory cytokines. The results indicated beneficial effects in the treatment of diabetes-associated carcinoma (Rahman et al., 2020).

Qian et al. developed RES-loaded polypeptide nanospheres to treat DM complicated by fatty liver. These nanospheres exhibit superior efficacy compared to RES alone in treating DM complicated by fatty liver, potentially offering valuable benefits for the therapeutic management of DM (Xiang et al., 2020).

However, despite the efficient potential to lower the DM, RES is still under investigation to find its way into clinical investigations.

12.3.4 QUERCETIN (QUR)

QUR, classified as a flavonoid under BCS class IV, is present in a diverse range of food sources, such as fruits, vegetables, nuts, wines, and seeds (Kim and Park, 2018). QUR can be found in two forms: as a glycoside, which is when it is attached to sugars, or as an aglycone, which is when it is not attached to sugars (Ulusoy and Sanlier, 2020). The bioavailability of QUR through the oral route is often limited (<10%) due to inadequate water solubility, chemical stability, and absorption characteristics (Kandemir et al., 2022).

QUR, a polyphenolic compound, displays various biological effects such as neuroprotective, anti-allergic, anticancer, antidiabetic, and anti-inflammatory properties (Bule et al., 2019).

Mahadev et al. synthesized and assessed a nanoemulsion of quercetin (CUR-NE) with ultrasonic assistance. The aim was to elevate the nanoemulsion's systemic availability and healing potential in addressing diabetes in rats. CUR-NE demonstrated notable protective and therapeutic impacts in regulating body weight, blood glucose levels, lipid profiles, and tissue injury markers. Consequently, the recently developed CUR-NE helps treat diabetes (Mahadev et al., 2022).

Tang et al. developed liposomes containing QUR labelled as QUR-PEGL to treat STZ-induced DN. The therapeutic effectiveness of QUR-PEGL surpassed that of free QUR. PEGylated QUR liposomes enabled the maintenance of higher concentrations of QUR in plasma compared to its non-encapsulated form. The administration of QUR liposomes reduced disease symptoms in a DN rat model (Tang et al., 2020).

Mukhopadhyay et al. fabricated QUR-succinylated chitosan-alginate core-shell-corona NPs for the treatment of diabetes. Compared to free QUR given orally, oral administration significantly reduced blood glucose levels and effectively regulated glucose balance. This indicates the development of a highly effective vehicle to deliver oral QUR for treating diabetes (Mukhopadhyay et al., 2018).

Badhwar et al. conducted a study investigating using QUR-loaded AgNPs in a hydrogel matrix (QUR-AgNP) as a combined treatment approach for diabetic wounds. *In vivo*, findings demonstrated that the QUR-AgNP hydrogel significantly decreased the wound gap and enhanced the percentage of re-epithelialization in a diabetic wound model. Ultimately, these results lay the groundwork for effectively managing diabetic wounds (Badhwar et al., 2021).

Ahmed et al. developed NPs using the polymer Eudragit L-100 to encapsulate QUR. These NPs were created explicitly for their potential anti-diabetic effects. Therefore, this technology provides a potent oral drug for managing diabetes. This data indicates that QT/EDLNP can effectively treat diabetes orally with a low dose and frequency that is also convenient for patients. (Ahmad et al., 2023).

12.3.5 NARINGENIN (NRG)

NRG is a flavonoid classified within the flavanones subclass. This compound is widely available in various citrus fruits, bergamot, tomatoes, and other fruits, predominantly in its glycosides, with NRG being particularly notable (Salehi et al., 2019). NRG exhibits high solubility in organic solvents such as ethanol, dimethyl formamide, and dimethyl sulfoxide. Nevertheless, its solubility in water-based buffers is sparingly soluble and weakly alkaline (Joshi et al., 2018). Additionally, NRG undergoes significant degradation in the gastrointestinal tract, is metabolized by the liver in the first pass, and has limited ability to pass through cell membranes. These factors collectively contribute to the low solubility and oral bioavailability of NRG (Bhia et al., 2021).

NRG inhibits the production of inflammatory cytokines through both transcriptional and post-transcriptional pathways. Remarkably, NRG not only inhibits the expression of cytokine mRNA but also increases the breakdown of cytokine proteins through lysosomes (Zeng et al., 2018).

Yeo et al. prepared a nanoemulgel containing tocotrienols-rich NRG to treat chronic wounds found in individuals with diabetes locally. The release of NRG in phosphate-buffered saline under laboratory conditions showed a sustained and prolonged release pattern. Research has revealed fascinating results that indicate a potential future in the field of wound healing, especially concerning the problems arising from diabetes (Yeo et al., 2021).

Maity et al. developed NRG-containing PLGA NPs to treat DM. The encapsulation process was an emulsion-diffusion-evaporation process. The group treated with NRG-PLGA nanoparticles exhibited a notable decrease in glycated hemoglobin levels, elevated insulin levels, and improvements in dyslipidemia and oxidative stress parameters. These results indicate the potential of NRG-PLGA nanoparticles in the treatment of diabetes (Maity and Chakraborti, 2020).

Zafar et al. formulated NRG-based polymeric NPs for the treatment of DM. They prepared matric using chitosan and sodium alginate to create polymeric NPs loaded with NRG as polymers. The results demonstrated a higher absorption profile and significant ($P < 0.05$) antidiabetic effectiveness compared to pure NRG-dispersion. The data suggested that using polymeric NRG-NPs could be a viable strategy to advance the effectiveness of DM management (Zafar et al., 2023).

Raina et al. created a novel hydrogel containing NRG, which promotes the regrowth of epithelial tissue in chronic diabetic wounds. Drug-loaded hydrogels demonstrated improved tissue adhesion and drug release for up to 12 hours. Histopathologic examination revealed that the drug-containing hydrogel had the potential to improve the healing of skin wounds. Accelerated healing and advanced antibacterial and antioxidant characteristics suggest that the drug-containing hydrogel is an ideal treatment for chronic diabetic wounds (Raina et al., 2023).

12.3.6 GLYCYRRHIZIN (GLZ)

GLZ, often called glycyrrhizic acid (18 β-GL), is a primary bioactive compound classified as a saponin found in the well-known herbal remedy liquorice (*Glycyrrhiza glabra*) (Bakr et al., 2022). GLZ, a triterpenoid saponin, possesses a sweetness approximately 50 times greater than sucrose. Following oral administration, GLZ undergoes metabolism facilitated by gut bacteria to produce 18-glycyrrhizic acid, 3-monoglucuronide and glycyrrhizic acid (GA) (Pastorino et al., 2018).

Due to its amphoteric properties, GLZ can self-associate in water- and non-water-based environments. It can also form water-soluble complexes with some lipophilic drugs (Selyutina and Polyakov, 2019). GLZ exhibits a broad antiviral effect against many RNA and DNA viruses and works as an antioxidant, antimicrobial, antiviral, anti-inflammatory, antiulcer, antitumor, antidiabetic, neuroprotective, hepatoprotective, and cardioprotective effects (Gomaa and Abdel-Wadood, 2021; Kowalska and Kalinowska-Lis, 2019).

GLZ exerts its effects through multiple molecular and cellular pathways, such as modulating the function of T-lymphocytes, mast cells, neutrophils and macrophages. GLZ and its derivatives, when applied directly to the affected areas, have great potential in treating inflammatory disorders of the mucous membranes and skin caused by bacteria, fungi, and viruses (Gromova et al., 2022).

Sen et al. used liposome-encapsulated GLZ on STZ-induced rats to treat diabetes. Administration of liposomal GLZ significantly improved hyperglycemia, glucose intolerance, and glycohemoglobin levels. Renal and liver problems were eliminated. It was discovered that liposome-encapsulated GLZ effectively suppresses diabetic complications by exerting antioxidant effects, thus treating diabetes (Sen et al., 2022).

Rani et al. fabricated GLZ-loaded NPs (GLZ-NPs) to evaluate their efficacy in reducing hyperglycaemia in rats with type II diabetes. GLZ-NPs demonstrated remarkable antidiabetic properties even when they contained only 25% of the dose compared to the pure-form (Rani et al., 2017).

Rastegari et al. developed chitosan lactate NPs encompassing siRNA to knock down the *CRTC2* gene, targeted explicitly by poly (ethylene glycol)-GLZ acid to suppress hepatic gluconeogenesis in diabetes. CT/PEG-GA NPs can be viable for delivering siRNA specifically to hepatocytes to control gluconeogenesis in diabetic individuals (Rastegari et al., 2019).

Duysak et al. reported the effect of a nanoemulsion (NE) formulation containing GLZ on streptozotocin-induced diabetic rats. Diabetic rats that received GLY-NE had lower blood sugar levels. The results showed that the NE formulations displayed superior antidiabetic and antioxidant properties. Additionally, these formulations reduced oxidative stress indicators in rats with diabetes caused by STZ. Thus, GLY NE can be given orally for the treatment of diabetes (Duysak et al., 2023).

Xu et al. synthesized ferrous sulphide (FeS) NPs through in-situ interaction between Fe2+ and S2− in GA solution to enhance the healing process of infected diabetic wounds. Notably, in a model of infected diabetic wounds, the FeS/GA hydrogel effectively eliminated pathogens and controlled inflammation, enhancing wound healing (Xu et al., 2023).

12.3.7 HESPERIDIN (HES)

HES is a glycoside of the flavanone class, abundantly available in citrus fruits like lemons and sweet oranges (Hajialyani et al., 2019). HES exhibits low aqueous solubility, inadequate absorption, and restricted bioavailability (Sa'Ayinzat et al., 2021). HES has demonstrated encouraging results in managing both inflammatory and allergic conditions. Research has shown that HES has antibacterial, anticarcinogenic, anti-inflammatory antioxidant, etc. properties and reduces capillary fragility (Musa et al., 2019).

HES has several advantages, including its favorable safety profile, non-cumulative properties, and limited adverse effects, even during pregnancy (Wdowiak et al., 2022). Administration of HES can reduce the effects of high blood sugar-induced oxidative stress and inhibit the production of inflammatory cytokines such as IL-6 and TNF-α (Gandhi et al., 2020).

Shahawy et al. demonstrated that a unique combination of layered double hydroxide-HES NPs had beneficial effects in diabetic rats. MgAl-layer double hydroxide (LDH) was used to encapsulate HES. The findings showed favorable effects on blood glucose, insulin, and lipid profile and significant reductions in MDA, IL-17, and TNF-α levels. It shows potential as an effective carrier to deliver drugs to treat type 2 diabetes (El-Shahawy et al., 2021).

Elmoghayer et al. Improved administration of HES-loaded sulfopropylether-β-cyclodextrin/chitosan NPs (HSD/CD/CS NPs) via mouth enhanced the ability to lower blood glucose levels. A significant synergistic reduction in blood glucose levels was observed after oral ingestion. Overall, HSD/CD/CS NPs can be considered a beneficial oral method of HSD, resulting in improved antidiabetic effects (Elmoghayer et al., 2023).

Saad et al. prepared SLNs encapsulating HES (HES-SLNs) to enhance oral administration of HES for treating diabetes. HES-SLNs significantly increased the solubility, apparent permeability, stability and bioavailability of HES. As a result, oral administration of HES can be used to treat diabetes (Saad et al., 2020).

Ren et al. synthesized core-shell Ag NPs (Ag-HES NPs) using HES to enhance the healing process in diabetes-infected wounds. Ag-HES NPs were encapsulated within electrospun nanofibers, resulting in the formation of a hydrogel known as Ag-HES@H. Ag-HES@H, specifically developed to have antibacterial and anti-inflammatory properties, shows significant promise in enhancing the healing of infected wounds in individuals with diabetes (Ren et al., 2022).

12.3.8 CHRYSIN (CHR)

CHR is a phytochemical originated from the flavonoid class. It is found naturally in propolis, honey, passion fruit, and mushrooms (Naz et al., 2019). CHR has very low water solubility and is not easily absorbed by the body, resulting in low bioavailability (Stompor-Gorący et al., 2021). The main factors contributing to its limited systemic bioavailability are its initial metabolic processing, uptake metabolism aided by UDP-glucuronosyltransferases and sulfotransferases, and effectual exclusion through efflux transporters like BCRP and MRP2. CHR has exhibited numerous therapeutic attributes, anti-asthmatic effects, immune-modulating, antidepressant, encompassing anti-cancer and anti-diabetic (Gao et al., 2021; Garg and Chaturvedi et al., 2022).

CHR exerts its effects on multiple molecular targets and regulates various signaling pathways involved in inflammation and cellular metabolism (Siddiqui et al., 2018). CHR exerts anxiolytic and antidepressant effects by engaging with distinct neurotransmitter systems, such as the GABAergic and serotonergic systems, and by triggering the activation of other neurotrophic factors (Rodríguez-Landa et al., 2022). CHR's antidiabetic efficacy operates through diverse mechanisms, which encompass stimulating insulin signaling, inhibiting endoplasmic reticulum stress and oxidative damage, enhancing skeletal glucose absorption, and modulating apoptosis and autophagy signaling (Dewi et al., 2022).

Hussien et al. developed polymeric CHR nanocapsules using PLGA as a base material. These nanocapsules have increased potential for oral therapeutic application in treating diabetes. The enhanced therapeutic

TABLE 12.2 Illustrating Various Recent Literature on Phyto-Nanotherapeutics in Treating DM

Drug	Nanocarrier	Animal Model	Inference	References
Curcumin (CUR)	Chitosan NPs	Adult male Wistar rats induced with STZ.	Karri et al. fabricated collagen-alginate scaffolds containing chitosan NPs loaded with CUR to facilitate diabetic wound healing. The findings showed that the nanohybrid scaffold group displayed complete epithelialization by forming thick granulation tissue.	Karri et al. (2016)
	CUR and zinc oxide NPs	Rats with STZ-induced hepatic inflammation	Abdulmalek et al. assessed the effect of CUR NPs on liver and pancreas damage caused by high-fat diet and STZ in individuals with type 2 DM. Cur-NPs reduce the oxidative stress and inflammation caused by diabetes in liver and pancreas tissues.	Abdulmalek et al. (2021)
Berberine (BER)	Nanosuspension	STZ-induced diabetic C57BL/6 mice.	Wang et al. created a nanosuspension of BER that improved the effectiveness of reducing blood glucose in rats with STZ-induced diabetes. Data show that administering low doses of BER-NPs reduces systemic glucose levels and increases lipid metabolism in rats with type 2 diabetes.	Wang et al. (2015)
	Solid lipid NPs	-	Xue et al. developed BER-loaded solid lipid NPs with a specific affinity for the liver, effectively improving diabetes-induced hepatosteatosis in rats. The findings showed that BBR-SLN has effectively treated hepatosteatosis in diabetic rats by inhibiting lipogenesis and lipolysis.	Xue et al. (2015)
	Liquid crystalline NPs	BER-LCNs in LPS-induced RAW264.7 mouse	Alnuqaydan et al. developed BER-loaded liquid crystalline NPs to reduce oxidative stress and inflammation in lipopolysaccharide-induced rats to treat diabetes. Results suggested their potential use in the treatment of DM.	Alnuqaydan et al. (2022)
Resveratrol (RES)	Chitosan NPs	DM rats induced by STZ	Du et al. synthesized chitosan-encapsulated nano RES to combat gestational DM in streptozotocin-produced rats. The CS–ZnO–RS compound effectively decreased the concentration of inflammatory markers and alleviated endoplasmic reticulum stress, providing diabetes treatment.	Du et al. (2020)
	Mesoporous silica nanoparticle	STZ induced rats	Tan et al. fabricated mesoporous silica NPs (MSNs) coated to regulate the immune system and reduce insulin resistance in treating diabetic periodontitis. This study aims to investigate the additional effect of MSN-RES in alleviating insulin resistance and regulating glucose metabolism.	Tan et al. (2022)

TABLE 12.2 *(Continued)*

Drug	Nanocarrier	Animal Model	Inference	References
Quercetin (QUR)	Superparamagnetic iron oxide NPs.	Alloxan-induced diabetic mice.	Alam et al. fabricated QUR nanorods (QCNRs) to investigate their antidiabetic properties in rats with alloxan-induced diabetes. The study indicates that QUR nanorods have antioxidant properties that may protect against diabetes-related damage.	Alam et al. (2016)
	Nanorods	STZ-induced male albino adult rats	Jameel et al. developed QUR NPs and administered them to male rats with streptozotocin-induced diabetes, targeting the kidneys. Their findings indicate that treating diabetic rats with QUNPs positively affects cell regeneration in injured kidneys.	Al-Jameel and Abd El-Rahman (2017)
Glycyrrhizin (GLY)	Chitosan-coated superparamagnetic iron oxide nanoparticle	Male Sprague Dawley (SD) rat, C57BL/6J mice and FVB mice of seven-week-old	Jang et al. constructed DAMP-modulating NPs for pancreas islet and stem cell transplantation in diabetic rats. The combined use of SPIO@Chitosan-GLY NPs can be employed in multimodal nanomedicine to reduce the inflammatory response in diabetic rats.	Jang et al., (2022)
Hesperidin (HES)	Gold NPs	Diabetes-induced cognitively impaired rats	Pradhan et al. prepared gold nanoparticles of HES (HSP-AuNP) to improve memory in diabetic rat models. Their work demonstrated the enhanced potency and effectiveness of HSP-AuNPs in protecting against cognitive decline in a diabetic rat model through their antioxidant properties.	Pradhan et al. (2022)

effects of CHR, achieved through its encapsulation in polymeric nano-capsules, demonstrate its potential as a viable treatment for diabetes when administered orally (El-Hussien et al., 2021).

Marasy et al. engineered nanovesicles containing CHR, demonstrating their effectiveness in ameliorating diabetic peripheral neuropathy. The research delves into the impact of CHY and CHY-loaded lipidic NPs (CHY-LNPs) on STZ-induced diabetic peripheral neuropathy in rats. CHY-LNPs mitigated STZ-induced diabetic peripheral neuropathy by lowering elevated blood glucose levels, showcasing antioxidant and anti-inflammatory properties. These findings provide valuable insights into diabetes treatment. (El-Marasy et al., 2023). The illustration of different recent advancements in Phyto-nanotherapeutics in the treatment of DM is shown in Table 12.2.

KEYWORDS

- **diabetes**
- **herbal medicines**
- **hesperidin**
- **nanoparticles**
- **phototherapeutic**

REFERENCES

Abdulmalek, S., Eldala, A., Awad, D., & Balbaa, M. (2021). Ameliorative effect of curcumin and zinc oxide nanoparticles on multiple mechanisms in obese rats with induced type 2 diabetes. *Scientific Reports, 11*(1), 20677. https://doi.org/10.1038/s41598-021-00108-w (accessed on 28th June 2025).

Abu-Taweel, G. M., Attia, M. F., Hussein, J., Mekawi, E. M., Galal, H. M., Ahmed, E. I., … El-Naggar, M. E. (2020). Curcumin nanoparticles have a potential antioxidant effect and restore tetrahydrobiopterin levels in experimental diabetes. *Biomedicine & Pharmacotherapy, 131*, 110688. https://doi.org/10.1016/j.biopha.2020.110688 (accessed on 28th June 2025).

Ahmad, M. Z., Pathak, K., Das, R. J., Saikia, R., Sarma, H., Gogoi, N., … Abdel-Wahab, B. A. (2023). Design and optimization of quercetin-loaded polymeric Eudragit L-100 nanoparticles for anti-diabetic activity with improved oral delivery: In vitro and in-vivo evaluation. *Journal of Inorganic and Organometallic Polymers and Materials*, 1–18. https://doi.org/10.1007/s10904-023-02694-w (accessed on 28th June 2025).

Al-Jameel, S. S., & Abd El-Rahman, S. N. (2017). Effect of quercetin nanoparticles on the kidney of streptozotocin-induced diabetes in male rats: A histological study and serum biochemical alterations. *African Journal of Biotechnology, 16*(39), 1944–1952. https://doi.org/10.1038/s41598-020-59411-7 (accessed on 28th June 2025).

Alam, M. M., Abdullah, K., Singh, B. R., Naqvi, A. H., & Naseem, I. (2016). Ameliorative effect of quercetin nanorods on diabetic mice: Mechanistic and therapeutic strategies. *RSC Advances, 6*(60), 55092–55103. https://doi.org/10.1039/C6RA04821H (accessed on 28th June 2025).

Alnuqaydan, A. M., Almutary, A. G., Azam, M., Manandhar, B., De Rubis, G., Madheswaran, T., … Dua, K. (2022). Phytantriol-based berberine-loaded liquid crystalline nanoparticles attenuate inflammation and oxidative stress in lipopolysaccharide-induced RAW264.7 macrophages. *Nanomaterials, 12*(23), 4312. https://doi.org/10.3390/nano12234312 (accessed on 28th June 2025).

Badhwar, R., Mangla, B., Neupane, Y. R., Khanna, K., & Popli, H. (2021). Quercetin-loaded silver nanoparticles in hydrogel matrices for diabetic wound healing. *Nanotechnology, 32*(50), 505102. https://doi.org/10.3390/nano12234312 (accessed on 28th June 2025).

Bakr, A. F., Shao, P., & Farag, M. A. (2022). Recent advances in glycyrrhizin metabolism, health benefits, clinical effects and drug delivery systems for efficacy improvement: A comprehensive review. *Phytomedicine, 99*, 153999. https://doi.org/10.1016/j.phymed.2022.153999 (accessed on 28th June 2025).

Banday, M. Z., Sameer, A. S., & Nissar, S. (2020). Pathophysiology of diabetes: An overview. *Avicenna Journal of Medicine, 10*(4), 174–188. https://doi.org/10.4103/ajm.ajm_53_20 (accessed on 28th June 2025).

Bhargava, S. K., Singh, T. G., Mannan, A., Singh, S., & Gupta, S. (2022). Pharmacological evaluation of *Thuja occidentalis* for the attenuation of nephropathy in streptozotocin-induced diabetes rats. *Obesity Medicine, 31*, 100391. https://doi.org/10.1016/j.obmed.2022.100391 (accessed on 28th June 2025).

Bhargava, S. K., Singh, T. G., Mannan, A., Singh, S., Singh, M., & Gupta, S. (2022). Pharmacological evaluation of *Thuja occidentalis* for the attenuation of neuropathy via AGEs and TNF-α inhibition in diabetic neuropathic rats. *Environmental Science and Pollution Research International, 29*(40), 60542–60557. https://doi.org/10.1007/s11356-022-20106-3 (accessed on 28th June 2025).

Bhawana, Basniwal, R. K., Buttar, H. S., Jain, V. K., & Jain, N. (2011). Curcumin nanoparticles: Preparation, characterisation, and antimicrobial study. *Journal of Agricultural and Food Chemistry, 59*(5), 2056–2061. https://doi.org/10.1021/jf104402t (accessed on 28th June 2025).

Bhia, M., Motallebi, M., Abadi, B., Zarepour, A., Pereira-Silva, M., Saremnejad, F., … Jafari, S. M. (2021). Naringenin nano-delivery systems and their therapeutic applications. *Pharmaceutics, 13*(2), 291. https://doi.org/10.3390/pharmaceutics13020291 (accessed on 28th June 2025).

Boarescu, P.-M., Boarescu, I., Bulboacă, A. E., Bocșan, I. C., Pop, R. M., Gheban, D., … Buzoianu, A. D. (2021). Multi-organ protective effects of curcumin nanoparticles on drug-induced acute myocardial infarction in rats with type 1 diabetes mellitus. *Applied*

Sciences, 11(12), 5497. https://doi.org/10.3390/app11125497 (accessed on 28th June 2025).

Bozkurt, O., Kocaadam-Bozkurt, B., & Yildiran, H. (2022). Effects of curcumin, a bioactive component of turmeric, on type 2 diabetes mellitus and its complications: An updated review. *Food & Function*. https://doi.org/10.1039/D2FO02625B (accessed on 28th June 2025).

Bule, M., Abdurahman, A., Nikfar, S., Abdollahi, M., & Amini, M. (2019). Antidiabetic effect of quercetin: A systematic review and meta-analysis of animal studies. *Food and Chemical Toxicology, 125*, 494–502. https://doi.org/10.1016/j.fct.2019.01.037 (accessed on 28th June 2025).

Cole, J. B., & Florez, J. C. (2020). Genetics of diabetes mellitus and diabetes complications. *Nature Reviews Nephrology, 16*(7), 377–390. https://doi.org/10.1038/s41581-020-0278-5 (accessed on 28th June 2025).

Devi, S., Chauhan, S., Mannan, A., & Singh, T. G. (2023). Targeting cardiovascular risk factors with eugenol: An anti-inflammatory perspective. *Inflammopharmacology*. https://doi.org/10.1007/s10787-023-01392-w (accessed on 28th June 2025).

Dewi, R. M., Megawati, M., & Antika, L. D. (2022). Antidiabetic properties of dietary chrysin: A cellular mechanism review. *Mini Reviews in Medicinal Chemistry, 22*(10), 1450–1457. https://doi.org/10.2174/1389557521666211101162449 (accessed on 28th June 2025).

Dhiman, S., & Thakur, G. S. (2011). Nanosuspension: A recent approach for nano drug delivery system. *International Journal of Current Pharmaceutical Research, 3*(4), 96–101.

Du, S., Lv, Y., Li, N., Huang, X., Liu, X., Li, H., … Jia, Y.-F. (2020). Biological investigations on therapeutic effect of chitosan encapsulated nano resveratrol against gestational diabetes mellitus rats induced by streptozotocin. *Drug Delivery, 27*(1), 953–963. https://doi.org/10.1080/10717544.2020.1775722 (accessed on 28th June 2025).

Duysak, L., Kaplan, A. B. U., Gulaboglu, M., Cetin, M., Kutlu, Z., & Demirci, T. (2023). Investigation of the effects of nanoemulsion formulation containing glycyrrhizin in streptozotocin-induced diabetic rats. *Food Bioscience, 56*, 103210. https://doi.org/10.1016/j.fbio.2023.103210 (accessed on 28th June 2025).

Ekta, Gupta, M., Kaur, A., Singh, T. G., & Bedi, O. (2020). Pathobiological and molecular connections involved in the high fructose and high fat diet induced diabetes associated nonalcoholic fatty liver disease. *Inflammation Research, 69*(9), 851–867. https://doi.org/10.1007/s00011-020-01373-7 (accessed on 28th June 2025).

El-Hussien, D., El-Zaafarany, G. M., Nasr, M., & Sammour, O. (2021). Chrysin nanocapsules with dual anti-glycemic and anti-hyperlipidemic effects: Chemometric optimisation, physicochemical characterisation and pharmacodynamic assessment. *International Journal of Pharmaceutics, 592*, 120044. https://doi.org/10.1016/j.ijpharm.2020.120044 (accessed on 28th June 2025).

El-Marasy, S. A., AbouSamra, M. M., El-Mosallamy, A. E., Emam, A. N., Mabrok, H. B., Galal, A. F., … Moustafa, P. E. (2023). Chrysin-loaded nanovesicles ameliorated diabetic peripheral neuropathy: Role of NGF/AKT/GSK-3β pathway. *Chemico-Biological Interactions, 375*, 110402. https://doi.org/10.1016/j.cbi.2023.110402 (accessed on 28th June 2025).

El-Shahawy, A. A., Abdel-Moneim, A., Ebeid, A. S., Eldin, Z. E., & Zanaty, M. I. (2021). Novel layered double hydroxide-hesperidin nanoparticles exert antidiabetic, antioxidant and anti-inflammatory effects in rats with diabetes. *Molecular Biology Reports, 48*, 5217–5232. https://doi.org/10.1007/s11033-021-06527-2 (accessed on 28th June 2025).

Elmoghayer, M. E., Saleh, N. M., & Abu Hashim, I. I. (2023). Enhanced oral delivery of hesperidin-loaded sulfobutylether-β-cyclodextrin/chitosan nanoparticles for augmenting its hypoglycemic activity: In vitro-in vivo assessment study. *Drug Delivery and Translational Research,* 1–23. https://doi.org/10.1007/s13346-023-01440-6 (accessed on 28th June 2025).

Gandhi, G. R., Vasconcelos, A. B. S., Wu, D.-T., Li, H.-B., Antony, P. J., Li, H., … Gan, R.-Y. (2020). Citrus flavonoids as promising phytochemicals targeting diabetes and related complications: A systematic review of in vitro and in vivo studies. *Nutrients, 12*(10), 2907. https://doi.org/10.3390/nu12102907 (accessed on 28th June 2025).

Gao, S., Siddiqui, N., Etim, I., Du, T., Zhang, Y., & Liang, D. (2021). Developing nutritional component chrysin as a therapeutic agent: Bioavailability and pharmacokinetics consideration, and ADME mechanisms. *Biomedicine & Pharmacotherapy, 142*, 112080. https://doi.org/10.1016/j.biopha.2021.112080 (accessed on 28th June 2025).

Garg, A., & Chaturvedi, S. (2022). A comprehensive review on chrysin: Emphasis on molecular targets, pharmacological actions and bio-pharmaceutical aspects. *Current Drug Targets, 23*(4), 420–436. https://doi.org/10.2174/1389450122666210824141044 (accessed on 28th June 2025).

Garg, N., Singh, T. G., Khan, H., Arora, S., Kaur, A., & Mannan, A. (2021). Mechanistic interventions of selected *Ocimum* species in management of diabetes, obesity and liver disorders: Transformative developments from preclinical to clinical approaches. *Biointerface Research in Applied Chemistry, 12*(1), 1304–1323. https://doi.org/10.33263/BRIAC121.13041323 (accessed on 28th June 2025).

Gomaa, A. A., & Abdel-Wadood, Y. A. (2021). The potential of glycyrrhizin and licorice extract in combating COVID-19 and associated conditions. *Phytomedicine Plus, 1*(3), 100043. https://doi.org/10.1016/j.phyplu.2021.100043 (accessed on 28th June 2025).

Gromova, O. A., Torshin, I. Y., & Tetruashvili, N. K. (2022). A systematic review of experimental and clinical studies on the pharmacology of glycyrrhizin and its derivatives. *Obstetrics and Gynecology*(4), 34–46. https://dx.doi.org/10.18565/aig.2022.4.34-46 (accessed on 28th June 2025).

Gupta, S., Khan, A., Vishwas, S., Gulati, M., Singh, T. G., Dua, K., Kumar Singh, S., Najda, A., Sayed, A. A., Almeer, R., & Abdel-Daim, M. M. (2021). Demethyleneberberine: A possible treatment for Huntington's disease. *Medical Hypotheses, 153*, 110639. https://doi.org/10.1016/j.mehy.2021.110639 (accessed on 28th June 2025).

Hajialyani, M., Hosein Farzaei, M., Echeverría, J., Nabavi, S. M., Uriarte, E., & Sobarzo-Sánchez, E. (2019). Hesperidin as a neuroprotective agent: A review of animal and clinical evidence. *Molecules, 24*(3), 648. https://doi.org/10.3390/molecules24030648 (accessed on 28th June 2025).

Hussain, Y., Khan, H., Alotaibi, G., Khan, F., Alam, W., Aschner, M., … Saso, L. (2022). How curcumin targets inflammatory mediators in diabetes: Therapeutic insights and possible solutions. *Molecules, 27*(13), 4058. https://doi.org/10.3390/molecules27134058 (accessed on 28th June 2025).

Imenshahidi, M., & Hosseinzadeh, H. (2019). Berberine and barberry (*Berberis vulgaris*): A clinical review. *Phytotherapy Research, 33*(3), 504–523. https://doi.org/10.1002/ptr.6252 (accessed on 28th June 2025).

Jang, S. B., Jin, S.-M., Kim, H. S., Jeong, Y. Y., Lee, S. J., Hahn, S., ... Lee, D. Y. (2022). DAMP-modulating nanoparticle for successful pancreatic islet and stem cell transplantation. *Biomaterials, 287*, 121679. https://doi.org/10.1016/j.biomaterials.2022.121679 (accessed on 28th June 2025).

Joshi, R., Kulkarni, Y. A., & Wairkar, S. (2018). Pharmacokinetic, pharmacodynamic and formulations aspects of naringenin: An update. *Life Sciences, 215*, 43–56. https://doi.org/10.1016/j.lfs.2018.10.066 (accessed on 28th June 2025).

Kandemir, K., Tomas, M., McClements, D. J., & Capanoglu, E. (2022). Recent advances in the improvement of quercetin bioavailability. *Trends in Food Science & Technology, 119*, 192–200. https://doi.org/10.1016/j.tifs.2021.11.032 (accessed on 28th June 2025).

Karri, V. V. S. R., Kuppusamy, G., Talluri, S. V., Mannemala, S. S., Kollipara, R., Wadhwani, A. D., ... Malayandi, R. (2016). Curcumin-loaded chitosan nanoparticles impregnated into collagen-alginate scaffolds for diabetic wound healing. *International Journal of Biological Macromolecules, 93*, 1519–1529. https://doi.org/10.1016/j.ijbiomac.2016.05.038 (accessed on 28th June 2025).

Kaur, N., Kishore, L., Farooq, S. A., Kajal, A., Singh, R., Agrawal, R., Mannan, A., & Singh, T. G. (2023). *Cucurbita pepo* seeds improve peripheral neuropathy in diabetic rats by modulating the inflammation and oxidative stress in rats. *Environmental Science and Pollution Research International.* https://doi.org/10.1007/s11356-023-28339-6 (accessed on 28th June 2025).

Kim, J. K., & Park, S. U. (2018). Quercetin and its role in biological functions: An updated review. *EXCLI Journal, 17*, 856. http://dx.doi.org/10.17179/excli2018-1538 (accessed on 28th June 2025).

Koushki, M., Amiri-Dashatan, N., Ahmadi, N., Abbaszadeh, H. A., & Rezaei-Tavirani, M. (2018). Resveratrol: A miraculous natural compound for disease treatment. *Food Science & Nutrition, 6*(8), 2473–2490. https://doi.org/10.1002/fsn3.855 (accessed on 28th June 2025).

Kowalska, A., & Kalinowska-Lis, U. (2019). 18β-Glycyrrhetinic acid: Its core biological properties and dermatological applications. *International Journal of Cosmetic Science, 41*(4), 325–331. https://doi.org/10.1111/ics.12548 (accessed on 28th June 2025).

Kumar, R., Saha, P., Kumar, Y., Sahana, S., Dubey, A., & Prakash, O. (2020). A review on diabetes mellitus: Type 1 & Type 2. *World Journal of Pharmacy and Pharmaceutical Sciences, 9*(10), 838–850. https://doi.org/10.20959/wjpps202010-17336 (accessed on 28th June 2025).

Laddha, U. D., Kshirsagar, S. J., Sayyad, L. S., Ahmed, M. T., Gaikwad, S. S., Udavant, P. B., & Kulkarni, A. D. (2022). Development of surface-modified nanoparticles of curcumin for topical treatment of diabetic retinopathy: In vitro, ex vivo and vivo investigation. *Journal of Drug Delivery Science and Technology, 76*, 103835. https://doi.org/10.1016/j.jddst.2022.103835 (accessed on 28th June 2025).

Liao, H. T., Lai, Y.-T., Kuo, C.-Y., & Chen, J.-P. (2021). A bioactive multi-functional heparin-grafted aligned poly (lactide-co-glycolide)/curcumin nanofiber membrane to accelerate diabetic wound healing. *Materials Science and Engineering: C, 120*, 111689. https://doi.org/10.1016/j.msec.2020.111689 (accessed on 28th June 2025).

Lim, C. L., Raju, C. S., Mahboob, T., Kayesth, S., Gupta, K. K., Jain, G. K., … Nissapatorn, V. (2022). Precision and advanced nano-phytopharmaceuticals for therapeutic applications. *Nanomaterials, 12*(2), 238. https://www.mdpi.com/2079-4991/12/2/238 (accessed on 28th June 2025).

Lovic, D., Piperidou, A., Zografou, I., Grassos, H., Pittaras, A., & Manolis, A. (2020). The growing epidemic of diabetes mellitus. *Current Vascular Pharmacology, 18*(2), 104–109. https://doi.org/10.2174/1570161117666190405165911 (accessed on 28th June 2025).

Mahadev, M., Nandini, H. S., Ramu, R., Gowda, D. V., Almarhoon, Z. M., Al-Ghorbani, M., & Mabkhot, Y. N. (2022). Fabrication and evaluation of quercetin nanoemulsion: A delivery system with improved bioavailability and therapeutic efficacy in diabetes mellitus. *Pharmaceuticals, 15*(1), 70. https://doi.org/10.3390/ph15010070 (accessed on 28th June 2025).

Maity, S., & Chakraborti, A. S. (2020). Formulation, physicochemical characterisation and antidiabetic potential of naringenin-loaded poly D,L lactide-co-glycolide (N-PLGA) nanoparticles. *European Polymer Journal, 134*, 109818. https://doi.org/10.1016/j.eurpolymj.2020.109818 (accessed on 28th June 2025).

Malaguarnera, L. (2019). Influence of resveratrol on the immune response. *Nutrients, 11*(5), 946. https://doi.org/10.3390/nu11050946 (accessed on 28th June 2025).

Marton, L. T., Pescinini-e-Salzedas, L. M., Camargo, M. E. C., Barbalho, S. M., Haber, J. F. d. S., Sinatora, R. V., … Cincotto dos Santos Bueno, P. (2021). The effects of curcumin on diabetes mellitus: A systematic review. *Frontiers in Endocrinology, 12*, 669448. https://doi.org/10.3389/fendo.2021.669448 (accessed on 28th June 2025).

Mehta, S., Nain, P., Agrawal, B. K., Singh, R. P., Kaur, J., Maity, S., Bhattacharjee, A., Peela, J., Nauhria, S., & Nauhria, S. (2021). Effectiveness of empagliflozin with vitamin D supplementation in peripheral neuropathy in type 2 diabetic patients. *Cureus, 13*(12), e20208. https://doi.org/10.7759/cureus.20208 (accessed on 28th June 2025).

Mezil, S. A., & Abed, B. A. (2021). A complication of diabetes mellitus. *Annals of the Romanian Society for Cell Biology*, 1546–1556.

Mirhadi, E., Rezaee, M., & Malaekeh-Nikouei, B. (2018). Nano strategies for berberine delivery, a natural alkaloid of *Berberis*. *Biomedicine & Pharmacotherapy, 104*, 465–473. https://doi.org/10.1016/j.biopha.2018.05.067 (accessed on 28th June 2025).

Mohseni, R., ArabSadeghabadi, Z., Ziamajidi, N., Abbasalipourkabir, R., & RezaeiFarimani, A. (2019). Oral administration of resveratrol-loaded solid lipid nanoparticles improves insulin resistance by targeting the expression of SNARE proteins in adipose and muscle tissue in rats with type 2 diabetes. *Nanoscale Research Letters, 14*, 1–9. https://doi.org/10.1186/s11671-019-3042-7 (accessed on 28th June 2025).

Mukhopadhyay, P., Maity, S., Mandal, S., Chakraborti, A. S., Prajapati, A., & Kundu, P. P. (2018). Preparation, characterisation and in vivo evaluation of pH-sensitive, safe quercetin-succinylated chitosan-alginate core-shell-corona nanoparticle for diabetes treatment. *Carbohydrate Polymers, 182*, 42–51. https://doi.org/10.1016/j.carbpol.2017.10.098 (accessed on 28th June 2025).

Murakami, T., Bodor, E., & Bodor, N. (2023). Approaching strategy to increase the oral bioavailability of berberine, a quaternary ammonium isoquinoline alkaloid: Part 1. Physicochemical and pharmacokinetic properties. *Expert Opinion on Drug Metabolism*

& *Toxicology, 19*(3), 129–137. https://doi.org/10.1080/17425255.2023.2203857 (accessed on 28th June 2025).

Musa, A. E., Omyan, G., Esmaely, F., & Shabeeb, D. (2019). Radioprotective effect of hesperidin: A systematic review. *Medicina, 55*(7), 370. https://doi.org/10.3390/medicina55070370 (accessed on 28th June 2025).

Najar, I. A., Bhat, M. H., Qadrie, Z. L., Amaldoss, M. J. N., Kushwah, A. S., Singh, T. G., Kabra, A., Khan, N., & Kumar, M. (2022). Cardioprotection by *Citrus grandis* (L.) peel ethanolic extract in alloxan-induced cardiotoxicity in diabetic rats. *BioMed Research International, 2022*, 2807337. https://doi.org/10.1155/2022/2807337 (accessed on 28th June 2025).

Nakrani, M. N., Wineland, R. H., & Anjum, F. (2020). Physiology, glucose metabolism.

Naz, S., Imran, M., Rauf, A., Orhan, I. E., Shariati, M. A., Shahbaz, M., ... Heydari, M. (2019). Chrysin: Pharmacological and therapeutic properties. *Life Sciences, 235*, 116797. https://doi.org/10.1016/j.lfs.2019.116797 (accessed on 28th June 2025).

Och, A., Podgórski, R., & Nowak, R. (2020). Biological activity of berberine—A summary update. *Toxins, 12*(11), 713. https://doi.org/10.3390/toxins12110713 (accessed on 28th June 2025).

Panda, D. S., Eid, H. M., Elkomy, M. H., Khames, A., Hassan, R. M., Abo El-Ela, F. I., & Yassin, H. A. (2021). Berberine encapsulated lecithin–chitosan nanoparticles as an innovative wound healing agent in type II diabetes. *Pharmaceutics, 13*(8), 1197. https://doi.org/10.3390/pharmaceutics13081197 (accessed on 28th June 2025).

Pastorino, G., Cornara, L., Soares, S., Rodrigues, F., & Oliveira, M. B. P. (2018). Liquorice (*Glycyrrhiza glabra*): A phytochemical and pharmacological review. *Phytotherapy Research, 32*(12), 2323–2339. https://doi.org/10.1002/ptr.6178 (accessed on 28th June 2025).

Pradhan, S. P., Sahoo, S., Behera, A., Sahoo, R., & Sahu, P. K. (2022). Memory amelioration by hesperidin conjugated gold nanoparticles in diabetes-induced cognitive impaired rats. *Journal of Drug Delivery Science and Technology, 69*, 103145. https://doi.org/10.1016/j.jddst.2022.103145 (accessed on 28th June 2025).

Rahman, M., Almalki, W. H., Afzal, O., Alfawaz Altamimi, A. S., Kazmi, I., Al-Abbasi, F. A., ... Beg, S. (2020). Cationic solid lipid nanoparticles of resveratrol for hepatocellular carcinoma treatment: Systematic optimisation, in vitro characterisation and preclinical investigation. *International Journal of Nanomedicine*, 9283–9299.

Raina, N., Haque, S., Tuli, H. S., Jain, A., Slama, P., & Gupta, M. (2023). Optimisation and characterization of a novel antioxidant naringenin-loaded hydrogel for encouraging re-epithelization in chronic diabetic wounds: A preclinical study. *ACS Omega, 8*(38), 34995–35011. https://doi.org/10.1021/acsomega.3c04441 (accessed on 28th June 2025).

Rani, R., Dahiya, S., Dhingra, D., Dilbaghi, N., Kim, K.-H., & Kumar, S. (2017). Evaluation of anti-diabetic activity of glycyrrhizin-loaded nanoparticles in nicotinamide-streptozotocin-induced diabetic rats. *European Journal of Pharmaceutical Sciences, 106*, 220–230. https://doi.org/10.1016/j.ejps.2017.05.068 (accessed on 28th June 2025).

Rastegari, A., Mottaghitalab, F., Dinarvand, R., Amini, M., Arefian, E., Gholami, M., & Atyabi, F. (2019). Inhibiting hepatic gluconeogenesis by chitosan lactate nanoparticles containing CRTC2 siRNA targeted by poly (ethylene glycol)-glycyrrhetinic acid. *Drug Delivery and Translational Research, 9*, 694–706. https://doi.org/10.1007/s13346-019-00618-1 (accessed on 28th June 2025).

Rathore, S., Mukim, M., Sharma, P., Devi, S., Nagar, J. C., & Khalid, M. (2020). Curcumin: A review for health benefits. *International Journal of Research and Review, 7*(1), 273–290.

Ren, X., Hu, Y., Chang, L., Xu, S., Mei, X., & Chen, Z. (2022). Electrospinning of antibacterial and anti-inflammatory Ag@ hesperidin core-shell nanoparticles into nanofibers promotes infected wound healing. *Regenerative Biomaterials, 9*, rbac012. https://doi.org/10.1093/rb/rbac012 (accessed on 28th June 2025).

Rodríguez-Landa, J. F., German-Ponciano, L. J., Puga-Olguín, A., & Olmos-Vázquez, O. J. (2022). Pharmacological, neurochemical, and behavioural mechanisms underlying the anxiolytic- and antidepressant-like effects of flavonoid chrysin. *Molecules, 27*(11), 3551. https://doi.org/10.3390/molecules27113551 (accessed on 28th June 2025).

Rohilla, M., Rishabh, B., Bansal, S., Garg, A., Dhiman, S., Dhankhar, S., Saini, M., Chauhan, S., Alsubaie, N., Batiha, G. E.-S., Albezrah, N. K. A., & Singh, T. G. (2023). Discussing pathologic mechanisms of diabetic retinopathy & therapeutic potentials of curcumin and β-glucogallin in the management of diabetic retinopathy. *Biomedicine & Pharmacotherapy = Biomedecine & Pharmacotherapie, 169*, 115881. https://doi.org/10.1016/j.biopha.2023.115881 (accessed on 28th June 2025).

Sa'Ayinzat, F., Bawa, E., Ogwu, D., & Ayo, J. (2021). Hesperidin—Sources, chemistry, extraction, measurement and biologic effects on reproduction in animals: A review. *International Journal of Veterinary Sciences and Animal Husbandry, 6*(4), 1–8. https://doi.org/10.22271/veterinary.2021.v6.i3a.360 (accessed on 28th June 2025).

Saad, S., Ahmad, I., Kawish, S. M., Khan, U. A., Ahmad, F. J., Ali, A., & Jain, G. K. (2020). Improved cardioprotective effects of hesperidin solid lipid nanoparticles prepared by supercritical antisolvent technology. *Colloids and Surfaces B: Biointerfaces, 187*, 110628. https://doi.org/10.1016/j.colsurfb.2019.110628 (accessed on 28th June 2025).

Salehi, B., Fokou, P. V. T., Sharifi-Rad, M., Zucca, P., Pezzani, R., Martins, N., & Sharifi-Rad, J. (2019). The therapeutic potential of naringenin: A review of clinical trials. *Pharmaceuticals, 12*(1), 11. https://doi.org/10.1016/j.colsurfb.2019.110628 (accessed on 28th June 2025).

Santos, A. C., Pereira, I., Pereira-Silva, M., Ferreira, L., Caldas, M., Magalhães, M., … Veiga, F. (2019). Nanocarriers for resveratrol delivery: Impact on stability and solubility concerns. *Trends in Food Science & Technology, 91*, 483–497. https://doi.org/10.1016/j.tifs.2019.07.048 (accessed on 28th June 2025).

Selyutina, O. Y., & Polyakov, N. (2019). Glycyrrhizic acid as a multifunctional drug carrier–From physicochemical properties to biomedical applications: A modern insight on the ancient drug. *International Journal of Pharmaceutics, 559*, 271–279. https://doi.org/10.1016/j.ijpharm.2019.01.047 (accessed on 28th June 2025).

Sen, S. (2022). Liposome-encapsulated glycyrrhizin alleviates hyperglycemia and glycation-induced iron-catalyzed oxidative reactions in streptozotocin-induced diabetic rats. *Journal of Liposome Research, 32*(4), 376–385. https://doi.org/10.1080/08982104.2022.2036756 (accessed on 28th June 2025).

Sharma, T., Kaur, D., Grewal, A. K., & Singh, T. G. (2021). Therapies modulating insulin resistance in Parkinson's disease: A cross talk. *Neuroscience Letters, 749*, 135754. https://doi.org/10.1016/j.neulet.2021.135754 (accessed on 28th June 2025).

Sharma, V. K., & Singh, T. G. (2020). Chronic stress and diabetes mellitus: Interwoven pathologies. *Current Diabetes Reviews, 16*(6), 546–556. https://doi.org/10.2174/1573399815666191111152248 (accessed on 28th June 2025).

Siddiqui, A., Badruddeen, A., J., U., MS, S., Khan, M. I., Khalid, M., & Ahmad, M. (2018). A naturally occurring flavone (chrysin): Chemistry, occurrence, pharmacokinetic, toxicity, molecular targets and medicinal properties. *Journal of Biologically Active Products from Nature, 8*(4), 208–227. https://doi.org/10.1080/22311866.2018.1498750 (accessed on 28th June 2025).

Sim, S., & Wong, N. K. (2021). Nanotechnology and its use in imaging and drug delivery. *Biomedical Reports, 14*(5), 1–9. https://doi.org/10.3892/br.2021.1418 (accessed on 28th June 2025).

Singh, M., Bhowal, R., Vishwakarma, R., & Chopra, D. (2020). Assessing the impact on aqueous solubility of berberine chloride via co-crystallization with different stoichiometric ratios of pyromellitic dianhydride. *Journal of Molecular Structure, 1200*, 127086. https://doi.org/10.1016/j.molstruc.2019.127086 (accessed on 28th June 2025).

Singh, R., Farooq, S. A., Mannan, A., Singh, T. G., Najda, A., Grażyna, Z., Albadrani, G. M., Sayed, A. A., & Abdel-Daim, M. M. (2022). Animal models of diabetic microvascular complications: Relevance to clinical features. *Biomedicine & Pharmacotherapy = Biomedecine & Pharmacotherapie, 145*, 112305. https://doi.org/10.1016/j.biopha.2021.112305 (accessed on 28th June 2025).

Song, D., Hao, J., & Fan, D. (2020). Biological properties and clinical applications of berberine. *Frontiers of Medicine, 14*(5), 564–582. https://doi.org/10.1007/s11684-019-0724-6 (accessed on 28th June 2025).

Stompor-Gorący, M., Bajek-Bil, A., & Machaczka, M. (2021). Chrysin: Perspectives on contemporary status and future possibilities as pro-health agent. *Nutrients, 13*(6), 2038. https://doi.org/10.3390/nu13062038 (accessed on 28th June 2025).

Tan, S. Y., Wong, J. L. M., Sim, Y. J., Wong, S. S., Elhassan, S. A. M., Tan, S. H., … Bhattamisra, S. K. (2019). Type 1 and 2 diabetes mellitus: A review of the current treatment approach and gene therapy as a potential intervention. *Diabetes & Metabolic Syndrome: Clinical Research & Reviews, 13*(1), 364–372. https://doi.org/10.1016/j.dsx.2018.10.008 (accessed on 28th June 2025).

Tan, Y., Feng, J., Xiao, Y., & Bao, C. (2022). Grafting resveratrol onto mesoporous silica nanoparticles towards efficient sustainable immunoregulation and insulin resistance alleviation for diabetic periodontitis therapy. *Journal of Materials Chemistry B, 10*(25), 4840–4855. https://doi.org/10.1039/D2TB00484D (accessed on 28th June 2025).

Tang, L., Li, K., Zhang, Y., Li, H., Li, A., Xu, Y., & Wei, B. (2020). Quercetin liposomes ameliorate streptozotocin-induced diabetic nephropathy in diabetic rats. *Scientific Reports, 10*(1), 2440. https://doi.org/10.1038/s41598-020-59411-7 (accessed on 28th June 2025).

Tesauro, M., & Mazzotta, F. A. (2020). Pathophysiology of diabetes. In *Transplantation, Bioengineering, and Regeneration of the Endocrine Pancreas* (pp. 37–47). Elsevier.

Ulusoy, H. G., & Sanlier, N. (2020). A minireview of quercetin: From its metabolism to possible mechanisms of its biological activities. *Critical Reviews in Food Science and Nutrition, 60*(19), 3290–3303. https://doi.org/10.1080/10408398.2019.1683810 (accessed on 28th June 2025).

Wachtel-Galor, S., & Benzie, I. F. (2011). Herbal medicine. In Lester Packer, Ph.D. (Ed.), *Herbal Medicine* (Vol. 1).

Wang, G., Song, X., Zhao, L., Li, Z., & Liu, B. (2018). Resveratrol prevents diabetic cardiomyopathy by increasing Nrf2 expression and transcriptional activity. *BioMed Research International, 2018*. https://doi.org/10.1155/2018/2150218 (accessed on 28th June 2025).

Wang, Z., Wu, J., Zhou, Q., Wang, Y., & Chen, T. (2015). Berberine nanosuspension enhances hypoglycemic efficacy in streptozotocin-induced diabetic C57BL/6 mice. *Evidence-Based Complementary and Alternative Medicine, 2015*. https://doi.org/10.1155/2015/239749 (accessed on 28th June 2025).

Wdowiak, K., Walkowiak, J., Pietrzak, R., Bazan-Woźniak, A., & Cielecka-Piontek, J. (2022). Bioavailability of hesperidin and its aglycone hesperetin—Compounds found in citrus fruits as a parameter conditioning the pro-health potential (neuroprotective and antidiabetic activity)—Mini-review. *Nutrients, 14*(13), 2647. https://doi.org/10.3390/nu14132647 (accessed on 28th June 2025).

Xiang, Q., Xiong, L., Chen, X., Chen, L., He, J., & Zhou, T. (2020). Effect of resveratrol-loaded polypeptide nanospheres on diabetes mellitus complicated with fatty liver. *Nanoscience and Nanotechnology Letters, 12*(6), 834–840. https://doi.org/10.1166/nnl.2020.3170 (accessed on 28th June 2025).

Xu, Z., Xu, Z., Gu, J., Zhou, J., Sha, G., Huang, Y., … Xi, J. (2023). In situ formation of ferrous sulphide in glycyrrhizic acid hydrogels to promote healing of multi-drug resistant *Staphylococcus aureus*-infected diabetic wounds. *Journal of Colloid and Interface Science, 650*, 1918–1929. https://doi.org/10.1016/j.jcis.2023.07.141 (accessed on 28th June 2025).

Xue, M., Zhang, L., Yang, M.-x., Zhang, W., Li, X.-m., Ou, Z.-m., … Yang, S.-y. (2015). Berberine-loaded solid lipid nanoparticles are concentrated in the liver and ameliorate hepatosteatosis in db/db mice. *International Journal of Nanomedicine*, 5049–5057.

Yeo, E., Chieng, C. J. Y., Choudhury, H., Pandey, M., & Gorain, B. (2021). Tocotrienols-rich naringenin nanoemulgel for the management of diabetic wound: Fabrication, characterisation and comparative in vitro evaluations. *Current Research in Pharmacology and Drug Discovery, 2*, 100019. https://doi.org/10.1016/j.crphar.2021.100019 (accessed on 28th June 2025).

Yücel, Ç., Karatoprak, G. Ş., & Aktaş, Y. (2018). Nanoliposomal resveratrol as a novel approach to treatment of diabetes mellitus. *Journal of Nanoscience and Nanotechnology, 18*(6), 3856–3864. https://doi.org/10.1166/jnn.2018.15247 (accessed on 28th June 2025).

Zafar, A., Alsaidan, O. A., Elkomy, M. H., Imam, S. S., Yasir, M., Alharbi, K. S., & Khalid, M. (2023). Formulation and optimisation of naringin polymeric nanoparticles: Optimization to in vivo evaluation. *Journal of Drug Delivery Science and Technology, 88*, 104978. https://doi.org/10.1016/j.jddst.2023.104978 (accessed on 28th June 2025).

Zeng, W., Jin, L., Zhang, F., Zhang, C., & Liang, W. (2018). Naringenin is a potential immunomodulator in therapeutics. *Pharmacological Research, 135*, 122–126. https://doi.org/10.1016/j.phrs.2018.08.002 (accessed on 28th June 2025).

Zhang, P., He, L., Zhang, J., Mei, X., Zhang, Y., Tian, H., & Chen, Z. (2020). Preparation of novel berberine nano-colloids for improving wound healing of diabetic rats by acting Sirt1/NF-κB pathway. *Colloids and Surfaces B: Biointerfaces, 187*, 110647. https://doi.org/10.1016/j.colsurfb.2019.110647 (accessed on 28th June 2025).

Zheng, D., Huang, C., Huang, H., Zhao, Y., Khan, M. R. U., Zhao, H., & Huang, L. (2020). Antibacterial mechanism of curcumin: A review. *Chemistry & Biodiversity, 17*(8), e2000171. https://doi.org/10.1002/cbdv.202000171 (accessed on 28th June 2025).

CHAPTER 13

Role of Natural Products in the Management of Chronic Kidney Disease

PRANALI B. YERAM,[1] AMISHA VORA,[1] YOGESH A. KULKARNI,[1,*] and NITIN CHITRANSHI[2]

[1]Shobhaben Pratapbhai Patel School of Pharmacy and Technology Management, SVKM's Narsee Monjee Institute of Management Studies (NMIMS) Deemed to Be University, Mumbai, Maharashtra, India

[2]Faculty of Medicine, Health and Human Sciences, Macquarie University, North Ryde, New South Wales, Australia

*Corresponding author

ABSTRACT

Chronic kidney disease (CKD) is represented by the gradual loss of kidney function due to various risk factors such as aging, diabetes, hypertension, genetics, etc. The prevalence of CKD is rising, highlighting the limitations of current therapeutic options. Inflammation, Oxidative stress, and fibrosis are the critical factors involved in the progression of chronic kidney disease. In recent years, natural products have demonstrated their potential as an alternative option to treat various diseases, and they are attracting greater attention. They are being explored for the management of CKD. Plant secondary metabolites, especially flavonoids, tannins, terpenes, etc., have various beneficial effects, such as anti-inflammatory, anti-oxidant, anti-fibrotic, anti-diabetic, and anti-hypertensive. Therefore, they may have a valuable role in the management of CKD. The chapter provides a comprehensive insight into scientific studies on different types of natural products and their possible use in CKD.

Precision Nutrition and Endocrine Health: Synthesis, Characterization, and Applications.
Thakur Gurjeet Singh and Sanjana Mehta (Eds.)

DOI: 10.1201/9781998511877-13

13.1 INTRODUCTION

13.1.1 NATURAL PRODUCTS AND THEIR CLASSIFICATION

Natural products are secondary metabolites produced by plants. They exert various pharmacological effects on plants and other organisms (Singh et al., 2020; Teoh, 2016). Plants show two types of chemicals: primary metabolites and secondary metabolites. Primary metabolites are compounds such as carbohydrates, proteins, nucleic acids, and lipids. They have a direct role in healthy growth, development, and reproduction. Secondary metabolites are the remaining chemicals, such as alkaloids, terpenoids, polyphenols, steroids, saponins, etc. They are not directly involved in plant growth, but they are engaged in ecological function. The restricted distribution of secondary metabolites within the plant kingdom sets them apart from primary metabolites. In other words, whereas primary metabolites are present across the plant kingdom, specific secondary metabolites are exclusive to a single plant or a closely related species group. Secondary metabolites have several protective properties for the human body. They can strengthen the immune system, shield the body from free radical damage, eradicate harmful bacteria, and much more, all while maintaining good health. (Anulika et al., 2016; Koche et al., 2016; Singh et al., 2020).

13.1.2 PATHOPHYSIOLOGY OF CHRONIC KIDNEY DISEASE

CKD is characterized by a gradual decline in kidney function, persistent inflammation, oxidative stress, changes in blood vessel structure, and scarring of the kidney's filtering units and surrounding tissues (Impellizzeri et al., 2014). In both developed and developing nations, diabetes and hypertension are the primary contributors to the onset of chronic kidney disease (Ahn and Lucia, 2017; Ekta et al., 2020). CKD is becoming the primary cause of mortality in the world. Recent studies indicate that 10% of the world's population may be suffering from CKD. Among individuals aged 75 years and older, the prevalence of CKD is even higher, affecting half of the population in this age group (Kovesdy, 2022). The National Kidney Federation categorizes CKD into several stages, per the estimated glomerular filtration rate (eGFR) and kidney damage on other tests, such as proteinuria and creatinine albumin ratio. It has been recently shown that inflammation and oxidative stress significantly impact the onset and progression of CKD (Tucker et al., 2015). Renal fibrosis is mainly initiated by inflammation. Alongside the activation of immune cells within the kidney, various cells with fibro genic potential, such as T cells, B cells, macrophages, dendritic cells, and mast cells, are drawn to both the glomerulus and renal interstitial. This recruitment results in an elevated production of pro-inflammatory cytokines (Lousa et al., 2022; Thapa et al., 2021). Activated leukocytes produce ROS, chlorine, and nitrogen species, intensifying and sustaining Oxidative stress (Khan et al., 2021; Rapa et al., 2020). Upon the activation of cells that produce matrix and the release of cytokines promoting fibrosis, an excessive extracellular matrix (ECM) accumulates. This accumulation leads to the gradual deterioration of renal structure and function, as depicted in Figure 13.1.

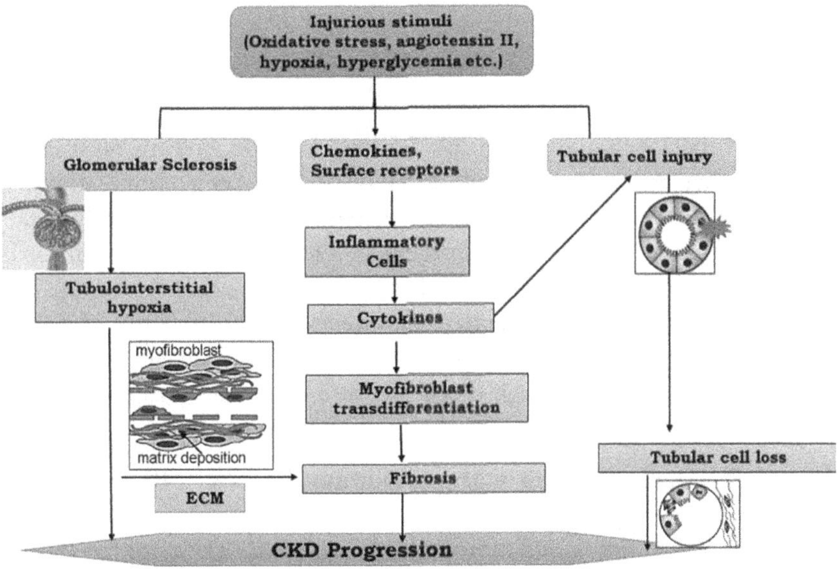

FIGURE 13.1 Pathophysiology of CKD.

In the initial stage, Stage 1, there is a normal eGFR more significant than 90 ml/min, but other test results reveal signs of kidney damage. Progressing to Stage 2, there is a mild decrease in kidney function with an eGFR of 60–90 ml/min, alongside evidence of kidney damage in other tests. Moving on to Stage 3, there is a mild to moderate reduction in kidney function, indicated by an eGFR of 45–59 ml/min. Stage 3, with an eGFR of 30–44 ml/min, signifies a moderate to severe reduction in kidney function. Finally, Stage 4 involves an eGFR of 15–29 ml/min, denoting a severe decrease in kidney function that necessitates additional medications to support specific kidney functions.

- **Diabetes and Chronic Kidney Disease:** Diabetes mellitus (DM) is one of the significant risk factors for non-communicable diseases, which affects many people worldwide. By 2030, the number of people with diabetes worldwide is expected to increase from 8.3% (366 million) in 2011 to 9.9% (522 million) (Whiting et al., 2011). Numerous factors, including genetic, environmental, socioeconomic situations, and demographics, impact diabetes. Hyperglycemia, or elevated blood sugar levels in the body as a result of either insufficient or inadequate insulin synthesis, is characteristic of diabetes mellitus. The leading cause of severe renal illness in type 2 diabetes mellitus (T2DM) is CKD, which is characterized by the presence of proteinuria and a progressive decline in kidney function (Bhargava et al., 2022; Hahr and Molitch, 2015; Sharma and Singh, 2023).
- **Hypertension and Chronic Kidney Disease:** Hypertension could either be a factor contributing to kidney disease or a result of it. While hypertension is more common and frequently addressed in individuals with CKD, its effective management is less probable. Hypertension is common in patients with CKD (Peralta et al., 2005). As a cause and outcome of CKD, hypertension affects the vast majority of people with a diagnosis of the illness. The increased occurrence of risk factors, including high blood pressure, is primarily responsible for the rising prevalence of CKD (Maranduca et al., 2023).
- **Inflammation and Chronic Kidney Disease:** Inflammation is acknowledged as an intricate biological response triggered by harmful stimuli and represents a significant risk factor for several diseases. Although acute inflammation has physiological roles in defense and repair, chronic inflammation can upset homeostasis when the regulating mechanisms change. The inflammatory reaction entails mobilizing innate immune cells that subsequently generate pro-inflammatory cytokines and chemokines, attracting lymphocytes to initiate tissue damage. ROS and various proteases are generated during the immune response to inflammation, all of which can play a role in fostering chronic inflammation (Shen et al., 2013; Thapa et al., 2022).
- **Oxidative Stress and Chronic Kidney Disease:** Oxidative stress is commonly linked to and plays a partial role in the development of

chronic renal failure. CKD development includes inflammation, renal fibrosis, and reduced antioxidant capacity in renal cells (Mohany et al., 2022; Singh et al., 2020). The body achieves homeostasis by preserving a balance between oxidants and antioxidants through its antioxidant defense systems. When these defense mechanisms are dysfunctional, reactive oxygen species (ROS) production rises. ROS interacts with molecules like lipids, proteins, or nucleic acids and induces oxidative stress. Specifically, lipid peroxidation initiated by ROS leads to damage in cellular membranes, ultimately resulting in cell death. (Brunetti et al., 2013). Owing to their antioxidant properties, natural products have demonstrated significant protective effects in various diseases affecting the liver, kidneys, nervous system, cardiovascular system, cancer, diabetes, and aging, especially under oxidative stress conditions.

- **Diabetic Nephropathy and Chronic Kidney Disease:** Diabetic nephropathy (DN) stands as the primary contributor to both CKD and renal failure. In addition to kidney damage, individuals with diabetes experience various complications, including retinopathy, neuropathy, and cardiovascular diseases (Kaur et al., 2023; Xiong and Zhou, 2019). DN is identified by elevated urine albumin excretion, glomerular lesions associated with diabetes, and a decline in glomerular filtration rate (GFR). Substantial evidence indicates that the pathogenesis and advancement of DN are primarily influenced by oxidative stress and inflammation induced by high blood sugar levels.

- **Glomerulonephritis and Chronic Kidney Disease:** Glomerulonephritis (GN) constitutes a diverse set of diseases, making up approximately 20% of CKD cases in many countries. It often impacts younger individuals and has a significant likelihood of progressing to end-stage renal disease (ESRD). Glomerulonephritis presents with diverse clinical symptoms that can encompass hypertension, proteinuria, hemorrhagic, and elevated levels of serum creatinine. Glomerulonephritis encompasses various types, including IgA nephropathy, membranous glomerulonephritis, minimal change disease, focal segmental glomerulosclerosis (FSGS), and membranoproliferative glomerulonephritis. Additionally, there are less common complement-associated types, such as dense deposit disease and C3 glomerulonephritis.

- **Terpenes and Chronic Kidney Disease:** Terpenes are a class of organic compounds mainly found in citrus fruits like lemon and mandarin and plants and trees like tea, hemp, and thyme. Isoprene units are linked together to form terpenoids, joining the head of one unit to the tail of another. A substance with five carbon atoms forms the basis of the terpene structure (Prado-audelo et al., 2021). Terpenes can be classified based on the number of isoprene units they contain. Hemiterpenes have one isoprene unit (C_5H_8), while monoterpenes have two isoprene units. There are various types of sesquiterpenes, diterpenes, tetraterpenes, and triterpenes. Sesquiterpenes have three isoprene units, triterpenes have six, and so on (Chiocchio et al., 2021). Terpenes are reported for their many pharmacological effects by various pathways, which may help manage CKD, as shown in Figure 13.2.

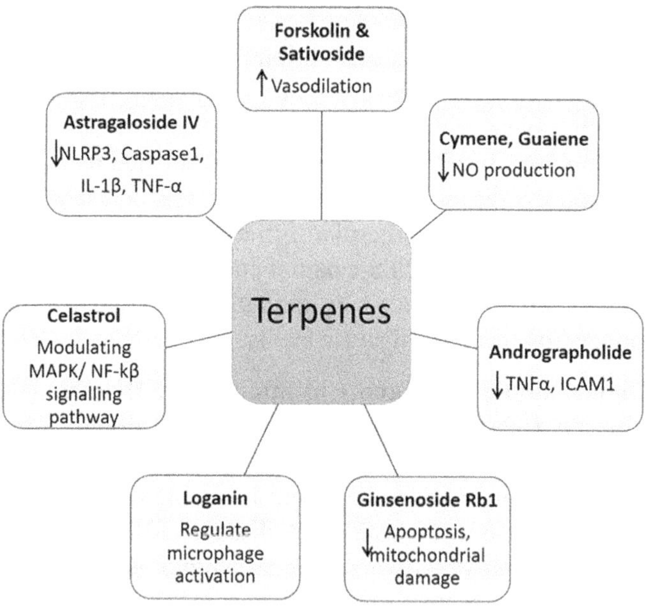

FIGURE 13.2 Terpenes in chronic kidney disease.

- **Terpenes in Chronic Kidney Disease:** Terpenes are widely explored compounds for their various pharmacological effects in managing diseases. In Chronic kidney disease, terpenes may be beneficial due to their antidiabetic, antihypertensive, anti-inflammatory, and antioxidant effects. Many terpenes have been reported to be effective in all these major causes of chronic kidney disease. Also, some terpenes were explored in the Animal modes of chronic kidney diseases and proven effective for managing chronic kidney disease. Acute kidney injury is the renal damage which further leads to chronic renal failure. Linalool is one of the widely explored terpene compounds. This compound is tested for treating acute renal injury in Doxorubicin-induced rats. Kidney biomarkers such as creatinine and BUN were measured, and the oxidative stress parameters were evaluated. This study demonstrated that linalool may act as a renoprotective by decreasing oxidative stress. It reduced the increased level of biomarkers in the experimental rats (Altinoz et al., 2022). D-Limonene is the monocyclic monoterpene commonly found in citrus fruits. D-limonene was explored for its potential in gentamicin-induced acute renal injury. This study predicted that D-limonene prevented acute renal injury by down-regulating proliferating cell nuclear antigens (PCNA). Upregulation of PCNA in renal cells causes intoxication and apoptosis. D-limonene also reduced oxidative stress and inflammation in the experimental rats (Babaeenezhad et al., 2021). Renal ischemia is one of the causes of CKD, in which the blood supply to the kidney suddenly stops. Geraniol is the acyclic monoterpene obtained from essential oils. Geraniol was explored for the treatment of renal ischemia. The study showed that geraniol safeguards against renal ischemia by suppressing the TLR2,4/MYD88/NF-kB pathway, leading to anti-inflammatory effects, activating the Nrf2 pathway, and enhancing antioxidative activities.

- **Antidiabetic Effects of Terpenes:** Medicinal plants have been suggested as a source of phytochemicals for managing type 2 diabetes, with terpenes being a significant component. Research was conducted on medicinal plants from Oriental Morocco to explore their potential for treating diabetes in rats. The findings revealed that the extracts from the studied plants predominantly consist of terpenes, terpene diols, and terpene diol glucosides (Mrabti et al., 2018).

- **Antihypertensive Effects of Terpenes:** Traditional remedies using medicinal plants have a history of effectively addressing hypertension and continue to be employed in the treatment of this condition. The research on the prominent and efficacious medicinal plants utilized in hypertension therapy based on Iran's ethnobotanical evidence revealed that most plants were rich in flavonoids and terpenes (IDM'HAND et al., 2022). Several naturally occurring diterpenes, such as forskolin and sativoside, have been observed to inhibit vascular constriction in experimental animal models. Forskolin, for instance, has been shown to lower intraocular pressure. Another diterpene, *Marrubium vulgare*, from the *Lamiaceae* family, is a widely used Traditional remedy for hypertension and has been demonstrated to induce vascular relaxation and reduce systolic blood pressure.

- **Anti-Inflammatory Effects of Terpenes:** Inflammation affects asthma, cancer, cardiovascular disease, diabetes, and neurodegenerative diseases (Devi et al., 2023; Mannan et al., 2022; Mohan et al., 2023). Terpenes demonstrate a reduction in the pro-inflammatory cytokines TNF-α and IL-1β and an increase in IL-10 production. Guaiene and m-cymene significantly inhibit NO production in a macrophage cell (Campos-xolalpa et al., 2022). *Filifolinone*, a semi-synthetic terpenoid derivative derived from *Heliotropium filifolium*, was identified as a significant contributor to the increased expression of interferon (IFN)-a1, IFN-g, IL-4/13A, and IL-17D in the kidney. Terpenoids inhibit COX and LOX enzymes and also inhibit albumin denaturation. Terpenoids also inhibit prostaglandin synthesis and regulate cytokines, which help reduce the effect of inflammation. In recent years, numerous studies have uncovered the anti-inflammatory properties of natural terpenoids and their derivatives. Terpenoids have demonstrated favorable characteristics in preclinical and clinical applications for treating inflammatory diseases. For example, andrographolide, identified as a diterpenic labdane compound, is a key active component in the traditional herb *Andrographis paniculata*. Moreover, andrographolide has found clinical use in addressing knee osteoarthritis and respiratory infections. Its efficacy has been attributed to the inhibition of TNFα-induced ICAM-1 and nitric oxide synthase (iNOS) expression, reducing nitric oxide production in human cells.
- **Anti-oxidant effects of Terpenes:** Monoterpenes and sesquiterpenes mostly show antioxidant activity. Monoterpene hydrocarbons

exhibit the highest activity level, particularly those containing highly activated methylene groups. They are structured in terpinolene, alpha-terpinene, and sabinene. In terms of antioxidant activity, oxygenated monoterpenes can be ranked with monoterpene phenols (thymol and carvacrol) being the most effective, followed by allylic alcohols (nerol, perillyl alcohol, geraniol, and cis-verbenol), and then monoterpene aldehydes and ketones (Matulja et al., 2021). Scientists are working on terpenes' antioxidant properties, which shows that terpenes are a promising treatment for CKD as antioxidants.

- **Terpenes in the Treatment of Diabetic Nephropathy:** Numerous research studies have examined the impact of terpenes on DN, with the majority indicating a favorable influence on renal function. The research explored the protective properties of astragaloside IV (AS-IV) against DN in db/db mice. AS-IV administration resulted in enhancements in weight, hyperglycemia, and lipid levels. On a mechanistic level, AS-IV suppressed NLRP3, caspase-1, and IL-1β pathways, reducing inflammation and TNF-α (Feng et al., 2021). *In vitro* experiments demonstrated that AS-IV shielded podocytes from injury induced by high glucose, indicating its potential to impede the progression of DN through its anti-NLRP3 inflammasome-mediated effects. Geniposide (GE) has effectively inhibited diabetic nephropathy (DN), yet its precise mechanism remains elusive. This study sought to investigate the anti-DN impact of GE in both high-fat diet/streptozotocin-induced DN mice and a high glucose-induced podocyte model. Evaluation of renal function in DN mice indicated that GE could significantly mitigate oxidative stress and inflammatory reactions, suppress pyroptosis, and hinder the advancement of DN (Zeng and Li, 2023). The proposed mechanism of action is associated with the AMPK/SIRT1/NF-κB pathway. Ginsenoside exhibits activity against diabetic nephropathy by investigating the effects of ginsenoside Rb1 (Rb1), the main active compound in Panax notoginseng, in alleviating podocyte injury in diabetic nephropathy and its related mechanisms. In cultured mouse podocyte cells, administering Rb1 at a concentration of 10 μM significantly impeded cell apoptosis and mitochondrial damage induced by high glucose (He et al., 2022). In this study, streptozotocin-induced diabetic mice served as the *in vivo* model. High glucose (HG) stimulated human proximal tubular HK-2 cells were used as the *in vitro* model. Renal changes were evaluated using hematoxylin-eosin and periodic acid-Schiff staining. The research examined the impact of β-amyrin on ameliorating kidney damage in DN mice and observed its ability to inhibit the inflammatory response in diabetes HK-2 cells. Loganin is a terpene that is seen as very useful for the treatment of DN. Loganin effectively inhibits macrophages' infiltration and activation by targeting CCR2 to regulate macrophage activation (Wu et al., 2023). Celastrol exhibits kidney-protective effects in diabetic rats by modulating the MAPK/NF-κB signaling pathway, suppressing inflammation, and slowing down renal injury (Xu et al., 2021).

- **Terpenes In Glomerulonephritis:** Triptolide, a terpene, is effective against glomerulonephritis. The study on the IgAN rat model concluded that it hinders the progression of IgA nephropathy by affecting the production of proinflammatory cytokines mediated by the inflammasome (Tong et al., 2022).

13.2 TANNINS AND CHRONIC KIDNEY DISEASE

Tannins are reported to have many pharmacological effects by various pathways, which may help manage CKD, as shown in Figure 13.3.

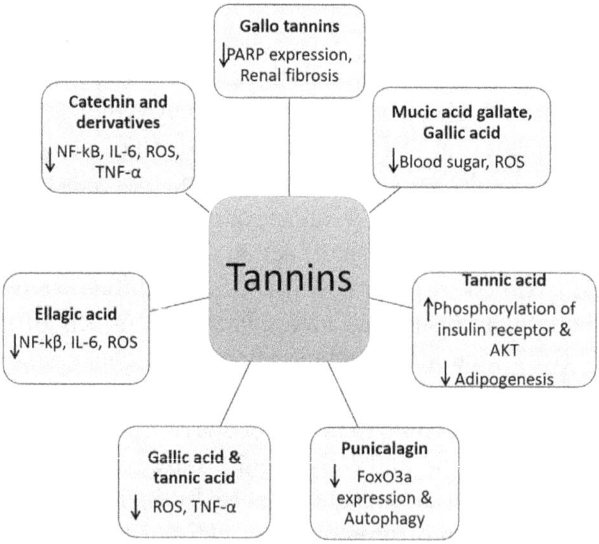

FIGURE 13.3 Tannins in chronic kidney disease.

13.2.1 TANNINS IN CKD

Tannins are proven effective in managing CKD by alleviating causes of renal damage such as hyperglycemia, oxidative stress, inflammation, diabetic nephropathy, etc. A few tannins were also explored in the various animal models of CKD. Renal fibrosis is a significant contributor to chronic kidney disease (CKD). Gallic acid was investigated for its protective properties against glyoxal-induced renal fibrosis in experimental rats. Markers of kidney damage, including serum blood urea nitrogen, creatinine, and alkaline phosphatase, were assessed to evaluate the impact of gallic acid. It notably mitigated renal damage through ROS quenching and anti-glycation activity (Yousuf and Vellaichamy, 2015). Ellagic acid is also a well-known tannin for its various beneficial effects. The effects of ellagic acid on chronic renal failure were investigated using a 5/6 nephrectomy model in rats. Ellagic acid treatment inhibited miR-182, TGF-β1, fibronectin, and Bax levels while promoting those of FOXO3a And Bcl-2 in rats with chronic renal failure. These findings suggest that ellagic acid may alleviate chronic renal failure in rats through the miR-182/FOXO3a pathway (Chen et al., 2021).

13.2.2 ANTIDIABETIC EFFECTS TANNINS

Tannins are widely used natural products for their various pharmacological effects. Catechins are the tannins that are explored for their anti-diabetic potential. Tea catechins are reported for antidiabetic activity by enhancing glucose metabolism and decreasing oxidative stress in rats (Samarghandian et al., 2017). Researchers worked on the plant fractions of the tannins for antidiabetic activity. *Ficus Asperifolia* plant extract contains tannins, which are reported for antidiabetic activity. It significantly Reduces blood glucose and lipid profile (Pwaniyibo et al., 2020). *Phyllanthus emblica* is a plant that contains hydrolysable tannins as the significant components. This plant is reported for its antidiabetic effects. Mucic acid gallate, mucic acid lactone gallate, monogalloylglucose, gallic acid, digalloylglucose, putranjivain A, galloyl-HHDP-glucose, elaeocarpusin, and chebulagic acid are the prominent hydrolysable tannins present in the *Phyllanthus emblica* plant as well as fruit. This extract ameliorates the blood sugar and the oxidative stress in the tissue (Yang and Liu, 2014). Tannic acid is the major component of hydrolysable tannin, also called gallo tannins.

Tannic acid and tannic acid-containing plant extract of *Banaba* worked as antidiabetic in 3T3-L1 cells by inducing phosphorylation of the insulin receptor (IR) and Akt. Also, it inhibited the expression of the critical genes of adipogenesis (Liu et al., 2005).

13.2.3 ANTIHYPERTENSIVE EFFECTS OF TANNINS

Tannins are reported for the treatment and management of metabolic disorders such as obesity, diabetes, and hypertension. *Terminalia bellirica* is a plant that contains tannins reported for antihypertensive activity in rats. These plant tannins reduce pulmonary arterial pressure, decrease oxidative stress during HAPH, and exert protective effects in rats with HAPH, and their mechanism of action is related to the regulation of the Nrf2/HO-1 signaling pathway (Aimaier et al., 2023). Pomegranate (*Punica granatum L.*) fruit and leaves also contain hydrolysable tannins, which are reported for their antihypertensive activity. *In vitro* and *in vivo* studies of these plant extracts and the active tannins showed decreased platelet aggregation and oxidative stress, decreased macrophage lipid uptake, improved endothelial cell function, and regulated blood pressure. (Wang et al., 2018). Grape seed extract (*Vitis vinifera*) was studied to treat and manage metabolic disorders. The study's findings demonstrate that grape polyphenols significantly affect blood pressure, lipid profiles, blood glucose levels, and the liver and heart through various pathways (Akaberi and Hosseinzadeh, 2016).

13.2.4 ANTI-INFLAMMATORY EFFECTS OF TANNINS

Inflammation is the leading cause of many diseases, and it leads to apoptosis of the cells. In renal diseases, inflammation leads to the progression of renal fibrosis, and it is interconnected with many of the cell degenerative mechanisms. Anti-inflammatory agents are the leading components in the management of renal dysfunction. Natural products are used to prevent inflammation and manage various diseases. Also, the extract containing tannins has proven to have anti-inflammatory effects. Tannic acid was reported for its anti-inflammatory activity in the rat model. It showed activity against myeloperoxidase enzyme activity in rats' paw edema models (Soyocak et al., 2019). Punicalagin is the active phytoconstituent of pomegranate juice and comes under tannins. The effect of Punicalagin was studied in lipopolysaccharide (LPS)-induced RAW264.7 macrophages. Punicalagin was found to be effective for anti-inflammatory effects by downregulating FoxO3a expression. Ultimately, it decreases autophagy (Cao et al., 2019). Tannin fractions of the bark extracts were also proven to have anti-inflammatory effects; for example, tannins isolated from the plant *Anacardium occidentale* L. showed anti-inflammatory effects (Mota et al., 1985).

13.2.5 ANTI-OXIDANT EFFECTS OF TANNINS

Tannins were reported to have beneficial effects in the treatment of various diseases. One of the major pathways involved in treating and preventing diseases is the antioxidant effect of tannins. Widely found tannins, such as catechins, gallic acid, ellagic acid, and other plant tannins, were studied for their antioxidant potential. The quantity and degree of hydroxyl group polymerization determine a compound's capacity to scavenge free radicals. Plant tannins have more antioxidant activity since they can be oxidized more readily than the hydroxyl groups they contain (Amarowicz et al., 2004; Tong et al., 2022). Also, the plant fractions of tannins have prevented the antioxidant potential. The research was performed to study the antioxidant potential of gallic acid and tannic acid in a cisplatin-induced nephrotoxicity model of rats. The study's results predicted that gallic acid and tannic acid suppressed the formation of reactive oxygen species, lipid peroxidation, and oxidative stress in kidney tissue (Akomolafe et al., 2014). The plant extract of *Piliostigma reticulatum (Dc) Hochst* and its tannin-containing fraction were studied for their antioxidant effects. The tannin fraction of the plant showed the highest antioxidant potential compared to the plant extract (Dieng et al., 2020).

13.2.6 TANNINS IN DIABETIC NEPHROPATHY

Gallo tannins were explored for the potential to treat diabetic nephropathy. Researchers found that gallo tannins ameliorate diabetic nephropathy by preventing the activation of PARP, an essential key factor in apoptotic cell death (Jang et al., 2008). Tannins from the pomegranate seed were reported for their effects against diabetic nephropathy in streptozotocin-induced diabetic rats by reducing renal fibrosis induced by hyperglycemia.

Also, it acts through the activation of microRNA-495 via regulating SMAD7 (Li et al., 2017). Gallic acid, ellagic acid catechins, etc., are reported to be used in the management of diabetic nephropathy by various mechanisms (Laddha and Kulkarni, 2019; Yokozawa et al., 2010). *Punica granatum* extract is rich in tannins and is proven to treat diabetic nephropathy in streptozotocin-induced diabetic rats (Mestry et al., 2017).

13.3 FLAVONOIDS AND CHRONIC KIDNEY DISEASE

Flavonoids are reported to have many pharmacological effects by various pathways, which may help manage CKD, as shown in Figure 13.4.

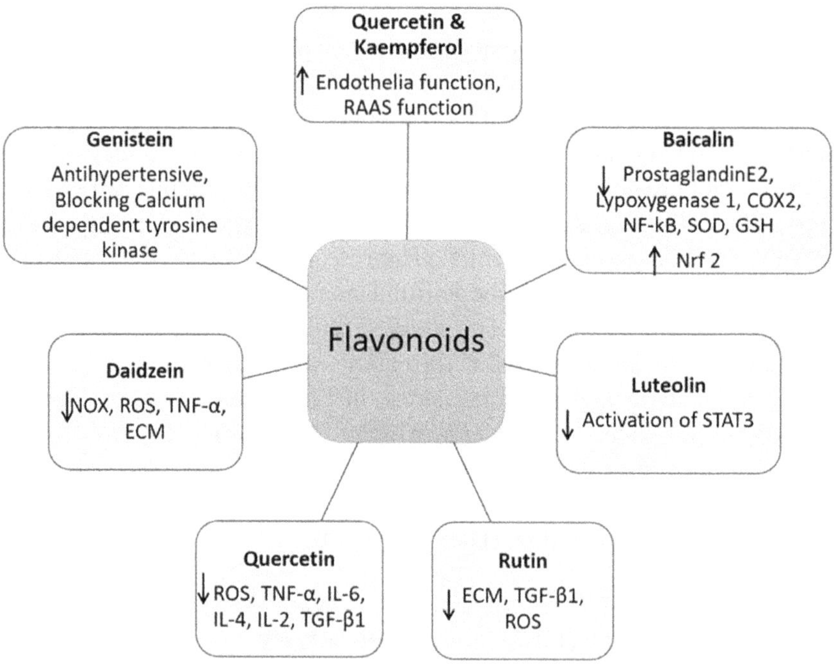

FIGURE 13.4 Flavonoids in chronic kidney disease.

13.3.1 FLAVONOIDS IN CHRONIC KIDNEY DISEASE

Flavonoids have been reported to be nephroprotective by acting as anti-diabetic antioxidants, anti-inflammatory, antifibrotic, etc. They also have studied the management of glomerulonephritis and diabetic nephropathy. Few studies of the flavonoids in the treatment were reported for managing CKD. Quercetin is a well-known flavonoid for its various pharmacological effects. This flavonoid is explored for its impact on the treatment of renal failure. This study is performed using the adenine-induced chronic renal failure model. All the urine parameters, such as Creatinine, Blood Urea Nitrogen, and Uric Acid, were measured. Researchers observed that quercetin minimizes renal fibrosis and apoptosis by inhibiting the PI3k/Akt pathway through targeting PIK3R1. Also, water retention and toxin accumulation were reduced in the quercetin-treated rats (Tu et al., 2021). An Invitro study was performed to check the effects of quercetin on chronic kidney disease. A CKD cell model was used for this study, and SV40 MES 13 cells were used with the glucose-induced medium. It found that quercetin reduced TNF-α, TGF-β1, and MDA, as well as the expression of the SMAD2, SMAD3, and SMAD4, and increased SMAD7 (Widowati et al., 2022). Quercetin and rutin were also studied for their effects in the doxorubicin-induced CKD model in rats. Quercetin and rutin significantly decreased renal amyloidosis and collagen deposition (Hsieh et al., 2013). Rutin is also explored in the adenine-induced CKD model in rats. By reducing oxidative stress and inflammation, Rutin shoved renoprotective and cardioprotective functions (Diwan et al., 2017).

13.3.2 ANTIDIABETIC EFFECTS OF FLAVONOIDS

Flavonoids are explored for their cytoprotective effects by antioxidant mechanisms. Flavonoids such as quercetin, rutin, kaempferol, baicalin, etc., are widely used for their antidiabetic effects. Rutin was reported for the antihyperglycemic effects. It decreases carbohydrate absorption in the small intestine, inhibits gluconeogenesis, increases tissue uptake of glucose, and stimulates insulin secretion from the pancreas. It is antidiabetic and has antioxidant and anti-inflammatory effects interconnected with the antidiabetic mechanism. The overall finding suggested that rutin is the potential molecule for hyperglycemia (Ghorbani, 2017). Quercetin has also been explored for its antidiabetic activity in a streptozotocin-induced rat model. It was proven that quercetin has antihyperglycemic potential (Vessal et al., 2003). Plants are the primary source of flavonoids. Plant extracts containing flavonoids were also reported to be beneficial for antidiabetic effects. The research was carried out on the *Sanguis Draconis* plant extract for its antidiabetic effects. This study shows that this plant has hypoglycemic and hypolipidemic effects in rats with type 2 diabetes, indicating that flavonoids are the main active components responsible for their anti-diabetic properties. It may have an anti-diabetic effect by reducing chronic inflammatory responses and protecting pancreatic islets. Similarly, other plant flavonoids have been reported to have antidiabetic effects, which ultimately help manage chronic kidney disease (Chen et al., 2013).

13.3.3 ANTIHYPERTENSIVE EFFECTS OF FLAVONOIDS

Various flavonoids are reported to have antihypertensive effects. They are used for the management of metabolic disorders that lead to hypertension, such as obesity. Naringenin comes in flavanones, significantly reducing BP and improving acetylcholine-mediated and sodium nitroprusside (SNP)-mediated relaxation in aortic rings. It also modulates nitric oxide levels and protects endothelial function. Isoflavones such as daidzein and genistein have also been explored for their antihypertensive effects. Daidzein acts as an antihypertensive compound by reducing NOX overproduction in humans by the PI3K/Akt/eNOS pathway. Genistein is also proven antihypertensive by blocking Pyk2, a Ca2+-dependent non-receptor tyrosine kinase (Callejo et al., 2020; Maaliki et al., 2019). Quercetin and kaempferol have an antihypertensive effect because of their capacity to enhance endothelial function, modify the renin-angiotensin-aldosterone system (RAAS), and alter the contractility of vascular smooth muscle cells. Human randomized controlled trials (RCTs) demonstrate that quercetin and catechins significantly decrease blood pressure. The mechanisms by which flavonoids exert their antihypertensive effects include enhancing the bioavailability of nitric oxide (NO), reducing oxidative stress in endothelial cells, and regulating the function of vascular ion channels (Serban et al., 2016).

13.3.4 ANTI-INFLAMMATORY EFFECTS OF FLAVONOIDS

New studies indicate flavonoids can suppress transcription factors or regulatory enzymes pivotal for controlling inflammatory mediators.

Additionally, flavonoids are potent antioxidants, potentially reducing fibrosis or tissue damage. It has been demonstrated that flavonoids have anti-inflammatory effects via various pathways, including immune cell modulation, enzyme and transcription factor inhibition, and inhibition. According to studies, flavonoids affect immune cell maturation, activation, and signaling transduction, which may hamper the synthesis and release of chemokines and cytokines. A class of protein kinases, including tyrosine kinase, phosphoinositol kinase, protein kinase C (PKC), and phosphatidylinositol kinase, is involved in inflammation. There have been reports of several flavonoid types inhibiting certain enzymes. Numerous investigations have discovered that flavonoids can also affect the metabolism of arachidonic acid by suppressing the production of prostaglandins, thromboxanes, and leukotrienes through the actions of enzymes, including phospholipase A2, cyclooxygenase, and lipoxygenase. Baicalin ameliorates the levels of prostaglandin E2 (PGE2), lipoxygenase-1 (LOX1), and cyclooxygenase-2 (COX) (Yuan et al., 2020). Additionally, flavonoids could affect protein kinases by blocking transcription factors like nuclear kappa-B (NF-κβ). NF-κβ regulates numerous cytokines, chemokines, and cell adhesion molecules involved in inflammation (Sharma et al., 2020).

13.3.5 ANTIOXIDANT EFFECTS OF FLAVONOIDS

It has been discovered that flavonoids, which function as exogenous antioxidants by giving electrons to peroxynitrite, hydroxyl, and peroxyl radicals, significantly help to stabilize these radicals and lower the body's levels of reactive oxygen species and other free radicals. It has been discovered that flavonoids activate intracellular antioxidant signaling pathways, which in turn inhibit ROS-generating enzymes like xanthine oxidase, myeloperoxidase (MDA), and nicotinamide adenine dinucleotide phosphate (NADPH) oxidase while also accelerating the production of endogenous antioxidants like glutathione (GSH), superoxide dismutase (SOD), and catalase (CAT) (Hamid et al., 2020). It has been observed that flavonoids, including quercetin, naringenin, baicalin, and genistein, protect against several diseases by activating the Nrf2 signaling pathway and reducing the rate at which the Nrf2 protein degrades by itself (Qin et al., 2014). In rats, baicalin significantly reduced oxidative stress by reducing MDA activity and raising SOD and GSH levels (Jiang, 2019).

13.3.6 FLAVONOIDS IN DIABETIC NEPHROPATHY

Flavonoids are proven to treat hyperglycemia by reducing factors responsible for the progression of diabetes. Quercetin was studied for its protective effect on glomerular and nephrotic damage. The study demonstrated that quercetin can potentially manage diabetic nephropathy by reducing lipid peroxidation and oxidative stress in streptozotocin-induced diabetic rats. Also, it prevents renal fibrosis by decreasing the expression of TGF-β1. Rutin was also reported for the treatment of diabetic nephropathy. It reduces renal fibrosis by suppressing oxidative stress, TGF-1/mothers against DPP homolog (Smad)/ECM, and TGF-β1/CTGF/ECM signaling pathways in STZ-induced DN rats, as well as affecting matrix metalloproteinases (MMPs) (Ganesan et al., 2018). In db/db mouse models, luteolin may reduce glomerulosclerosis and interstitial fibrosis by reducing oxidative stress and the inflammatory response by suppressing the activation of signal transducer and activator of transcription 3 (STAT3) (Zhou, 2020).

13.4 CONCLUSION

Natural products are accepted worldwide for managing chronic diseases due to their beneficial effects and fewer side effects. Flavonoids, tannins, and terpenes are the widely available compounds that have been explored for their potential in various diseases. The prevalence of chronic kidney disease is increasing worldwide due to limited treatment options in allopathic medicine. Natural products are the hope for managing chronic kidney disease due to their beneficial effects in the treatment of diabetes, diabetic nephropathy, glomerulonephritis, acute renal injury, and nephrotoxicity, which are the major causes of the progression of chronic kidney disease. Flavonoids, tannins, and terpenes act as antioxidants, anti-inflammatory and anti-fibrotic and are effective in managing diabetic nephropathy, glomerulonephritis and acute renal injury by modulating various pathways. Detailed investigations, including clinical studies, need to be done to establish the effects of natural products on chronic kidney disease.

KEYWORDS

- **anti-inflammatory**
- **chronic kidney disease**
- **flavonoids**
- **natural products**
- **tannins**
- **terpenes**

REFERENCES

Ahn, H., & Lucia, M. S. H. K. C., & Kim, T. J. K. D. C. (2017). Chronic kidney disease diagnosis and management. *Physiology & Behavior, 176*(10), 139–148. https://doi.org/10.1001/jama.2019.14745.Chronic (accessed on 28th June 2025).

Aimaier, S., Tao, Y., Lei, F., Yupeng, Z., Wenhui, S., Aikemu, A., & Maimaitiyiming, D. (2023). Protective effects of the *Terminalia bellirica* tannin-induced Nrf2/HO-1 signaling pathway in rats with high-altitude pulmonary hypertension. *BMC Complementary Medicine and Therapies, 23*(1), 1–11. https://doi.org/10.1186/s12906-023-03981-2 (accessed on 28th June 2025).

Akaberi, M., & Hosseinzadeh, H. (2016). Ptr5570. *556*(October 2015), 540–556.

Akomolafe, S. F., Akinyemi, A. J., & Anadozie, S. O. (2014). Phenolic acids (gallic and tannic acids) modulate antioxidant status and cisplatin-induced nephrotoxicity in rats. *International Scholarly Research Notices, 2014*, 1–8. https://doi.org/10.1155/2014/984709 (accessed on 28th June 2025).

Altinoz, E., Oner, Z., Elbe, H., Uremis, N., & Uremis, M. (2022). Linalool exhibits therapeutic and protective effects in a rat model of doxorubicin-induced kidney injury by modulating oxidative stress. *Drug and Chemical Toxicology, 45*(5), 2024–2030. https://doi.org/10.1080/01480545.2021.1894751 (accessed on 28th June 2025).

Amarowicz, R., Troszyńska, A., Baryłko-Pikielna, N., & Shahidi, F. (2004). Polyphenolics extracts from legume seeds: Correlations between total antioxidant activity, total phenolics content, tannins content and astringency. *Journal of Food Lipids, 11*(4), 278–286. https://doi.org/10.1111/j.1745-4522.2004.01143.x (accessed on 28th June 2025).

Anulika, N. P., Ignatius, E. O., Raymond, E. S., Osasere, O. I., & Abiola, A. H. (2016). The chemistry of natural product: Plant secondary metabolites. *International Journal of Technology Enhancements and Emerging Engineering Research, 4*(8), 1–8.

Babaeenezhad, E., Hadipour Moradi, F., Rahimi Monfared, S., Fattahi, M. D., Nasri, M., Amini, A., Dezfoulian, O., & Ahmadvand, H. (2021). D-limonene alleviates acute kidney injury following gentamicin administration in rats: Role of NF-κB pathway, mitochondrial apoptosis, oxidative stress, and PCNA. *Oxidative Medicine and Cellular Longevity, 2021*. https://doi.org/10.1155/2021/6670007 (accessed on 28th June 2025).

Bhargava, S. K., Singh, T. G., Mannan, A., Singh, S., & Gupta, S. (2022). Pharmacological evaluation of *Thuja occidentalis* for the attenuation of nephropathy in streptozotocin-induced diabetes rats. *Obesity Medicine, 31*, 100391. https://doi.org/10.1016/j.obmed.2022.100391 (accessed on 28th June 2025).

Brunetti, C., Di Ferdinando, M., Fini, A., & Pollastri, S. (2013). Flavonoids as antioxidants and developmental regulators: Relative significance in plants and humans. *International Journal of Molecular Sciences, 14*, 3540–3555. https://doi.org/10.3390/ijms14023540 (accessed on 28th June 2025).

Callejo, M., Barberá, J. A., Duarte, J., & Perez-Vizcaino, F. (2020). Impact of nutrition on pulmonary arterial hypertension. *Nutrients, 12*(1), 1–18. https://doi.org/10.3390/nu12010169 (accessed on 28th June 2025).

Campos-Xolalpa, N., Esquivel-Campos, A. L., Martínez-Casares, R. M., Pérez-Gutiérrez, S., Pérez-Ramos, J., & Sánchez-Mendoza, E. (2022). Anti-inflammatory activity of piquerol isolated from *Piqueria trinervia* Cav. *Pharmaceuticals, 15*(7). https://doi.org/10.3390/ph15070771 (accessed on 28th June 2025).

Cao, Y., Chen, J., Ren, G., Zhang, Y., Tan, X., & Yang, L. (2019). Punicalagin prevents inflammation in LPS-induced RAW264.7 macrophages by inhibiting FOXO3a/autophagy signaling pathway. *Nutrients, 11*(11), 1–14. https://doi.org/10.3390/nu11112794 (accessed on 28th June 2025).

Chen, F., Xiong, H., Wang, J., Ding, X., Shu, G., & Mei, Z. (2013). Antidiabetic effect of total flavonoids from *Sanguis draxonis* in type 2 diabetic rats. *Journal of Ethnopharmacology, 149*(3), 729–736. https://doi.org/10.1016/j.jep.2013.07.035 (accessed on 28th June 2025).

Chen, S., Zhou, M., Ying, X., & Zhou, C. (2021). Ellagic acid protects rats from chronic renal failure via miR-182/FOXO3a axis. *Molecular Immunology, 138*(251), 150–160. https://doi.org/10.1016/j.molimm.2021.08.007 (accessed on 28th June 2025).

Chiocchio, I., Mandrone, M., Tomasi, P., Marincich, L., & Poli, F. (2021). Plant secondary metabolites: An opportunity for circular economy. *Molecules, 26*(2). https://doi.org/10.3390/molecules26020495 (accessed on 28th June 2025).

Devi, S., Chauhan, S., Mannan, A., & Singh, T. G. (2023). Targeting cardiovascular risk factors with eugenol: An anti-inflammatory perspective. *Inflammopharmacology*. https://doi.org/10.1007/s10787-023-01392-w (accessed on 28th June 2025).

Dieng, S. I. M., Mathieu, C., Sarr, A., Diatta-Badji, K., & Fall, A. D. (2020). Condensed tannins content and their influence on the antioxidant activity of bark hydroethanol extract of *Piliostigma reticulatum* (DC) Hochst and its fractions. *Pharmacognosy Journal, 12*(2), 361–368. https://doi.org/10.5530/pj.2020.12.57 (accessed on 28th June 2025).

Diwan, V., Brown, L., & Gobe, G. C. (2017). The flavonoid rutin improves kidney and heart structure and function in an adenine-induced rat model of chronic kidney disease. *Journal of Functional Foods, 33*, 85–93. https://doi.org/10.1016/j.jff.2017.03.012 (accessed on 28th June 2025).

Ekta, Gupta, M., Kaur, A., Singh, T. G., & Bedi, O. (2020). Pathobiological and molecular connections involved in the high fructose and high fat diet induced diabetes-associated nonalcoholic fatty liver disease. *Inflammation Research, 69*(9), 851–867. https://doi.org/10.1007/s00011-020-01373-7 (accessed on 28th June 2025).

Feng, H., Zhu, X., Tang, Y., Fu, S., Kong, B., & Liu, X. (2021). Astragaloside IV ameliorates diabetic nephropathy in db/db mice by inhibiting NLRP3 inflammasome-mediated inflammation. *International Journal of Molecular Medicine, 48*(2), 1–12. https://doi.org/10.3892/ijmm.2021.4996 (accessed on 28th June 2025).

Ganesan, D., Holkar, A., Albert, A., Paul, E., & Mariakuttikan, J. (2018). Combination of ramipril and rutin alleviate alloxan-induced diabetic nephropathy targeting multiple stress pathways *in vivo*. *Biomedicine & Pharmacotherapy, 108*, 1338–1346. https://doi.org/10.1016/j.biopha.2018.09.142 (accessed on 28th June 2025).

Ghorbani, A. (2017). Mechanisms of antidiabetic effects of flavonoid rutin. *Biomedicine & Pharmacotherapy, 96*, 305–312. https://doi.org/10.1016/j.biopha.2017.10.001 (accessed on 28th June 2025).

Hahr, A. J., & Molitch, M. E. (2015). Management of diabetes mellitus in patients with chronic kidney disease. *Clinical Diabetes and Endocrinology, 1*(1), 1–9. https://doi.org/10.1186/s40842-015-0001-9 (accessed on 28th June 2025).

Hamid, A. A., Aminuddin, A., Yunus, M. H. M., Murthy, J. K., Hui, C. K., & Ugusman, A. (2020). Antioxidative and anti-inflammatory activities of *Polygonum minus*: A review of literature. *Reviews in Cardiovascular Medicine, 21*(2), 275–288. https://doi.org/10.31083/J.RCM.2020.02.50 (accessed on 28th June 2025).

He, J. Y., Hong, Q., Chen, B. X., Cui, S. Y., Liu, R., Cai, G. Y., Guo, J., & Chen, X. M. (2022). Ginsenoside Rb1 alleviates diabetic kidney podocyte injury by inhibiting aldose reductase activity. *Acta Pharmacologica Sinica, 43*(2), 342–353. https://doi.org/10.1038/s41401-021-00788-0 (accessed on 28th June 2025).

Hsieh, C. L., Peng, C. C., Chen, K. C., & Peng, R. Y. (2013). Rutin (quercetin rutinoside) induced protein-energy malnutrition in chronic kidney disease, but quercetin acted beneficially. *Journal of Agricultural and Food Chemistry, 61*(30), 7258–7267. https://doi.org/10.1021/jf304595p (accessed on 28th June 2025).

Idm'hand, E., Msanda, F., & Cherifi, K. (2022). A review of Moroccan medicinal plants used in the treatment of hypertension. *International Journal of Nature and Life Sciences, 6*(1), 48–78. https://doi.org/10.47947/ijnls.1010197 (accessed on 28th June 2025).

Impellizzeri, D., Esposito, E., Attley, J., & Cuzzocrea, S. (2014). Targeting inflammation: New therapeutic approaches in chronic kidney disease (CKD). *Pharmacological Research, 81*, 91–102. https://doi.org/10.1016/j.phrs.2014.02.007 (accessed on 28th June 2025).

Jang, M. H., Piao, X. L., Kim, J. M., Kwon, S. W., & Park, J. H. (2008). Inhibition of cholinesterase and amyloid-β aggregation by resveratrol oligomers from *Vitis amurensis*. *Phytotherapy Research, 22*(4), 544–549. https://doi.org/10.1002/ptr (accessed on 28th June 2025).

Jiang, K. (2019). Enteral baicalin, a flavone glycoside, reduces indicators of cardiac surgery-associated acute kidney injury in rats. *Kidney & Blood Pressure Research, 28*, 31–40. https://doi.org/10.1159/000492159 (accessed on 28th June 2025).

Kaur, N., Kishore, L., Farooq, S. A., Kajal, A., Singh, R., Agrawal, R., Mannan, A., & Singh, T. G. (2023). *Cucurbita pepo* seeds improve peripheral neuropathy in diabetic rats by modulating the inflammation and oxidative stress in rats. *Environmental Science and Pollution Research International.* https://doi.org/10.1007/s11356-023-28339-6 (accessed on 28th June 2025).

Khan, H., Gupta, A., Singh, T. G., & Kaur, A. (2021). Mechanistic insight on the role of leukotriene receptors in ischemic-reperfusion injury. *Pharmacological Reports, 73*(5), 1240–1254. https://doi.org/10.1007/s43440-021-00258-8 (accessed on 28th June 2025).

Koche, D., Shirsat, R., & Kawale, M. (2016). An overview of major classes of phytochemicals: Their types and role in disease prevention. *Hislopia Journal, 9*(1/2), 1–11.

Kovesdy, C. P. (2022). Epidemiology of chronic kidney disease: An update 2022. *Kidney International Supplements, 12*(1), 7–11. https://doi.org/10.1016/j.kisu.2021.11.003 (accessed on 28th June 2025).

Laddha, A. P., & Kulkarni, Y. A. (2019). Tannins and vascular complications of diabetes: An update. *Phytomedicine, 56*, 229–245. https://doi.org/10.1016/j.phymed.2018.10.026 (accessed on 28th June 2025).

Li, H. J., Shen, H. R., Shao, G. F., & Shi, B. M. (2017). Tannins from pomegranate seeds ameliorate renal injury in streptozotocin-induced diabetic rats through the activation of microRNA-495 via regulating SMAD7. *International Journal of Clinical and Experimental Medicine, 10*(2), 2532–2540.

Liu, X., Kim, J. K., Li, Y., Li, J., Liu, F., & Chen, X. (2005). Tannic acid stimulates glucose transport and inhibits adipocyte differentiation in 3T3-L1 cells. *Journal of Nutrition, 135*(2), 165–171. https://doi.org/10.1093/jn/135.2.165 (accessed on 28th June 2025).

Lousa, I., Reis, F., Santos-Silva, A., & Belo, L. (2022). The signaling pathway of TNF receptors: Linking animal models of renal disease to human CKD. *International Journal of Molecular Sciences, 23*(6). https://doi.org/10.3390/ijms23063284 (accessed on 28th June 2025).

Maaliki, D., Shaito, A. A., Pintus, G., El-Yazbi, A., & Eid, A. H. (2019). Flavonoids in hypertension: A brief review of the underlying mechanisms. *Current Opinion in Pharmacology, 45*, 57–65. https://doi.org/10.1016/j.coph.2019.04.014 (accessed on 28th June 2025).

Mannan, A., Singh, T. G., Singh, V., Garg, N., Kaur, A., & Singh, M. (2022). Insights into the mechanism of the therapeutic potential of herbal monoamine oxidase inhibitors in neurological diseases. *Current Drug Targets, 23*(3), 286–310. https://doi.org/10.2174/1389450122666210707120256 (accessed on 28th June 2025).

Maranduca, M., Clim, A., Pinzariu, A., Statescu, C., Sascau, R., Tanase, D., Serban, D., Branisteanu, D., Branisteanu, D., Huzum, B., & Serban, I. (2023). Role of arterial hypertension and angiotensin II in chronic kidney disease (Review). *Experimental and Therapeutic Medicine, 25*(4), 1–5. https://doi.org/10.3892/etm.2023.11852 (accessed on 28th June 2025).

Matulja, D., Grbčić, P., Bojanić, K., Topić-Popović, N., Čož-Rakovac, R., Laclef, S., Šmuc, T., Jović, O., Marković, D., & Pavelić, S. K. (2021). Chemical evaluation, antioxidant, antiproliferative, anti-inflammatory and antibacterial activities of organic extract and semi-purified fractions of the Adriatic sea fan, *Eunicella cavolini. Molecules, 26*(19), 1–21. https://doi.org/10.3390/molecules26195751 (accessed on 28th June 2025).

Mestry, S. N., Dhodi, J. B., Kumbhar, S. B., & Juvekar, A. R. (2017). Attenuation of diabetic nephropathy in streptozotocin-induced diabetic rats by *Punica granatum* Linn.

leaves extract. *Journal of Traditional and Complementary Medicine, 7*(3), 273–280. https://doi.org/10.1016/j.jtcme.2016.06.008 (accessed on 28th June 2025).

Mohan, M., Mannan, A., & Singh, T. G. (2023). Therapeutic implication of Sonic Hedgehog as a potential modulator in ischemic injury. *Pharmacological Reports, 75*(4), Article 4. https://doi.org/10.1007/s43440-023-00505-0 (accessed on 28th June 2025).

Mohany, M., Ahmed, M. M., & Al-Rejaie, S. S. (2022). Antioxidants molecular mechanistic pathways targeted by natural antioxidants in the prevention and treatment of chronic kidney disease. *Oxidative Medicine and Cellular Longevity*. [Details incomplete; DOI/ link missing]

Mota, M., Thomas, G., & Filho, J. B. (1985). Anti-inflammatory bark of. *Journal/Volume/ Page details missing.*

Mrabti, H. N., Jaradat, N., Fichtali, I., Ouedrhiri, W., Jodeh, S., Ayesh, S., Cherrah, Y., & Faouzi, M. E. A. (2018). Separation, identification, and antidiabetic activity of catechin isolated from *Arbutus unedo* L. plant roots. *Plants, 7*(2). https://doi.org/10.3390/plants7020031 (accessed on 28th June 2025).

Peralta, C. A., Hicks, L. S., Chertow, G. M., Ayanian, J. Z., Vittinghoff, E., Lin, F., & Shlipak, M. G. (2005). Control of hypertension in adults with chronic kidney disease in the United States. *Hypertension, 45*(6), 1119–1124. https://doi.org/10.1161/01.HYP.0000164577.81087.70 (accessed on 28th June 2025).

Prado-Audelo, M. L. del, Cortés, H., Caballero-Florán, I. H., González-Torres, M., Escutia-Guadarrama, L., & Bernal-Chávez, S. A. (2021). Therapeutic applications of terpenes on inflammatory diseases. *Frontiers in Pharmacology, 12*(August), 1–7. https://doi.org/10.3389/fphar.2021.704197 (accessed on 28th June 2025).

Pwaniyibo, S. F., Teru, P. A., Samuel, N. M., & Jahng, W. J. (2020). Anti-diabetic effects of *Ficus asperifolia* in streptozotocin-induced diabetic rats. *Journal of Diabetes and Metabolic Disorders, 19*(1), 605–616. https://doi.org/10.1007/s40200-020-00524-1 (accessed on 28th June 2025).

Qin, S., Deng, F., Wu, W., Jiang, L., Yamashiro, T., Yano, S., & Hou, D. (2014). Baicalein modulates Nrf2/Keap1 system in both Keap1-dependent and Keap1-independent mechanisms. *Archives of Biochemistry and Biophysics*, 1–9. https://doi.org/10.1016/j.abb.2014.03.011 (accessed on 28th June 2025).

Rapa, S. F., Di Iorio, B. R., Campiglia, P., Heidland, A., & Marzocco, S. (2020). Inflammation and oxidative stress in chronic kidney disease—Potential therapeutic role of minerals, vitamins and plant-derived metabolites. *International Journal of Molecular Sciences, 21*(1). https://doi.org/10.3390/ijms21010263 (accessed on 28th June 2025).

Samarghandian, S., Azimi-Nezhad, M., & Farkhondeh, T. (2017). Catechin treatment ameliorates diabetes and its complications in streptozotocin-induced diabetic rats. *Dose-Response, 15*(1), 1–7. https://doi.org/10.1177/1559325817691158 (accessed on 28th June 2025).

Serban, M. C., Sahebkar, A., Zanchetti, A., Mikhailidis, D. P., Howard, G., Antal, D., Andrica, F., Ahmed, A., Aronow, W. S., Muntner, P., Lip, G. Y. H., Graham, I., Wong, N., Rysz, J., & Banach, M. (2016). Effects of quercetin on blood pressure: A systematic review and meta-analysis of randomized controlled trials. *Journal of the American Heart Association, 5*(7), 1–15. https://doi.org/10.1161/JAHA.115.002713 (accessed on 28th June 2025).

Sharma, S., Baboota, S., Amin, S., & Mir, S. R. (2020). Ameliorative effect of a standardized polyherbal combination in methotrexate-induced nephrotoxicity in the rat. *Pharmaceutical Biology, 58*(1), 184–199. https://doi.org/10.1080/13880209.2020.1717549 (accessed on 28th June 2025).

Sharma, V., & Singh, T. G. (2023). Drug induced nephrotoxicity—A mechanistic approach. *Molecular Biology Reports, 50*(8), 6975–6986. https://doi.org/10.1007/s11033-023-08573-4 (accessed on 28th June 2025).

Shen, H., Kreisel, D., & Goldstein, D. R. (2013). Processes of sterile inflammation. *The Journal of Immunology*. https://doi.org/10.4049/jimmunol.1301539 (accessed on 28th June 2025).

Singh, H. P., Singh, T. G., & Singh, R. (2020). Sinapic acid attenuates cisplatin-induced nephrotoxicity through peroxisome proliferator-activated receptor gamma agonism in rats. *Journal of Pharmacy & Bioallied Sciences, 12*(2), Article 2. https://doi.org/10.4103/jpbs.JPBS_220_19 (accessed on 28th June 2025).

Singh, M., Sharma, P., Singh, P. K., Singh, T. G., & Saini, B. (2020). Medicinal potential of heterocyclic compounds from diverse natural sources for the management of cancer. *Mini Reviews in Medicinal Chemistry, 20*(11), 942–957. https://doi.org/10.2174/1389557520666200212104742 (accessed on 28th June 2025).

Singh, S., Singh, T. G., Mahajan, K., & Dhiman, S. (2020). Medicinal plants used against various inflammatory biomarkers for the management of rheumatoid arthritis. *The Journal of Pharmacy and Pharmacology, 72*(10), 1306–1327. https://doi.org/10.1111/jphp.13326 (accessed on 28th June 2025).

Soyocak, A., Kurt, H., Cosan, D. T., Saydam, F., Calis, I. U., Kolac, U. K., Koroglu, Z. O., Degirmenci, I., Mutlu, F. S., & Gunes, H. V. (2019). Tannic acid exhibits anti-inflammatory effects on formalin-induced paw edema model of inflammation in rats. *Human and Experimental Toxicology, 38*(11), 1296–1301. https://doi.org/10.1177/0960327119864154 (accessed on 28th June 2025).

Teoh, E. S. (2016). *Medicinal Orchids of Asia*, 1–752. https://doi.org/10.1007/978-3-319-24274-3 (accessed on 28th June 2025).

Thapa, K., Singh, T. G., & Kaur, A. (2021). Cyclic nucleotide phosphodiesterase inhibition as a potential therapeutic target in renal ischemia reperfusion injury. *Life Sciences, 282*, 119843. https://doi.org/10.1016/j.lfs.2021.119843 (accessed on 28th June 2025).

Thapa, K., Singh, T. G., & Kaur, A. (2022). Targeting ferroptosis in ischemia/reperfusion renal injury. *Naunyn-Schmiedeberg's Archives of Pharmacology, 395*(11), Article 11. https://doi.org/10.1007/s00210-022-02277-5 (accessed on 28th June 2025).

Tong, X., Qiao, Y., Yang, Y., Liu, H., Cao, Z., Yang, B., Wei, L., & Yang, H. (2022). Applications and mechanisms of *Tripterygium wilfordii* Hook. F. and its preparations in kidney diseases. *Frontiers in Pharmacology, 13*(March), 1–15. https://doi.org/10.3389/fphar.2022.846746 (accessed on 28th June 2025).

Tong, Z., He, W., Fan, X., & Guo, A. (2022). Biological function of plant tannin and its application in animal health. *Frontiers in Veterinary Science, 8*(January), 1–7. https://doi.org/10.3389/fvets.2021.803657 (accessed on 28th June 2025).

Tu, H., Ma, D., Luo, Y., Tang, S., Li, Y., Chen, G., Wang, L., Hou, Z., Shen, C., Lu, H., Zhuang, X., & Zhang, L. (2021). Quercetin alleviates chronic renal failure by targeting the PI3K/Akt pathway. *Bioengineered, 12*(1), 6538–6558. https://doi.org/10.1080/21655979.2021.1973877 (accessed on 28th June 2025).

Tucker, P. S., Scanlan, A. T., & Dalbo, V. J. (2015). Chronic kidney disease influences multiple systems: Describing the relationship between oxidative stress, inflammation, kidney damage, and concomitant disease. *Oxidative Medicine and Cellular Longevity, 2015*, Article ID 806358. https://doi.org/10.1155/2015/806358 (accessed on 28th June 2025).

Vessal, M., Hemmati, M., & Vasei, M. (2003). Antidiabetic effects of quercetin in streptozotocin-induced diabetic rats. *Comparative Biochemistry and Physiology – C Toxicology and Pharmacology, 135*(3), 357–364. https://doi.org/10.1016/S1532-0456(03)00140-6 (accessed on 28th June 2025).

Wang, D., Özen, C., Abu-Reidah, I. M., Chigurupati, S., Patra, J. K., Horbanczuk, J. O., Jóźwik, A., Tzvetkov, N. T., Uhrin, P., & Atanasov, A. G. (2018). Vasculoprotective effects of pomegranate (*Punica granatum* L.). *Frontiers in Pharmacology, 9*(May), 1–15. https://doi.org/10.3389/fphar.2018.00544 (accessed on 28th June 2025).

Whiting, D. R., Guariguata, L., Weil, C., & Shaw, J. (2011). IDF Diabetes Atlas: Global estimates of the prevalence of diabetes for 2011 and 2030. *Diabetes Research and Clinical Practice, 94*(3), 311–321. https://doi.org/10.1016/j.diabres.2011.10.029 (accessed on 28th June 2025).

Widowati, W., Prahastuti, S., Tjokropranoto, R., Onggowidjaja, P., Kusuma, H. S. W., Afifah, E., Arumwardana, S., Maulana, M. A., & Rizal, R. (2022). Quercetin prevents chronic kidney disease on mesangial cells model by regulating inflammation, oxidative stress, and TGF-β1/SMADs pathway. *PeerJ, 10*, e13257. https://doi.org/10.7717/peerj.13257 (accessed on 28th June 2025).

Wu, C., Wang, J., Zhang, R., Zhao, H., Li, X., Wang, L., Liu, P., & Li, P. (2023). Research progress on *Cornus officinalis* and its active compounds in the treatment of diabetic nephropathy. *Frontiers in Pharmacology, 14*(July), 1–5. https://doi.org/10.3389/fphar.2023.1207777 (accessed on 28th June 2025).

Xiong, Y., & Zhou, L. (2019). The signaling of cellular senescence in diabetic nephropathy. *Oxidative Medicine and Cellular Longevity, 2019*, Article ID 7495629. https://doi.org/10.1155/2019/7495629 (accessed on 28th June 2025).

Xu, Q., Chen, G., Xu, H., Xia, G., Zhu, M., Zhan, H., Zhang, B., Dai, M., Fan, H., & Liu, X. (2021). Celastrol attenuates RANKL-induced osteoclastogenesis in vitro and reduces titanium particle-induced osteolysis and ovariectomy-induced bone loss in vivo. *Frontiers in Pharmacology, 12*(June), 1–13. https://doi.org/10.3389/fphar.2021.682541 (accessed on 28th June 2025).

Yang, B., & Liu, P. (2014). Composition and biological activities of hydrolyzable tannins of fruits of *Phyllanthus emblica. Journal of Agricultural and Food Chemistry, 62*(3), 529–541. https://doi.org/10.1021/jf404703k (accessed on 28th June 2025).

Yokozawa, T., Nakagawa, T., Oya, T., Okubo, T., & Juneja, L. R. (2010). Green tea polyphenols and dietary fibre protect against kidney damage in rats with diabetic nephropathy. *Journal of Pharmacy and Pharmacology, 57*(6), 773–780. https://doi.org/10.1211/0022357056154 (accessed on 28th June 2025).

Yousuf, M. J., & Vellaichamy, E. (2015). Protective activity of gallic acid against glyoxal-induced renal fibrosis in experimental rats. *Toxicology Reports, 2*, 1246–1254. https://doi.org/10.1016/j.toxrep.2015.07.007 (accessed on 28th June 2025).

Yuan, Y., Men, W., Shan, X., Zhai, H., Qiao, X., Geng, L., & Li, C. (2020). Baicalein exerts neuroprotective effect against ischaemic/reperfusion injury via alteration of NF-κB and

LOX and AMPK/Nrf2 pathway. *Inflammopharmacology, 28*(5), 1327–1341. https://doi.org/10.1007/s10787-020-00714-6 (accessed on 28th June 2025).

Zeng, S., & Li, Y. (2023). Research progress of autophagy in pathogenesis of diabetes nephropathy. *Diabetes & Metabolic Syndrome, 3*(May), 51–57. https://doi.org/10.1515/dine-2023-0006 (accessed on 28th June 2025).

Zhou, L. (2020). Luteolin attenuates diabetic nephropathy through suppressing inflammatory response and oxidative stress by inhibiting STAT3 pathway. *Exp Clin Endocrinol Diabetes, doi: 10.1055/a-0998-7985.*

CHAPTER 14

Nutritional Intervention in the Management of Metabolic Syndrome

UJJWAL KAUSHIK,[1,*] PARGAT SINGH,[1] RANIYA MALIK,[2,3] THAKUR GURJEET SINGH,[1] RAJWINDER KAUR,[1] RUPINDER KAUR,[1] SANJANA MEHTA,[1] and SHOWKAT R. MIR[4]

[1]*Chitkara College of Pharmacy, Chitkara University, Punjab, India*

[2]*Discipline of Pharmacy, Graduate School of Health, University of Technology Sydney, Sydney, New South Wales, Australia*

[3]*Faculty of Health, Australian Research Center in Complementary and Integrative Medicine, University of Technology Sydney, Ultimo, New South Wales, Australia*

[4]*School of Pharmaceutical Education and Research, Jamia Hamdard, New Delhi, India*

*Corresponding author

ABSTRACT

Due to the sedentary lifestyle and hectic work culture, metabolic syndrome has risen exponentially worldwide. Though the Western world (USA, Europe) is more affected by this syndrome, its prevalence has gained impetus in Southeast Asian countries as well. In addition to central obesity, insulin resistance, atherogenic dyslipidemia, hypertension, and other cardiovascular abnormalities, it is frequently recognized as a cluster of metabolic abnormalities. Restoring the body's equilibrium is greatly aided by proper food and nutrition. The chapter discusses nutritional

Precision Nutrition and Endocrine Health: Synthesis, Characterization, and Applications.
Thakur Gurjeet Singh and Sanjana Mehta (Eds.)

DOI: 10.1201/9781998511877-14

interventions, such as dietary patterns and herbal remedies for managing metabolic syndrome.

14.1 INTRODUCTION

A collection of metabolic disorders known as metabolic syndrome comprises hypertension, atherogenic dyslipidemia, insulin resistance, central obesity, and other anomalies related to the cardiovascular system (Devi et al., 2024; Garg et al., 2022; Mehta et al., 2021). Reaven's syndrome, insulin resistance syndrome, dysmetabolic syndrome X, syndrome X, multiple metabolic syndrome, and metabolic cardiovascular syndrome are other names for metabolic syndrome (Khosravi et al., 2013; Silveira Rossi et al., 2022). It is associated with an increased risk of atherosclerotic cardiovascular diseases. Five diagnostic criteria have been established by the Adult Treatment Panel-III (ATPIII). Any three of these symptoms—dyslipidemia, hypertension, impaired fasting glucose (FG) and central obesity—are considered sufficient to diagnose the condition, as shown in Figure 14.1 (Devaraj et al., 2009; Sharma et al., 2020).

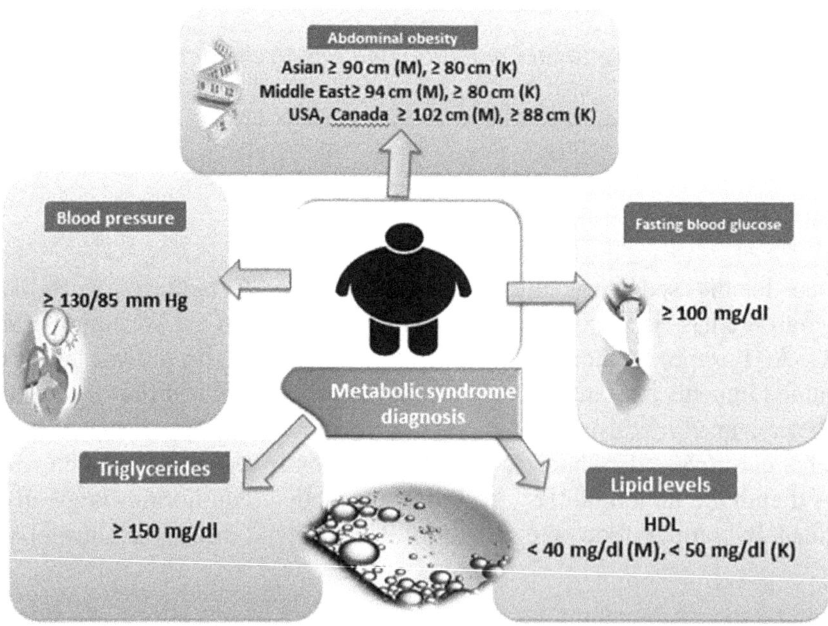

FIGURE 14.1 Diagnostic criteria for Metabolic syndrome established by the adult treatment panel-III (M = men; K = Women).

Depending on the geography, urban/rural settings, and the demographics of the research population, the prevalence of metabolic syndrome (MetS) varies from less than 10% to 80%. All Western civilizations have high rates of MetS prevalence, independent of any criterion, which is believed to be caused by central obesity (Noubiap et al., 2022).

14.2 DIETARY INTERVENTION IN THE MANAGEMENT OF METABOLIC SYNDROME

Different dietary patterns have been followed in vivid regions of the globe to combat metabolic syndrome and its related consequences. Distinct dietary patterns with their multifocal targets have been demonstrated to control the symptoms of metabolic syndrome, as shown in Figure 14.2.

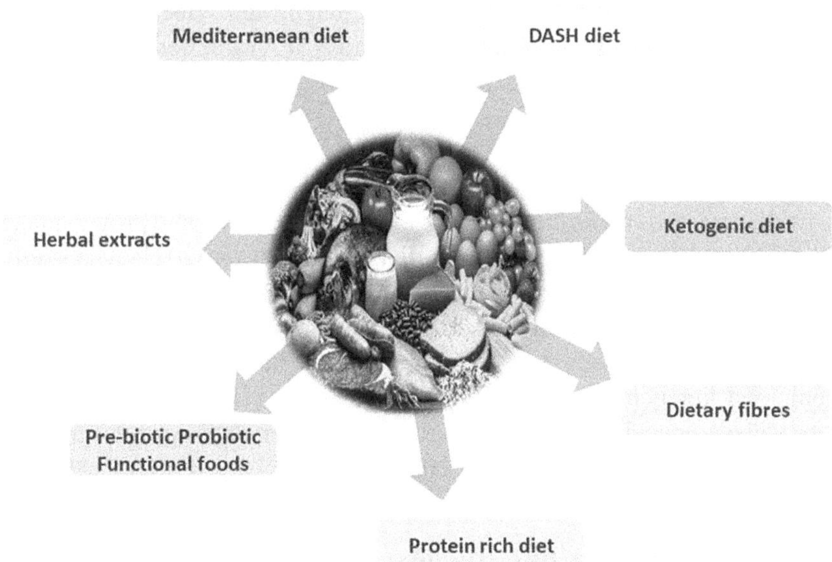

FIGURE 14.2 Different dietary patterns recommended for metabolic syndrome.

14.2.1 MEDITERRANEAN DIET

Based on the Seven Countries Study, the Mediterranean diet (MedDiet) concept was conceived in the 1950s, highlighting the positive associations of Mediterranean food patterns with low chronic illness rates (Guasch-Ferre, 2021; Toshima et al., 2012). The MedDiet is a plant-based diet with a high nut intake, olive oil, and moderate wine consumption, particularly red wine, distinguishing it from other healthy diets. Extra-virgin olive oil and nuts, as specific MedDiet components, offer numerous health benefits. Low rates of MetS incidence are linked to increased biomarkers in Mediterranean diet foods, specifically oleic and -linolenic acids.

14.2.2 DIETARY APPROACH TO STOP HYPERTENSION (DASH) DIET

In the 1990s, this diet plan was created for the DASH experiment, a randomized controlled study in which over 400 people were randomly assigned to follow the DASH diet, an "American" diet high in fruits and vegetables, or the control diet (Harrison et al., 2020). The modern-day DASH diet encourages the consumption of fruits, vegetables, whole grains, legumes, fish, poultry, and nuts. It also recommends avoiding trans fats, high amounts of potassium, calcium, magnesium, fiber, and protein, and limiting sodium and saturated fatty acids (SFA) and trans fats (Appel, 1997; National et al., 2020).

14.2.3 KETOGENIC DIET

Low dietary carbs combined with variable amounts of fat and protein make up the foundation of the ketogenic diet (Kumar et al., 2021; McGaugh, 2022). Insulin has been shown to impede lipolysis, and reduced insulin in low-carb diets is thought to enhance the breakdown of fat. When a deliberate carbohydrate reduction is consumed, the body uses the gluconeogenic and ketogenic metabolic pathways. Because ketone bodies create more adenosine triphosphate than glucose, this "metabolic shift" may be advantageous (Di Raimond et al., 2021).

14.2.4 ROLE OF DIETARY FIBERS

By modifying the makeup and function of the gut microbiota, various forms of dietary fiber can differently affect how fat and glucose are metabolized (Cronin et al., 2021). Because soluble fiber increases the viscosity of luminal contents, it positively affects the metabolism of fats and carbohydrates. Due to their gelling qualities, soluble dietary fibers such as guar gum and psyllium are linked to decreased postprandial glucose levels and enhanced insulin sensitivity (Papathanasopoulos and Camilleri et al., 2010).

14.2.5 PROTEIN-RICH DIET

Consuming protein is linked to several benefits that may help manage metabolic syndrome, including a decreased loss of lean tissue, a lower glycemic, improved satiety, a slower rate of stomach emptying, and enhanced insulin secretion (Jamshidi et al., 2022). Enzymatic hydrolysis is a commonly employed technique for generating bioactive peptides from dietary proteins. These multifunctional hydrolysates show promising effects in preventing or treating multifactorial disorders such as metabolic syndrome (Garcés-Rimón et al., 2022). Through the protective fibroblast growth factor, plant proteins with lower methionine and branched-chain amino acid content, in contrast to animal proteins, have been shown to avert the development of insulin resistance and metabolic syndrome in animal studies (Markova et al., 2017).

14.2.6 PRE-BIOTIC AND PROBIOTIC FUNCTIONAL FOODS IN THE MANAGEMENT OF METABOLIC SYNDROME

Prebiotic supplementation boosts gut microorganisms' proliferation and raises dietary fiber levels. Prebiotics also actively improve the surrounding food matrix's physiochemical characteristics, which permits a decrease in fat, sugar, and energy content without compromising the flavor or texture of the final product (Gupta et al., 2021). Prebiotics are highly effective in reorganizing and stabilizing the host microbiome and addressing several pathogenic pathways linked to the onset and metabolic effects of obesity (Green et al., 2020).

14.3 ROLE OF HERBS IN TREATMENT OF METABOLIC SYNDROME

Studies have depicted the effectiveness of herbal medicines in metabolic syndrome-associated complications. With few to no adverse effects, medicinal plants and their extracts are beneficial in treating patients with metabolic syndrome (Arozal et al., 2020; Garg et al., 2021; Kaur et al., 2023). The naturally occurring aporphine alkaloids have shown protective effects on the risks characterizing metabolic syndrome (Wang et al., 2021). Table 14.1 below provides the study insights of a few frequently used medicinal herbs in underdeveloped nations that have been researched and proven to have some effects on metabolic syndrome.

TABLE 14.1 Herbal Extracts Have Beneficial Effects in Managing Symptoms of Metabolic Syndrome

Sr. No.	Name	Model/Study Design	Dose/Duration	Outcome	References
1.	*Green tea (Camellia sinensi)s*	Healthy participants n–16 Rats fed high cholesterol and high sucrose diet	300, 400, 870, 928, 1,000, and 6,000 milligrams of green tea each day 150, 300, 458, 468, 886, and 1,200 mg/day of catechins for a period of 8 to 12 weeks functional beverages containing catechins and EGCG for 56 days	Both body weight and BMI were reduced. Notable decrease in hip and waist circumference Notable reductions in LDL and cholesterol. Decrease of LDL and cholesterol Decrease in BW, Attenuation of insulin and blood glucose levels	Vieira Senger et al. (2012) Ahmad et al. (2015)
2.	*White tea*	streptozotocin-induced diabetic rats n-32 Rats were administered an HFD. STZ inducted diabetic rats	1.5% aqueous extract of white tea for 30 days For six weeks, white tea 400 or 800 mg/kg of polyphenol and polysaccharide Catechin was administered for 28 days at 2550 mg/kg and 50 mg/kg doses.	Low blood levels of glucose, LDL, cholesterol, and triglycerides but higher levels of HDL in contrast to the control group. Suppressed weight gain and fat storage in the body. Additionally, polyphenols and polysaccharides enhanced blood lipid and antioxidant levels, decreased serum leptin levels, and decreased *TNF-α* and *IL-6* gene expression levels. Shown a dual impact of lowering serum leptin levels and anti-inflammatory action. Decreased body weight and decreased MMP-9 levels, plasma glucose levels, and cardiac hypertrophy. Enhanced measures of oxidative stress in the nerves	Amanzadeh et al. (2020) Xu et al. (2015) Addepalli et al. (2018)
3.	*Phaseolus vulgaris*	Healthy participants n–3 Male mice given HFD, n–6	445, 1,000, and 3,000 mg/day for 4–12 weeks *P. vulgaris* extract at a dose level of 500 mg/kg daily for 19 weeks	Notable reduction in BMI and body weight. There is a noticeable decrease in hip and waist diameter and reductions in LDL and cholesterol. Decreased levels of total cholesterol	Udani Spadafranca et al. (2018) Micheli et al. (2019)
4.	*Garcinia cambogia*	overweight/obese patients randomised controlled trials. obese women n–30	*G. cambogia* (500 mg), twice a day for six months 2.4 g (800 mg 3×/day) of garcinia extract For two months	Glucose, triglycerides and cholesterol levels are reduced. TG was significantly reduced.	Maia-Landim et al. (2021) Vasques et al. (2014)

TABLE 14.1 *(Continued)*

Sr. No.	Name	Model/Study Design	Dose/Duration	Outcome	References
5.	*Nigella sativa*	Double-masked placebo-controlled randomised clinical trial in women with obesity n–84 healthy volunteer n–70 Metabolic syndrome n-80 Mice n-50 Obese and overweight women Patients with metabolic syndrome n–99	For eight weeks at 3 g each day. Take 2.5 mL of N. Sativa oil twice a day for eight weeks. 0.5 g of powder daily for eight weeks For 30 days, provide 200 and 300 mg/kg of *N. sativa* hydrochloric and hexane extract. *N. sativa* 1,000 mg/day capsules for eight weeks Oral black seed oil (1.5 and 3 millilitres each day) for 20 days	Tumor necrosis factor-alpha and high-sensitivity C-reactive protein were shown to be reduced in blood levels by *N. Sativa* oil. Notable blood pressure control without any negative consequences Considerable control over HbA1c, PPBG, and FPG raised HDL, decreased TG, LDL, and cholesterol, and improved UCP-1 Decreased TNF-α, adiponectin, and PPAR-γ expression in obese women Lower levels of HbA1c	Chakraborty et al. (2023) Alizadeh et al. (2018) Mahmoudi et al. (2018) Razmpoosh et al., (2019)
6.	*Puerh Tea*	The Male patients (*N*=70)	For 12 weeks, use 1000 mg of puerh tea extract capsules daily	Notable decrease in BMI and body weight. There was a significant decrease in waist diameter but no change in hip circumference , with notable reductions in LDL and cholesterol.	Yang et al. (2014)
7.	*Irvingia gabonensis*	Healthy, overweight and obese volunteer n-102 A clinical study using randomisation, double blinding, and placebo control for patients with metabolic syndrome, n = 24	150, 300, 3150 mg/day for 4–10 weeks 150 mg twice daily for 90 days	Substantial loss of body weight. And a discernible reduction in waist circumference. Notable reductions in LDL and cholesterol. It significantly decreased waist diameter, glucose levels, triglycerides and VLDL.	Ngondi et al. (2009) Méndez-del Villar et al. (2014)
8.	*Caralluma Fimbriata*	A double-blind, randomised clinical study including 43 adults Overweight and obese individuals n-89	For 8 to 12 weeks, 1000 mg daily was administered. For 12 weeks, we administered 500 mg twice a day.	A significant drop in body weight without a corresponding reduction in BMI. No discernible variations were found.	Astell et al. (2013) Arora et al. (2015)

TABLE 14.1 *(Continued)*

Sr. No.	Name	Model/Study Design	Dose/Duration	Outcome	References
9.	*Hibiscus Sabdariffa*	Salt-induced hypertensive rats Male volunteers n–32 Adult patients with Metabolic syndrome, n-40	Aqueous extract at doses of 100, 200, and 400 mg/kg, once daily for six weeks For 14 days, extract 1000 mg/day. We administered 500 mg of H. sabdariffa calyx powder daily or a placebo for four weeks. For 4–6 weeks, administered 75, 500, or 1000 mg daily	decreased HR, diastolic, mean arterial and systolic pressure. Serum levels of TC, LDL, and VLDL were also significantly lowered. There is a notable drop in TC, LDL, and HDL values in the blood. Markedly lower serum TG and SBP Notable BMI and body weight decrease, decreased waist diameter, and reduced LDL and cholesterol.	Balogun et al. (2019) Tazoho et al. (2016) Asgary et al., (2016)
10.	*Curcuma longa*	Overweight individuals affected by MetS n–44 Healthy males positive for MetS n = 250 Individuals with MetS. n–120 Men with MetS n-10	The animal was treated for 30 days with 800 mg/dose of a mixture of sunflower phospholipids and Curcuma longa extract, then combined with piperine from a Piper nigrum extract at a dose level of 8 mg. 2.4 grams of turmeric every day for eight weeks. Phospholipidated curcumin (PC) and unformulated curcumin (UC) capsules (1 g/day) for six weeks Curcumin supplement 20 mg/kg for eight weeks	Notable decrease in BMI and body weight Notable decrease in hip diameter, waist circumference, and body fat Following four weeks of improvement in BMI, waist diameter, and Body fat percentage, all metrics except HDL cholesterol showed improvement, with lower FBG and LDL cholesterol levels. Following eight weeks, turmeric lowered CRP and LDL cholesterol. Enhanced every aspect. Reduction in severe anxiety post-treatment with PC and UC Notable decrease in BMI and body weight. Notable decrease in hip and waist Diameter Notable reductions in LDL and cholesterol.	Di Pierro et al., 2015 Amin et al. (2015); Saberi-Karimian et al. (2018) Salimi Avansar (2017)
11.	*Allium sativum*	Metabolic syndrome patients n-40 Male Sprague-Dawley rats n-32 Hyperlipidemic patients n-112	Raw, crushed garlic was given twice daily for four weeks at a 100 mg/kg dose based on body weight. Five weeks of using 0.5% or 1.5% black garlic extract Daily garlic plus one tablespoon (20 g) of lemon juice for eight weeks	Substantial rise in serum HDL cholesterol and significantly decreased FBG, triglycerides, systolic and diastolic blood pressure, and waist diameter. Decreased metabolism of fat and cholesterol. Reduced TG, cholesterol, and total lipid levels. Reductions in LDL and total cholesterol. Decreased blood pressure, both diastole and systole	Choudhary et al. (2018) Ha et al. (2015) Aslani et al. (2016).

TABLE 14.1 *(Continued)*

Sr. No.	Name	Model/Study Design	Dose/Duration	Outcome	References
12.	*Cinnamomum verum*	A double-blind, placebo-controlled, randomised study including 130 participants with T2DM Individuals with metabolic syndrome (n = 116) in a double-blind randomised control experiment	For 90 days, 3 g of cinnamon per day 3 g cinnamon for 16 weeks	Reduction in glycemic levels (HbA1c and fasting venous glucose) Lowering of total cholesterol, triglycerides, and LDL cholesterol levels. Raised the amount of HDL cholesterol. Reduction in BMI, central adiposity index, waist, thigh, neck and hip diameter and weight, among other anthropometric parameters. Significantly more significant decreases in FBG, glycosylated hemoglobin, waist circumference, and BMI Numerous additional parameters, such as the waist-to-hip ratio, blood pressure, serum total cholesterol, serum triglycerides, LDL cholesterol, and HDL cholesterol, showed a discernible decline.	Neto et al. (2020) Gupta et al. (2017)
13.	*Berberis vulgaris*	*In vivo*, rats *In vivo*, in-vitro models n-60 *In vivo*, hypertensive rats n-48 DM type 2-induced mice *In vivo*, high-fat diet rats n-48 Diabetes hamsters produced by a high-fat and high-glucose diet *in vivo* Grade 1 essential hypertension and HCh patients in humans, n-66 HFD-induced female mice	300 mg/kg IP of *B. vulgaris* extracts for 21 days BBR at dose levels 50, 100, and 150 mg/kg intraperitoneally for eight weeks BBR (100 mg/kg/d) Two weeks of berberine (100 mg/kg/d). *B. vulgaris* extract (p.o. for six weeks; 0.2 g/Kg) BBR (injection for six weeks; 50 and 100 mg/kg) BBR (500 mg) orally every day for six months) BBR for 12 weeks at 160 mg/kg/d	Lipid levels were decreased, including triglycerides, LDL cholesterol, and total cholesterol. Raised the amount of HDL cholesterol. Decreased levels of serum cholesterol and the rate of dietary cholesterol absorption Decrease in the absorption of cholesterol and *acyl-coenzyme* gene and protein acyltransferase-2 expression for cholesterol. Reduction of aldosterone, angiotensin II, IL6, IL17, and IL23 in addition to SBP. Decrease in FBG and MDA Elevation in SOD and CAT activity. Decrease in body mass, serum insulin levels, and glucose levels. Reduction of insulin, glucose, TBARS, free fatty acid, LDL-C, MDA, and body weight Elevation of mRNA and plasma superoxide dismutase activity Decreases in TG, LDL-C, PP, TC, and SBP Notably, decreased systolic cardiac function elevated pancreatic islets' glucose-stimulated insulin release and significantly decreased body weight.	Changizi Ashtiyani et al. (2013) Wang et al. (2014) Guo et al. (2015) Chatuphonprasert et al. (2014) El-Sayed et al., 2013 Liu et al., 2015 Mazza et al., (2015) Cole et al. (2021)

TABLE 14.1 *(Continued)*

Sr. No.	Name	Model/Study Design	Dose/Duration	Outcome	References
14.	*Lagenaria siceraria*	Healthy volunteer n–50 Obese individuals n-32	200 ml juice for 90 days 200 ml of fresh fruit juice for 45 days	Reduction in levels of total cholesterol, TG, LDL Significant change in weight, waist diameter, and body mass index observed	Katare et al., (2013) Vaibhav et al., (2016)
15.	*Trigonella foenum-graecum*	Male Wistar rats fed with a diet heavy in fat and sugar (n-60) alloxan-induced type-II diabetic rat model streptozotocin-induced diabetes rats Overweight (OW) and type 2 DM subjects n-40 ovariectomised rats n-49 high fructose-fed in rats with insulin resistance Type II diabetic patients n-114	2g/kg bw/day fenugreek seed flour for six weeks Fenugreek seeds hydroalcoholic extract for 30 days at dose levels of 500, 1000, and 1000 mg/kg Diosgenin for 45 days at doses of 15, 30, and 60 mg/kg body weight For 12 weeks, 5.45 g (6 days per week) of a fenugreek/*N. sativa* combination *T. foenum-graecum* seeds were extracted hexanic and ethanolic at dosage levels of 50 and 150 mg/kg for 42 days For eight weeks, TFG extract (1000 mg/kg/day) For one month, take 25 g of powder solution twice a day.	Reduction in glutathione reductase activity and plasma glutathione levels Increased body weight and glucose absorption, decreased levels of pancreatic enzymes, hepatic glucose transport, plasma glucose, glycosylated hemoglobin (HbA1c), and depleted muscle and liver glycogen were all recovered. the substantial rise in plasma insulin level and a considerable decrease in blood glucose level Triglycerides (TG), very low-density lipoprotein (VLDL), high-density lipoprotein (HDL) cholesterol, and total cholesterol (TC) were all reduced. CRS, fatty liver index, lipid accumulation product, and HSI all improved. A significant decrease in these cytokines in the serum resulted in a rise in glucose and body weight—a significant reduction in lipids, insulin, and adiponectin. Moreover, the expression of the *PPARγ* gene was enhanced. notably reduced levels of triglycerides, low-density lipoprotein cholesterol, and total cholesterol Notably, increased amount of HDL cholesterol	Szabó et al. (2018) Joshi et al. (2015) Saravanan et al. (2014) Rao et al. (2020) Abedinzade et al. (2015) Mohammadi et al. (2016) Geberemeskel et al. (2019)

BMI: Body mass index, LDL: Low density lipoproteins; HD: High density lipoproteins; BW: Body weight; HFD: High fat diet; TNF: Tissue necrosis factor; IL: Interleukin; MMP: metallopeptidase; STZ: Streptozotocin; TG: Triglycerides; HbA1c: Hemoglobin A1c; PPBG: Postparandial blood glucose; FPG: Fasting plasma glucose; UCP-1: Uncoupling protein-1; PPAR-γ: Peroxisome proliferator-activated receptor gamma; VLDL: Very low density Lipoproteins; HR: Heart rate; CRP: C-reactive protein; TC:Total cholesterol.

14.4 CONCLUSION

There has been ample evidence that a healthy dietary pattern has been associated with a decreased risk of metabolic ailments and helps prevent debilitating symptoms of metabolic syndrome. A rich diet of fruits, grains (whole), proteins, omega fatty acids, and dietary fibers helps prevent many metabolic-related health problems. Because a good diet positively impacts blood pressure, cholesterol, insulin resistance, and inflammatory processes, it can even eliminate or reverse metabolic syndrome.

KEYWORDS

- **hypertension**
- **insulin resistance**
- **keto diet**
- **Mediterranean diet**
- **metabolic syndrome**
- **obesity**

REFERENCES

Abedinzade, M., Nasri, S., Jamal Omodi, M., Ghasemi, E., & Ghorbani, A. (2015). Efficacy of *Trigonella foenum-graecum* seed extract in reducing metabolic and inflammatory alterations associated with menopause. *Iranian Red Crescent Medical Journal, 17*(11), e26685. https://doi.org/10.5812/ircmj.26685 (accessed on 28th June 2025).

Addepalli, V., & Suryavanshi, S. V. (2018). Catechin attenuates diabetic autonomic neuropathy in streptozotocin-induced diabetic rats. *Biomedicine & Pharmacotherapy, 108*, 1517–1523. https://doi.org/10.1016/j.biopha.2018.09.179 (accessed on 28th June 2025).

Ahmad, R. S., Butt, M. S., Sultan, M. T., Mushtaq, Z., Ahmad, S., Dewanjee, S., De Feo, V., & Zia-Ul-Haq, M. (2015). Preventive role of green tea catechins from obesity and related disorders especially hypercholesterolemia and hyperglycemia. *Journal of Translational Medicine, 13*, 79. https://doi.org/10.1186/s12967-015-0436-x (accessed on 28th June 2025).

Alizadeh, M., Namazi, N., Mirtaheri, E., Sargheini, N., & Kheirouri, S. (2018). Changes of insulin resistance and adipokines following supplementation with *Glycyrrhiza glabra*

L. extract in combination with a low-calorie diet in overweight and obese subjects: A randomized double blind clinical trial. *Advanced Pharmaceutical Bulletin, 8*(1), 123–130. https://doi.org/10.15171/apb.2018.015 (accessed on 28th June 2025).

Amanzadeh, Z., Zargari, F., & Khalilaria, A. (2020). The effect of aqueous extract of white tea on amount of glucose and lipid profile in diabetic rats. *Experimental Animal Biology, 8*(4), 123–130.

Amin, F., Islam, N., Anila, N., & Gilani, A. H. (2015). Clinical efficacy of the co-administration of turmeric and black seeds (Kalongi) in metabolic syndrome – a double blind randomized controlled trial – TAK-MetS trial. *Complementary Therapies in Medicine, 23*(2), 165–174. https://doi.org/10.1016/j.ctim.2015.01.008 (accessed on 28th June 2025).

Appel, L. J., Moore, T. J., Obarzanek, E., Vollmer, W. M., Svetkey, L. P., Sacks, F. M., Bray, G. A., Vogt, T. M., Cutler, J. A., Windhauser, M. M., Lin, P. H., & Karanja, N. (1997). A clinical trial of the effects of dietary patterns on blood pressure. DASH Collaborative Research Group. *The New England Journal of Medicine, 336*(16), 1117–1124. https://doi.org/10.1056/NEJM199704173361601 (accessed on 28th June 2025).

Arora, E., Khajuria, V., Tandon, V. R., Sharma, A., Mahajan, A., Gillani, Z. H., & Choudhary, N. (2015). To evaluate efficacy and safety of *Caralluma fimbriata* in overweight and obese patients: A randomized, single blinded, placebo control trial. *Perspectives in Clinical Research, 6*(1), 39–44. https://doi.org/10.4103/2229-3485.148812 (accessed on 28th June 2025).

Asgary, S., Soltani, R., Zolghadr, M., Keshvari, M., & Sarrafzadegan, N. (2016). Evaluation of the effects of roselle (*Hibiscus sabdariffa* L.) on oxidative stress and serum levels of lipids, insulin and hs-CRP in adult patients with metabolic syndrome: A double-blind placebo-controlled clinical trial. *Journal of Complementary & Integrative Medicine, 13*(2), 175–180. https://doi.org/10.1515/jcim-2015-0030 (accessed on 28th June 2025).

Aslani, N., Entezari, M. H., Askari, G., Maghsoudi, Z., & Maracy, M. R. (2016). Effect of garlic and lemon juice mixture on lipid profile and some cardiovascular risk factors in people 30–60 years old with moderate hyperlipidaemia: A randomized clinical trial. *International Journal of Preventive Medicine, 7*, 95. https://doi.org/10.4103/2008-7802.187248 (accessed on 28th June 2025).

Astell, K. J., Mathai, M. L., McAinch, A. J., Stathis, C. G., & Su, X. Q. (2013). A pilot study investigating the effect of *Caralluma fimbriata* extract on the risk factors of metabolic syndrome in overweight and obese subjects: A randomised controlled clinical trial. *Complementary Therapies in Medicine, 21*(3), 180–189. https://doi.org/10.1016/j.ctim.2013.01.004 (accessed on 28th June 2025).

Balogun, M. E., Besong, E. E., Obimma, J. N., Iyare, E. E., & Nwachukwu, D. C. (2019). Ameliorative effect of aqueous *Hibiscus sabdariffa* extract (roselle) on salt-induced hypertension in Wistar rats. *Pharmacologyonline, 2*, 247–258.

Chakraborty, S., Bogadi, S., Pamu, D., Karri, V. V. S. R., Booker, A., Rolfe, V., & Mohankumar, S. (2023). Role of herbs at the crossroads of metabolic syndrome and mental illness. *Indian Journal of Biochemistry and Biophysics (IJBB), 60*(2), 129–140. https://doi.org/10.56042/ijbb.v60i2.70738 (accessed on 28th June 2025).

Changizi, A. S., Zarei, A., Taheri, S., Rezaei, A., Golshan, M., & Ghafarzadegan, R. (2013). A comparative study of hypolipidemic activities of the extracts of *Melissa officinalis* and *Berberis vulgaris* in rats. *(Journal details not provided).*

Chatuphonprasert, W., Lao-Ong, T., & Jarukamjorn, K. (2013). Improvement of superoxide dismutase and catalase in streptozotocin-nicotinamide-induced type 2 diabetes in mice by berberine and glibenclamide. *Pharmaceutical Biology*. Advance online publication. https://doi.org/10.3109/13880209.2013.839714 (accessed on 28th June 2025).

Choudhary, P. R., Jani, R. D., & Sharma, M. S. (2018). Effect of raw crushed garlic (*Allium* et al.) on components of metabolic syndrome. *Journal of Dietary Supplements, 15*(4), 499–506. https://doi.org/10.1080/19390211.2017.1358233 (accessed on 28th June 2025).

Cole, L. K., Zhang, M., Chen, L., Sparagna, G. C., Vandel, M., Xiang, B., Dolinsky, V. W., & Hatch, G. M. (2021). Supplemental berberine in a high-fat diet reduces adiposity and cardiac dysfunction in offspring of mouse dams with gestational diabetes mellitus. *The Journal of Nutrition, 151*(4), 892–901. https://doi.org/10.1093/jn/nxaa408 (accessed on 28th June 2025).

Cronin, P., Joyce, S. A., O'Toole, P. W., & O'Connor, E. M. (2021). Dietary fibre modulates the gut microbiota. *Nutrients, 13*(5), 1655. https://doi.org/10.3390/nu13051655 (accessed on 28th June 2025).

Devaraj, S., Singh, U., & Jialal, I. (2009). Human C-reactive protein and the metabolic syndrome. *Current Opinion in Lipidology, 20*(3), 182–189. https://doi.org/10.1097/MOL.0b013e32832ac03e (accessed on 28th June 2025).

Devi, S., Chauhan, S., Mannan, A., & Singh, T. G. (2024). Targeting cardiovascular risk factors with eugenol: An anti-inflammatory perspective. *Inflammopharmacology, 32*(1), 307–317. https://doi.org/10.1007/s10787-023-01392-w (accessed on 28th June 2025).

Di Pierro, F., Bressan, A., Ranaldi, D., Rapacioli, G., Giacomelli, L., & Bertuccioli, A. (2015). Potential role of bioavailable curcumin in weight loss and omental adipose tissue decrease: Preliminary data of a randomised, controlled trial in overweight people with metabolic syndrome. *European Review for Medical and Pharmacological Sciences, 19*(21), 4195–4202.

Di Raimondo, D., Buscemi, S., Musiari, G., Rizzo, G., Pirera, E., Corleo, D., Pinto, A., & Tuttolomondo, A. (2021). Ketogenic diet, physical activity, and hypertension—a narrative review. *Nutrients, 13*(8), 2567. https://doi.org/10.3390/nu13082567 (accessed on 28th June 2025).

El-Sayed, M. M., Ghareeb, D. A., Talat, H. A., & Sarhan, E. M. (2013). High-fat diet-induced insulin resistance and elevated retinol-binding protein 4 in female rats; treatment and protection with *Berberis vulgaris* extract and vitamin A. *Pakistan Journal of Pharmaceutical Sciences, 26*(6), 1189–1195.

Garcés-Rimón, M., Morales, D., & Miguel-Castro, M. (2022). Potential role of bioactive proteins and peptides derived from legumes towards metabolic syndrome. *Nutrients, 14*(24), 5271. https://doi.org/10.3390/nu14245271 (accessed on 28th June 2025).

Garg, C., Khan, H., Kaur, A., Singh, T. G., Sharma, V. K., & Singh, S. K. (2022). Therapeutic implications of sonic hedgehog pathway in metabolic disorders: Novel target for effective treatment. *Pharmacological Research, 179*, 106194. https://doi.org/10.1016/j.phrs.2022.106194 (accessed on 28th June 2025).

Garg, N., Singh, T. G., Khan, H., Arora, S., Kaur, A., & Mannan, A. (2021). Mechanistic interventions of selected *Ocimum* species in management of diabetes, obesity and liver disorders: Transformative developments from preclinical to clinical approaches. *Biointerface Research in Applied Chemistry, 12*(1), 1304–1323.

Geberemeskel, G. A., Debebe, Y. G., & Nguse, N. A. (2019). Antidiabetic effect of fenugreek seed powder solution (*Trigonella foenum-graecum* L.) on hyperlipidemia in diabetic patients. *Journal of Diabetes Research, 2019*, 8507453. https://doi.org/10.1155/2019/8507453 (accessed on 28th June 2025).

Green, M., Arora, K., & Prakash, S. (2020). Microbial medicine: Prebiotic and probiotic functional foods to target obesity and metabolic syndrome. *International Journal of Molecular Sciences, 21*(8), 2890. https://doi.org/10.3390/ijms21082890 (accessed on 28th June 2025).

Guasch-Ferré, M., & Willett, W. C. (2021). The Mediterranean diet and health: A comprehensive overview. *Journal of Internal Medicine, 290*(3), 549–566. https://doi.org/10.1111/joim.13333 (accessed on 28th June 2025).

Guo, Z., Sun, H., Zhang, H., & Zhang, Y. (2015). Anti-hypertensive and renoprotective effects of berberine in spontaneously hypertensive rats. *Clinical and Experimental Hypertension, 37*(4), 332–339. https://doi.org/10.3109/10641963.2014.972560 (accessed on 28th June 2025).

Gupta Jain, S., Puri, S., Misra, A., Gulati, S., & Mani, K. (2017). Effect of oral cinnamon intervention on metabolic profile and body composition of Asian Indians with metabolic syndrome: A randomised double-blind control trial. *Lipids in Health and Disease, 16*(1), 113. https://doi.org/10.1186/s12944-017-0504-8 (accessed on 28th June 2025).

Gupta, M., Krishan, P., Kaur, A., Arora, S., Trehanpati, N., Singh, T. G., & Bedi, O. (2021). Mechanistic and physiological approaches of fecal microbiota transplantation in the management of NAFLD. *Inflammation Research, 70*(7), 765–776. https://doi.org/10.1007/s00011-021-01480-z (accessed on 28th June 2025).

Ha, A. W., Ying, T., & Kim, W. K. (2015). The effects of black garlic (*Allium sativum*) extracts on lipid metabolism in rats fed a high-fat diet. *Nutrition Research and Practice, 9*(1), 30–36. https://doi.org/10.4162/nrp.2015.9.1.30 (accessed on 28th June 2025).

Harrison, S., Couture, P., & Lamarche, B. (2020). Diet quality, saturated fat and metabolic syndrome. *Nutrients, 12*(11), 3232. https://doi.org/10.3390/nu12113232 (accessed on 28th June 2025).

Jamshidi, A., Farjam, M., Ekramzadeh, M., & Homayounfar, R. (2022). Evaluating type and amount of dietary protein in relation to metabolic syndrome among Iranian adults: Cross-sectional analysis of Fasa Persian cohort study. *Diabetology & Metabolic Syndrome, 14*(1), 42. https://doi.org/10.1186/s13098-022-00813-0 (accessed on 28th June 2025).

Jean Jacques Noubiap, Nansseu, J. R., Lontchi-Yimagou, E., Nkeck, J. R., Nyaga, U. F., Ngouo, A. T., Tounouga, D. N., Tianyi, F. L., Foka, A. J., Ndoadoumgue, A. L., & Bigna, J. J. (2022). Geographic distribution of metabolic syndrome and its components in the general adult population: A meta-analysis of global data from 28 million individuals. *Diabetes Research and Clinical Practice, 188*, 109924. https://doi.org/10.1016/j.diabres.2022.109924 (accessed on 28th June 2025).

Joshi, D. V., Patil, R. R., & Naik, S. R. (2015). Hydroalcoholic extract of *Trigonella foenum-graecum* seed attenuates inflammation and oxidative stress markers while improving exocrine function in diabetic rats. *Pharmaceutical Biology, 53*(2), 201–211. https://doi.org/10.3109/13880209.2014.913296 (accessed on 28th June 2025).

Katare, C., Saxena, S., Agrawal, S., & Prasad, G. B. K. S. (2013). Alleviation of diabetes-induced dyslipidemia by *Lagenaria siceraria* fruit extract in human type 2 diabetes.

Journal of Herbal Medicine, 3(1), 1–8. https://doi.org/10.1016/j.hermed.2012.11.002 (accessed on 28th June 2025).

Kaur, N., Kishore, L., Farooq, S. A., Kajal, A., Singh, R., Agrawal, R., ... & Singh, T. G. (2023). *Cucurbita pepo* seeds improve peripheral neuropathy in diabetic rats by modulating the inflammation and oxidative stress in rats. *Environmental Science and Pollution Research, 30*(36), 85910–85919. https://doi.org/10.1007/s11356-023-28339-6 (accessed on 28th June 2025).

Khosravi, R., Ka, K., Huang, T., Khalili, S., Nguyen, B. H., Nicolau, B., & Tran, S. D. (2013). Tumour necrosis factor-α and interleukin-6: Potential interorgan inflammatory mediators contributing to destructive periodontal disease in obesity or metabolic syndrome. *Mediators of Inflammation, 2013*, 728987. https://doi.org/10.1155/2013/728987 (accessed on 28th June 2025).

Kumar, S., Behl, T., Sachdeva, M., Sehgal, A., Kumari, S., Kumar, A., Kaur, G., Yadav, H. N., & Bungau, S. (2021). Implicating the effect of ketogenic diet as a preventive measure to obesity and diabetes mellitus. *Life Sciences, 264*, 118661. https://doi.org/10.1016/j.lfs.2020.118661 (accessed on 28th June 2025).

Liu, C., Wang, Z., Song, Y., Wu, D., Zheng, X., Li, P., Jin, J., Xu, N., & Li, L. (2015). Effects of berberine on ameliorating hyperglycemia and oxidative stress in high glucose and high fat diet-induced diabetic hamsters in vivo. *BioMed Research International, 2015*, 313808. https://doi.org/10.1155/2015/313808 (accessed on 28th June 2025).

Mahmoudi, A., Ghatreh Samani, K., Farrokhi, E., & Heidarian, E. (2018). Effects of *Nigella sativa* extracts on the lipid profile and uncoupling protein-1 gene expression in brown adipose tissue of mice. *Advanced Biomedical Research, 7*, 121. https://doi.org/10.4103/abr.abr_91_18 (accessed on 28th June 2025).

Maia-Landim, A., Lancho, C., Poblador, M. S., Lancho, J. L., & Ramírez, J. M. (2021). *Garcinia cambogia* and glucomannan reduce weight, change body composition, and ameliorate lipid and glucose blood profiles in overweight/obese patients. *Journal of Herbal Medicine, 26*, 100424. https://doi.org/10.1016/j.hermed.2021.100424 (accessed on 28th June 2025).

Markova, M., Pivovarova, O., Hornemann, S., Sucher, S., Frahnow, T., Wegner, K., Machann, J., Petzke, K. J., Hierholzer, J., Lichtinghagen, R., Herder, C., Carstensen-Kirberg, M., Roden, M., Rudovich, N., Klaus, S., Thomann, R., Schneeweiss, R., Rohn, S., & Pfeiffer, A. F. (2017). Isocaloric diets high in animal or plant protein reduce liver fat and inflammation in individuals with type 2 diabetes. *Gastroenterology, 152*(3), 571–585.e8. https://doi.org/10.1053/j.gastro.2016.10.007 (accessed on 28th June 2025).

Mazza, A., Lenti, S., Schiavon, L., Zuin, M., D'Avino, M., Ramazzina, E., & Casiglia, E. (2015). Nutraceuticals for serum lipid and blood pressure control in hypertensive and hypercholesterolemic subjects at low cardiovascular risk. *Advances in Therapy, 32*(7), 680–690. https://doi.org/10.1007/s12325-015-0229-x (accessed on 28th June 2025).

McGaugh, E., & Barthel, B. (2022). A review of ketogenic diet and lifestyle. *Missouri Medicine, 119*(1), 84–88.

Mehta, S., Nain, P., Agrawal, B. K., Singh, R. P., Kaur, J., Maity, S., Bhattacharjee, A., Peela, J., Nauhria, S., & Nauhria, S. (2021). Effectiveness of empagliflozin with vitamin D supplementation in peripheral neuropathy in type 2 diabetic patients. *Cureus, 13*(12), e20208. https://doi.org/10.7759/cureus.20208 (accessed on 28th June 2025).

Méndez-del Villar, M., González-Ortiz, M., Martínez-Abundis, E., Pérez-Rubio, K. G., & Lizárraga-Valdez, R. (2014). Effect of resveratrol administration on metabolic syndrome, insulin sensitivity, and insulin secretion. *Metabolic Syndrome and Related Disorders, 12*(10), 497–501. https://doi.org/10.1089/met.2014.0082 (accessed on 28th June 2025).

Micheli, L., Lucarini, E., Trallori, E., Avagliano, C., De Caro, C., Russo, R., ... & Di Cesare Mannelli, L. (2019). *Phaseolus vulgaris* L. extract: Alpha-amylase inhibition against metabolic syndrome in mice. *Nutrients, 11*(8), 1778. https://doi.org/10.3390/nu11081778 (accessed on 28th June 2025).

Mohammadi, A., Gholamhosseinian, A., & Fallah, H. (2016). *Trigonella foenum-graecum* water extract improves insulin sensitivity and stimulates PPAR and γ gene expression in high fructose-fed insulin-resistant rats. *Advanced Biomedical Research, 5*, 54. https://doi.org/10.4103/2277-9175.178799 (accessed on 28th June 2025).

National Heart Lung and Blood Institute. (2020). *DASH Eating Plan*. National Heart Lung and Blood Institute: Bethesda, MD, USA.

Neto, J. C. G. L., Damasceno, M. M. C., Ciol, M. A., de Freitas, R. W. J. F., de Araújo, M. F. M., de Souza Teixeira, C. R., Carvalho, G. C. N., de Siqueira Coelho Lisboa, K. W., de Souza, D. F., de Menezes Nogueira, J., Marques, R. L. L., & Alencar, A. M. P. G. (2020). Analysis of the effectiveness of cinnamon (*Cinnamomum verum*) in reducing glycemic and lipidic levels of adults with type 2 diabetes: A study protocol. *Medicine, 99*(1), e18553. https://doi.org/10.1097/MD.0000000000018553 (accessed on 28th June 2025).

Ngondi, J. L., Etoundi, B. C., Nyangono, C. B., Mbofung, C. M., & Oben, J. E. (2009). IGOB131, a novel seed extract of the West African plant *Irvingia gabonensis*, significantly reduces body weight and improves metabolic parameters in overweight humans in a randomized double-blind placebo controlled investigation. *Lipids in Health and Disease, 8*, 7. https://doi.org/10.1186/1476-511X-8-7 (accessed on 28th June 2025).

Papathanasopoulos, A., & Camilleri, M. (2010). Dietary fiber supplements: Effects in obesity and metabolic syndrome and relationship to gastrointestinal functions. *Gastroenterology, 138*(1), 65–72.e722. https://doi.org/10.1053/j.gastro.2009.11.045 (accessed on 28th June 2025).

Rao, A. S., Hegde, S., Pacioretty, L. M., DeBenedetto, J., & Babish, J. G. (2020). *Nigella sativa* and *Trigonella foenum-graecum* supplemented chapatis safely improve HbA1c, body weight, waist circumference, blood lipids, and fatty liver in overweight and diabetic subjects: A twelve-week safety and efficacy study. *Journal of Medicinal Food, 23*(9), 905–919. https://doi.org/10.1089/jmf.2020.0075 (accessed on 28th June 2025).

Razmpoosh, E., Safi, S., Mazaheri, M., Salehi-Abargouei, A., Abdollahi, N., Nazari, M., Fallahzadeh, H., & Nadjarzadeh, A. (2019). Effects of oral *Nigella sativa* oil on the expression levels and serum concentrations of adiponectin, PPAR-γ, and TNF-α in overweight and obese women: A study protocol for a crossover-designed, double-blind, placebo-controlled randomized clinical trial. *Trials, 20*(1), 512. https://doi.org/10.1186/s13063-019-3568-0 (accessed on 28th June 2025).

Saberi-Karimian, M., Parizadeh, S. M. R., Ghayour-Mobarhan, M., Salahshooh, M. M., Dizaji, B. F., Safarian, H., ... & Ahmadinejad, M. (2018). Evaluation of the effects of curcumin in patients with metabolic syndrome. *Comparative Clinical Pathology, 27*, 555–563. https://doi.org/10.1007/s00580-017-2624-y (accessed on 28th June 2025).

Salimi Avansar, M. (2017). The effects of eight weeks' interval training and curcumin consumption on TNF-α and BDNF levels in men with metabolic syndrome. *Journal of Ardabil University of Medical Sciences, 17*(3), 299–310.

Saravanan, G., Ponmurugan, P., Deepa, M. A., & Senthilkumar, B. (2014). Modulatory effects of diosgenin on attenuating the key enzyme activities of carbohydrate metabolism and glycogen content in streptozotocin-induced diabetic rats. *Canadian Journal of Diabetes, 38*(6), 409–414. https://doi.org/10.1016/j.jcjd.2014.02.004 (accessed on 28th June 2025).

Sharma, V. K., & Singh, T. G. (2020). Chronic stress and diabetes mellitus: Interwoven pathologies. *Current Diabetes Reviews, 16*(6), 546–556. https://doi.org/10.2174/157339981566619111152248 (accessed on 28th June 2025).

Silveira Rossi, J. L., Barbalho, S. M., Reverete de Araujo, R., Bechara, M. D., Sloan, K. P., & Sloan, L. A. (2022). Metabolic syndrome and cardiovascular diseases: Going beyond traditional risk factors. *Diabetes/Metabolism Research and Reviews, 38*(3), e3502. https://doi.org/10.1002/dmrr.3502 (accessed on 28th June 2025).

Szabó, K., Gesztelyi, R., Lampé, N., Kiss, R., Remenyik, J., Pesti-Asbóth, G., Priksz, D., Szilvássy, Z., & Juhász, B. (2018). Fenugreek (*Trigonella foenum-graecum*) seed flour and diosgenin preserve endothelium-dependent arterial relaxation in a rat model of early-stage metabolic syndrome. *International Journal of Molecular Sciences, 19*(3), 798. https://doi.org/10.3390/ijms19030798 (accessed on 28th June 2025).

Tazoho, G. M., Gouado, I., Ndomou, M., Bonsi, S. T., Wamba, Y. M., & Agbor, E. E. (2016). Clinical, hematological and biochemical health benefits of *Hibiscus sabdariffa* Lin dried calyx's beverage in humans. *Food and Nutrition Sciences, 7*(5), 383. https://doi.org/10.4236/fns.2016.75040 (accessed on 28th June 2025).

Toshima, H., Keys, A., Koga, Y., & Blackburn, H. (Eds.). (2012). *Lessons for science from the Seven Countries Study: A 35-year collaborative experience in cardiovascular disease epidemiology*. Springer Science & Business Media. http://dx.doi.org/10.1007/978-4-431-68269-1 (accessed on 28th June 2025).

Udani, J., Tan, O., & Molina, J. (2018). Systematic review and meta-analysis of a proprietary alpha-amylase inhibitor from white bean (*Phaseolus vulgaris* L.) on human weight and fat loss. *Foods, 7*(4), 63. https://doi.org/10.3390/foods7040063 (accessed on 28th June 2025).

Vaibhav, A., Singh, J. P., & Singh, O. P. (2016). Role of *Lagenaria siceraria* fruit juice in overweight and obesity. *International Journal of Research and Review, 3*, 6–11.

Vasques, C. A., Schneider, R., Klein-Júnior, L. C., Falavigna, A., Piazza, I., & Rossetto, S. (2014). Hypolipemic effect of *Garcinia cambogia* in obese women. *Phytotherapy Research, 28*(6), 887–891. https://doi.org/10.1002/ptr.5076 (accessed on 28th June 2025).

Vieira Senger, A. E., Schwanke, C. H., Gomes, I., & Valle Gottlieb, M. G. (2012). Effect of green tea (*Camellia sinensis*) consumption on the components of metabolic syndrome in elderly. *The Journal of Nutrition, Health & Aging, 16*, 738–742. https://doi.org/10.1007/s12603-012-0081-5 (accessed on 28th June 2025).

Wang, F. X., Zhu, N., Zhou, F., & Lin, D. X. (2021). Natural aporphine alkaloids with potential to impact metabolic syndrome. *Molecules, 26*(20), 6117. https://doi.org/10.3390/molecules26206117 (accessed on 28th June 2025).

Wang, Y., Yi, X., Ghanam, K., Zhang, S., Zhao, T., & Zhu, X. (2014). Berberine decreases cholesterol levels in rats through multiple mechanisms, including inhibition of cholesterol absorption. *Metabolism: Clinical and Experimental, 63*(9), 1167–1177. https://doi.org/10.1016/j.metabol.2014.05.013 (accessed on 28th June 2025).

Xu, Y., Zhang, M., Wu, T., Dai, S., Xu, J., & Zhou, Z. (2015). The anti-obesity effect of green tea polysaccharides, polyphenols and caffeine in rats fed a high-fat diet. *Food & Function, 6*(1), 297–304. https://doi.org/10.1039/C4FO00970C (accessed on 28th June 2025).

Yang, T. Y., Chou, J. I., Ueng, K. C., Chou, M. Y., Yang, J. J., Lin-Shiau, S. Y., ... & Lin, J. K. (2014). Weight reduction effect of *Puerh* tea in male patients with metabolic syndrome. *Phytotherapy Research, 28*(7), 1096–1101. https://doi.org/10.1002/ptr.5111 (accessed on 28th June 2025).

CHAPTER 15

Antioxidant Effects of Natural Phytochemicals in Thyroid Disorders

DEEPIKA JOSHI,[1,*] DEEPIKA RAINA,[2] BHAVANA SINGH,[3] ALOK BHATT,[2] and SOFIA KOKKINIS[4,5]

[1]*Siddhartha Institute of Pharmacy, Dehradun, Uttarakhand, India*

[2]*School of Pharmacy, Graphic Era Hill University, Dehradun, Uttarakhand, India*

[3]*School of Pharmacy, Sharda University, Greater Noida, Uttar Pradesh, India*

[4]*Discipline of Pharmacy, Graduate School of Health, University of Technology Sydney, Sydney, New South Wales, Australia*

[5]*Faculty of Health, Australian Research Center in Complementary and Integrative Medicine, University of Technology Sydney, Ultimo, New South Wales, Australia*

*Corresponding author

ABSTRACT

Among various endocrine disorders, thyroid disease is one of the most prevalent, and its occurrence rises with age. Thyroid hormones (THs) secreted by the gland control several physiological processes, including cell division, development, metabolism, homeostasis and proliferation. Some of the different thyroid diseases include Goiter (thyroid gland enlargement/swelling), Hyperthyroidism, Hypothyroidism, thyroiditis (thyroid swelling), thyroid cancer, and thyroid nodules (lumps/masses in the thyroid gland). Among clinical thyroid dysfunctions, hypothyroidism is

Precision Nutrition and Endocrine Health: Synthesis, Characterization, and Applications.
Thakur Gurjeet Singh and Sanjana Mehta (Eds.)

DOI: 10.1201/9781998511877-15

the most prevalent, which refers to thyroid deficiency to produce sufficient amounts of TH or reduced Thyroid stimulating hormones (TSH) activation of the thyroid as a result of hypopituitarism or hypothalamic illness. Hyperthyroidism, a thyroid dysfunction, describes an excess metabolic condition brought on by an excessive amount of TH being synthesized and secreted. The prevalence of hyperthyroidism and hypothyroidism is more significant in women compared to men. The choice of treatment for thyroid disease includes long-term antithyroid drug treatment and invasive methods. Various adverse effects in prolonged use accompany antithyroid drugs. Thus, in search of therapy with fewer side effects, the authors focused on reviewing various herbal plants rich in phytochemicals that are a significant source of natural antioxidants with anti-inflammatory, anti-microbial, and anti-proliferative qualities. Thyroid disorders can be treated with medicinal plants. Numerous plant components can potentially disrupt thyroid function or cause anomalies in thyroid function. Numerous plant components, including polyphenols and alkaloids, may have an anti-proliferative effect on thyroid cancer cells and interfere with the synthesis or metabolism of thyroid hormones.

15.1 INTRODUCTION

The butterfly-shaped thyroid gland is an endocrine gland that resides in the center of the human neck. For average growth and development, as well as the maintenance of baseline metabolic rate, triiodothyronine (T3) and thyroxine (T4) are secreted by the thyroid gland (Wu et al., 2000). Thyroid hormones work at the cellular level and are carried through the bloodstream. Thyroid hormones boost the rate of cell respiration in tissues, stimulate protein synthesis, and support the maturation of the neurological system by activating genes. Thyroid signaling homeostasis disruptions are typically the hallmark of thyroid disorders (Astapova et al., 2016). Goiter, hyperthyroidism, hypothyroidism, and thyroid cancer are among the various thyroid conditions. A goiter is characterized by a lump or swelling at the front of the neck due to iodine deficiency or inflammation of the thyroid gland. Hyperthyroidism is the outcome of producing too much thyroid hormone, whereas hypothyroidism is the result of producing insufficient amounts of the hormone. The most prevalent thyroid conditions include various forms of thyroid cancer, hyperthyroidism, and hypothyroidism. Around 1 in 10 women aged 60 and over suffers from thyroid disease. There are several metabolic factors related to thyroid disease. Oxidative stress has a growing correlation with thyroid disorders. Subclinical thyroid diseases are prevalent. However, they are frequently misdiagnosed.

Long-term thyroid drug administration causes drug resistance and side effects and results in a higher recurrence rate. Therefore, more safe anti-thyroid therapies still need to be introduced. This study aims to review phytochemicals as an antithyroid therapy. Phytochemicals are naturally occurring chemical substances produced in medicinal plants and have diverse physiological activities (Groves et al., 1994; Singh et al., 2020). Their physiological functions include anti-inflammation, hormone metabolism, immune system stimulation, oxidant scavenging, gene regulation, cell proliferation and death, antiviral, antibacterial activities, and anti-cancer effects with fewer side effects. Certain phytochemicals, such as cyanogenic glucosides, polyphenols, phenolic acids, and alkaloids, act as antithyroid agents and obstruct proper thyroid function.

15.2 METHODS

This study's details were reviewed in Science Direct, PubMed, and Google Scholar using keywords such as "thyroid disorder," "medicinal plants," "phytochemicals," "hypothyroidism," and "hyperthyroidism." All articles mentioned were searched from the last 10 years until 2023. The outcomes of this study mainly concentrated on the results or conclusions of phytochemicals' antithyroid activity.

15.3 THYROID GLAND RELATED DISEASES

The following are the common thyroid diseases:

- **Hyperthyroidism:** The thyroid gland secretes more thyroid hormones than the body requires when it has an overactive thyroid disease. Hyperthyroidism has several causes, such as an autoimmune disorder (Graves' disease), overactive thyroid nodules, thyroiditis, and high iodine intake (Oetting et al., 2007).
- **Hypothyroidism:** It is a condition of the thyroid gland producing inadequate thyroid hormones to meet the body's needs.

Hypothyroidism has several causes, such as an autoimmune disorder (Hashimoto's disease), Congenital hypothyroidism, thyroiditis, surgical thyroidectomy, either in whole or in part and various medicines.

- **Goiter and Iodine Deficiency Disorders:** A goiter might result from one or more thyroid nodules or an overall thyroid enlargement caused by abnormal cell proliferation. Thyroid hormone levels may rise or fall with a goiter, or there may be no change in thyroid function.
- **Thyroid cancer:** Cancer affecting the tissues of the thyroid gland is known as thyroid cancer. The symptoms include nodules in the neck, trouble breathing, trouble swallowing, and changes in voice, such as hoarseness.

15.4 OXIDATIVE STRESS (OS)

Oxidative stress (OS) is a disparity between the production of prooxidant molecules and antioxidant molecules in the body. Reactive oxygen species (ROS) and reactive nitrogen species (RNS) are the two most significant prooxidants (Lancaster et al., 1992; Rehni et al., 2009; Sharma and Singh, 2020). The ROS family members are the superoxide anion, hydroxyl radical, hydrogen peroxide, and hypochlorous acid (Singh et al., 2020). The oxidative metabolism of energy substrates occurs when the mitochondria's respiratory chain produces the first three compounds *in vivo* (Kang and Hamasaki, 2003; Littarru et al.,1994; Mehta et al., 2021). In addition to influencing the natural antioxidant pool (Brass et al., 2005; Wink et al., 2011), they function as regulators of redox-sensitive pathways that maintain the homeostasis of cells. (Valko, 2007). They also have an impact on certain transcription factors. RNS are nitric oxide (NO) and superoxide. NO reacts to make peroxynitrite, and carbon dioxide reacts to form nitrosoperoxycarbonate. ROS and RNS are significant pathogenetic agents in some disorders (Halliwell et al., 1979; Mannan et al., 2022; Rehni et al., 2009). The hydroxyl radical and superoxide anion, two molecules with high chemical reactivity because of one unpaired electron in the outermost orbital, have a particular pathogenetic function (Carmeli et al., 2008).

An imbalance of ROS generation and antioxidant defense systems leads to oxidative stress that disrupts intracellular signal transmission and physiologic response, causing oxidative DNA damage and lipid peroxidation. As a result of the changing intracellular redox status, protein kinases such as tyrosine kinase and protein kinase C are activated, which can result in alterations to cellular activities through the mitogen-activated protein kinase cascade (Mannan et al., 2021). Reduced antioxidative defense capability and elevated free radical generation combine to cause hypothyroidism-associated ROS. It is known that excess TSH directly causes OS (Dardano et al., 2006). Additional research verified the existence of lipid peroxidation in both overt and subclinical hypothyroidism, as seen by elevated malondialdehyde (MDA) levels. Additionally, protein oxidation has been documented, accompanied by elevated protein carbonyls (Haribabu et al., 2013).

It has been demonstrated that oxidative stress is linked to hypothyroidism (less antioxidant availability) and hyperthyroidism (produces more ROS). OS can cause harm to the thyroid itself when there is an excess of iodine in the body (Vitale et al., 2000; Zhang et al., 2015). In thyroid slices, iodide stimulates the production of hydrogen peroxide and, at high doses, causes thyroid cell death (Corvilain et al., 2000). Thyroid inflammation caused by oxidative stress impairs self-tolerance and ultimately results in autoimmune thyroid dysfunction.

In this investigation, we initially focus on the relationship between thyroid hormones and the parameters of OS. Next, we summarize the information that is currently known about the regulation of antioxidants and thyroid hormones. Lastly, we present our findings of phytochemical investigations and their influence on thyroid disorders. Thus, our review aims to discuss ROS deregulation in hyper- and hypothyroidism, which could be targeted using redox-active phyto-substances that may affect the thyroid glands physiology or pathology.

The lipid risk factors associated with atherosclerosis correlate with OS's prevalence in hypothyroidism (Nanda et al., 2008). Oxidative stress can also be exacerbated by a metabolic imbalance resulting from autoimmune-based hypothyroidism (Komosinska-Vassev et al., 2000). In Hashimoto's thyroiditis, low-grade chronic inflammation increases OS by impairing nitric oxide availability and causing endothelial dysfunction (Taddei et al., 2006).

12.5 PHYTOCHEMICAL ANTIOXIDANT ACTIVITY

Thyroid pathogenic diseases are linked to oxidative stress, which causes the body to produce excessive amounts of reactive oxygen species, which are not removed by the body's natural antioxidant defenses. Antioxidative substances like phytochemicals, particularly phenolic ones, may enhance these processes (Paunkov et al., 2019). Plants are considered a significant source of secondary metabolites, such as polyphenols, which have biological solid antioxidative properties (Wu et al., 2019). The most prevalent class of natural antioxidants is represented by phenolic chemicals, which have direct and indirect antioxidant activity and lower oxidative stress (Montane et al., 2020). Polyphenols function as solid antioxidants by giving reactive oxygen, nitrogen, and chlorine species electrons or hydrogen that prevent the production of unstable radicals (Tsao et al., 2012) and act as powerful hydroperoxide neutralizers and radical scavengers. Moreover, they can act as metal chelators, changing metal prooxidants into stable substances.

Phytochemicals with antioxidant activity are divided into three groups based on the mechanisms of action they use to protect against reactive oxygen species (ROS): (i) direct antioxidants are characterized by their redox activity and brief half-lives; (ii) indirect antioxidants are those that initiate intracellular pathways that can protect against oxidative stress in the long run; and (iii) bifunctional antioxidants are those that have both characteristics (Yang et al., 2020).

15.5.1 TANNINS (PHENOLIC ACIDS)

With its diverse range of pharmacological activities, including antiviral, antibacterial, anticancer, hypolipidemic, antioxidant, and chemopreventive qualities, tannins are the pharmacodynamic foundation of many widely used medicinal plants (Jiang et al., 2008; Liu et al., 2006). They work primarily by destroying thyroid cancer cells in the papillary (PTC) cell line, inhibiting carcinogenesis and progression of cellular signaling (Han et al., 2019), decreasing proliferation and invasiveness, inducing apoptosis, reducing aldehyde dehydrogenases (ALDH) associated cancer cell stemness, and upregulating thyroid differentiation markers Thyroid transcription factor 1 (TTF-1) and Na+/I-symporter (NIS) (Costa et al., 2018).

15.5.2 FLAVONOIDS (PHENOLIC ANTIOXIDANTS)

Flavonoids, which resemble estrogen in structure, have weak or negligible estrogenic effects. These include soy genistein, naringenin, phloretin, and chrysin (Mittal et al., 2023; Ye, 2019). Such phytoestrogens affect the synthesis and metabolism of thyroid hormone (De Souza et al., 2011; Gonçalves et al., 2017; Messina et al., 2006) by preventing cell viability, migration, and invasion and by activating the adenosine-monophosphate-activated protein kinase (AMPK). Numerous investigations have demonstrated the anticancer effects of the AMPK/mammalian target of the rapamycin (mTOR) pathway. They exhibit substantial toxicity to cells by causing ROS-mediated apoptotic and autophagic cell death in various tumor cells.

15.5.3 SAPONINS (STEROID OR TRITERPENOID GLYCOSIDES)

Pharmacological actions exhibited by saponins include anticancer, anti-inflammatory, hypoglycemic, immunomodulatory, and vasoprotective characteristics (Singh et al., 2017). Ginsenosides are the significant active component of the ginseng genus with a triterpenoid dammarane skeleton. They cause hemolysis and are cytotoxic. Its ability to suppress PTC cell proliferation at low concentrations (10~100 μM) suggests it has multidirectional effects on cancer cells (Koczurkiewicz et al., 2015). Table 15.1 explains the list of essential plants that act as antithyroid agents in hypo- and hyperthyroidism.

TABLE 15.1 The Following is a list of Essential Plants that Act as Antithyroid Agents in Hypo- and Hyperthyroidism.

S. No.	Name of Plant	Diseases	Activity
1.	*Withania somnifera*	Hypothyroidism	Stimulate TH function increases both T3 and T4 (Sharma, 2018)
2.	*Commiphora Mukul*	Hypothyroidism	Increasing iodine absorption, enhancing the activity of peroxidase (Stansbury, 2012)
3.	*Zingiber officinale* (Rosc.)	Hypothyroidism	Anti-inflammatory properties (Mahassni, 2019)

TABLE 15.1 *(Continued)*

S. No.	Name of Plant	Diseases	Activity
4.	*Bacopa monnieri*	Hypothyroidism	Increasing the amount of T4 (Vishwakarma, 2016)
5.	*Coleus forskohlii*	Hypothyroidism	Enhances the hormone's synthesis and secretion (Laurberg, 1984)
6.	*Linum usitatissimum*	Hypothyroidism	Promote TH production (Bhardawaj, 2021)
7.	*Melissa officinalis*	Hyperthyroidism	Raises TSH and TRH secretion levels, which in turn raises T3 and T4 levels (Santini, 2003)
8.	*Lemon balm*	Hyperthyroidism	It is effective on both the hormone and the receptor by blocking TSH from attaching itself to it (Santini, 2003)
9.	*Rauvolfia serpentine*	Hyperthyroidism	Decreased T3 and T4 serum concentrations (Panda, 2010)
10.	*Leonurus cardiac*	Hyperthyroidism	Anti-inflammatory drugs inhibit 5-deiodinase, which is the hormone that stimulates the thyroid and decreases the overproduction of thyroid hormones (Shokri, 2018)
11.	*Curcuma longa*	Thyroid cancer	Apoptosis can be instigated by four different pathways: Initiation of ATM-activated Chk2-Cdc25C-Cdc2 pathway-mediated ROS-independent DNA damage; ER stress activation through intracellular calcium homeostasis disturbance; Suppression of the β-catenin pathway; and Modification of the mitochondrial Bcl-2/Bax pathway (Sharifi, 2020)
12.	*Punicalagin*	Thyroid cancer	It causes the ATM-mediated DNA damage response, which kills the PTC cell line BCPAP (Yao, 2017).
13.	*Epimedium davidii*	Thyroid cancer	SW579 and TPC1 cells suppress cell growth, migration, and invasion by downregulating PI3K/AKT, miR-625-3p, and epithelial-mesenchymal transition (ERK) pathways (Shen, 2018).
14.	*Panax ginseng*	Thyroid cancer	It prevents PTC cells' migration, invasion, and proliferation (Pan, 2018).

TSH: Thyroid-stimulating hormone, TH: Thyroid hormones.

15.6 CONCLUSION

Thyroid disorders are treated with a variety of herbs containing phytochemicals. Thyroid hormones can protect by regulating antioxidant levels; tissue hypothyroidism can exacerbate OS. In this review, we have discussed the phytoconstituents, primarily in food or dietary supplements, that have antithyroid effects. Dietary phytochemicals have several medicinal qualities, such as anti-inflammatory, antioxidant, and anti-cancer actions, and they may also modify immune status. Their recognized mechanisms of action on thyroid hormone metabolism and cells have mostly been presented in tabular form. The ability of phytochemicals to defend against ROS and consequently lower the risk of several pathological processes and diseases associated with oxidative stress is one likely contributory mechanism.

KEYWORDS

- **hormone regulation**
- **hyperthyroidism**
- **hypothyroidism**
- **medicinal plants**
- **phytochemicals**
- **thyroid gland**

REFERENCES

Astapova, I. (2016). Role of co-regulators in metabolic and transcriptional actions of thyroid hormone. *Journal of Molecular Endocrinology, 56*(3), 73–97. https://doi.org/10.1530/JME-15-0246 (accessed on 28th June 2025).

Bharadwaj, N., & Siddiqui, N. (2021). Phytochemical screening and nanosynthesis of *Linum usitatissimum* [flax seeds] used in hypothyroid treatment. *Oriental Journal of Chemistry, 37*(3), 1–6.

Carmeli, E., Bachar, A., Barchad, S., Morad, M., & Merrick, J. (2008). Antioxidant status in the serum of persons with intellectual disability and hypothyroidism: A pilot study. *Research in Developmental Disabilities, 29*(5), 431–438. https://doi.org/10.1016/j.ridd.2007.08.001 (accessed on 28th June 2025).

Corvilain, B., Collyn, L., van Sande, J., & Dumont, J. E. (2000). Stimulation by iodide of H_2O_2 generation in thyroid slices from several species. *American Journal of Physiology. Endocrinology and Metabolism, 278*(4), E692–E699. https://doi.org/10.1152/ajpendo.2000.278.4.E692 (accessed on 28th June 2025).

Costa, M., Alves, S. P., Cappucci, A., Cook, S. R., Duarte, A., Caldeira, R. M., McAllister, T. A., & Bessa, R. J. B. (2018). Effects of condensed and hydrolyzable tannins on rumen metabolism with emphasis on the biohydrogenation of unsaturated fatty acids. *Journal of Agricultural and Food Chemistry, 66*(13), 3367–3377. https://doi.org/10.1021/acs.jafc.7b04770 (accessed on 28th June 2025).

Dardano, A., Ghiadoni, L., Plantinga, Y., Caraccio, N., Bemi, A., Duranti, E., Taddei, S., Ferrannini, E., Salvetti, A., & Monzani, F. (2006). Recombinant human thyrotropin reduces endothelium-dependent vasodilation in patients monitored for differentiated thyroid carcinoma. *The Journal of Clinical Endocrinology and Metabolism, 91*(10), 4175–4178. https://doi.org/10.1210/jc.2006-0440 (accessed on 28th June 2025).

Gonçalves, C. F. L., de Freitas, M. L., & Ferreira, A. C. F. (2017). Flavonoids, thyroid iodide uptake and thyroid cancer—a review. *International Journal of Molecular Sciences, 18*(6), 1247. https://doi.org/10.3390/ijms18061247 (accessed on 28th June 2025).

Groves, M. N. (1994). *Endocrine class 3: Natural thyroid support.* Wintergreen Botanicals.

Halliwell, B., & Gutteridge, J. M. C. (1979). *Free radical in biology and medicine* (2nd ed.). Clarendon Press, Oxford, UK.

Han, Y., Jo, H., Cho, J. H., Dhanasekaran, D. N., & Song, Y. S. (2019). Resveratrol as a tumor-suppressive nutraceutical modulating tumor microenvironment and malignant behaviors of cancer. *International Journal of Molecular Sciences, 20*(4), 925. https://doi.org/10.3390/ijms20040925 (accessed on 28th June 2025).

Haribabu, A., Reddy, V. S., Pallavi, C. H., Bitla, A. R., Sachan, A., Pullaiah, P., Suresh, V., Rao, P. V., & Suchitra, M. M. (2013). Evaluation of protein oxidation and its association with lipid peroxidation and thyrotropin levels in overt and subclinical hypothyroidism. *Endocrine, 44*(1), 152–157. https://doi.org/10.1007/s12020-012-9849-y (accessed on 28th June 2025).

Jiang, Z. H., Wen, X. Y., Tanaka, T., et al. (2008). Cytotoxic hydrolysable tannins from *Balanophora japonica. Journal of Natural Products, 71*(4), 719–723.

Kang, D., & Hamasaki, N. (2003). Mitochondrial oxidative stress and mitochondrial DNA. *Clinical Chemistry and Laboratory Medicine, 41*(10), 1281–1288. https://doi.org/10.1515/CCLM.2003.195 (accessed on 28th June 2025).

Koczurkiewicz, P., Czyż, J., Podolak, I., Wójcik, K., Galanty, A., Janeczko, Z., & Michalik, M. (2015). Multidirectional effects of triterpene saponins on cancer cells: Mini-review of in vitro studies. *Acta Biochimica Polonica, 62*(3), 383–393. https://doi.org/10.18388/abp.2015_1089 (accessed on 28th June 2025).

Komosinska-Vassev, K., Olczyk, K., Kucharz, E. J., Marcisz, C., Winsz-Szczotka, K., & Kotulska, A. (2000). Free radical activity and antioxidant defense mechanisms in patients with hyperthyroidism due to Graves' disease during therapy. *Clinica Chimica Acta, 300*(1–2), 107–117. https://doi.org/10.1016/s0009-8981(00)00306-5 (accessed on 28th June 2025).

Lancaster, J. R. (1992). Nitric oxide in cells. *American Scientist, 80*, 249–259.

Laurberg, P. (1984). Forskolin stimulation of thyroid secretion of T4 and T3. *FEBS Letters, 170*(2), 273–276.

Le, M. B., Clement, M. V., Pervaiz, S., & Brenner, C. (2005). Reactive oxygen species and the mitochondrial signalling pathway of cell death. *Histology and Histopathology, 20*(1), 205–220.

Littarru, G. P. (1994). *Energy and defence*. CESI, Roma, Italy.

Liu, C., Cai, D., Zhang, L., Tang, W., Yan, R., Guo, H., & Chen, X. (2016). Identification of hydrolyzable tannins (punicalagin, punicalin and geraniin) as novel inhibitors of hepatitis B virus covalently closed circular DNA. *Antiviral Research, 134*, 97–107. https://doi.org/10.1016/j.antiviral.2016.08.026 (accessed on 28th June 2025).

Mahassni, S. H., & Bukhari, O. A. (2019). Beneficial effects of an aqueous ginger extract on the immune system cells and antibodies, hematology, and thyroid hormones in male smokers and non-smokers. *Journal of Nutrition & Intermediary Metabolism, 15*, 10–17. https://doi.org/10.1016/j.jnim.2018.10.001 (accessed on 28th June 2025).

Mangge, H., Becker, K., Fuchs, D., & Gostner, J. M. (2014). Antioxidants, inflammation and cardiovascular disease. *World Journal of Cardiology, 6*(6), 462–477. https://doi.org/10.4330/wjc.v6.i6.462 (accessed on 28th June 2025).

Mannan, A., Garg, N., Singh, T. G., & Kang, H. K. (2021). Peroxisome proliferator-activated receptor-gamma (PPAR-γ): Molecular effects and its importance as a novel therapeutic target for cerebral ischemic injury. *Neurochemical Research, 46*(11), 2800–2831. https://doi.org/10.1007/s11064-021-03402-1 (accessed on 28th June 2025).

Mannan, A., Singh, T. G., Singh, V., Garg, N., Kaur, A., & Singh, M. (2022). Insights into the mechanism of the therapeutic potential of herbal monoamine oxidase inhibitors in neurological diseases. *Current Drug Targets, 23*(3), 286–310. https://doi.org/10.2174/1389450122666210707120256 (accessed on 28th June 2025).

Mehta, S., Nain, P., Agrawal, B. K., Singh, R. P., Kaur, J., Maity, S., Bhattacharjee, A., Peela, J., Nauhria, S., & Nauhria, S. (2021). Effectiveness of empagliflozin with vitamin D supplementation in peripheral neuropathy in type 2 diabetic patients. *Cureus, 13*(12), e20208. https://doi.org/10.7759/cureus.20208 (accessed on 28th June 2025).

Mendoza, A., & Hollenberg, A. N. (2017). New insights into thyroid hormone action. *Pharmacology & Therapeutics, 173*, 135–145. https://doi.org/10.1016/j.pharmthera.2017.02.012 (accessed on 28th June 2025).

Messina, M., & Redmond, G. (2006). Effects of soy protein and soybean isoflavones on thyroid function in healthy adults and hypothyroid patients: A review of the relevant literature. *Thyroid, 16*(3), 249–258. https://doi.org/10.1089/thy.2006.16.249 (accessed on 28th June 2025).

Mittal, P., Dhankhar, S., Chauhan, S., Garg, N., Bhattacharya, T., Ali, M., Chaudhary, A. A., Rudayni, H. A., Al-Zharani, M., Ahmad, W., Khan, S. U., Singh, T. G., & Mujwar, S. (2023). A review on natural antioxidants for their role in the treatment of Parkinson's disease. *Pharmaceuticals (Basel, Switzerland), 16*(7), 908. https://doi.org/10.3390/ph16070908 (accessed on 28th June 2025).

Montane, X., Kowalczyk, O., Reig-Vano, B., Bajek, A., Roszkowski, K., Tomczyk, R., et al. (2020). Current perspectives of the applications of polyphenols and flavonoids in cancer therapy. *Molecules, 25*(15), 3342. https://doi.org/10.3390/molecules25153342 (accessed on 28th June 2025).

Nanda, N., Bobby, Z., & Hamide, A. (2008). Oxidative stress and protein glycation in primary hypothyroidism: Male/female difference. *Clinical and Experimental Medicine,*

8(2), 101–108. https://doi.org/10.1007/s10238-008-0164-0 (accessed on 28th June 2025).

Pan, W., Xue, B., Yang, C., Miao, L., Zhou, L., Chen, Q., Cai, Q., Liu, Y., Liu, D., He, H., Zhang, Y., Yin, T., & Tang, X. (2018). Biopharmaceutical characters and bioavailability improving strategies of ginsenosides. *Fitoterapia, 129*, 272–282. https://doi.org/10.1016/j.fitote.2018.06.001 (accessed on 28th June 2025).

Panda, S., & Kar, A. (2010). Regulation of hyperthyroidism by *Rauwolfia serpentina* root extract in mice. *Pharmacy and Pharmacology Communications, 6*(11), 517–520. https://doi.org/10.1211/146080800128735629 (accessed on 28th June 2025).

Paunkov, A., Chartoumpekis, D. V., Ziros, P. G., Chondrogianni, N., Kensler, T. W., & Sykiotis, G. P. (2019). Impact of antioxidant natural compounds on the thyroid gland and implication of the Keap1/Nrf2 signalling pathway. *Current Pharmaceutical Design, 25*(16), 1828–1846. https://doi.org/10.2174/1381612825666190701165821 (accessed on 28th June 2025).

Rehni, A. K., Singh, T. G., Kalra, R., & Singh, N. (2009). Pharmacological inhibition of inducible nitric oxide synthase attenuates the development of seizures in mice. *Nitric Oxide: Biology and Chemistry, 21*(2), 120–125. https://doi.org/10.1016/j.niox.2009.06.001 (accessed on 28th June 2025).

Santini, F., Vitti, P., Ceccarini, G., Mammoli, C., Rosellini, V., Pelosini, C., et al. (2003). In vitro assay of thyroid disruptors affecting TSH-stimulated adenylate cyclase activity. *Journal of Endocrinological Investigation, 26*(10), 950–955. https://doi.org/10.2174/1381612825666190701165821 (accessed on 28th June 2025).

Sharifi-Rad, J., Rajabi, S., Martorell, M., López, M. D., Toro, M. T., Barollo, S., Armanini, D., Fokou, P. V. T., Zagotto, G., Ribaudo, G., & Pezzani, R. (2020). Plant natural products with anti-thyroid cancer activity. *Fitoterapia, 146*, 104640. https://doi.org/10.1016/j.fitote.2020.104640 (accessed on 28th June 2025).

Sharma, A. K., Basu, I., & Singh, S. (2018). Efficacy and safety of Ashwagandha root extract in subclinical hypothyroid patients: A double-blind, randomized placebo-controlled trial. *Journal of Alternative and Complementary Medicine (New York, N.Y.), 24*(3), 243–248. https://doi.org/10.1089/acm.2017.0183 (accessed on 28th June 2025).

Sharma, V. K., & Singh, T. G. (2020). Navigating Alzheimer's disease via chronic stress: The role of glucocorticoids. *Current Drug Targets, 21*(5), 433–444. https://doi.org/10.2174/1389450120666191017114735 (accessed on 28th June 2025).

Shen, R., & Wang, J. H. (2018). The effect of icariin on immunity and its potential application. *American Journal of Clinical and Experimental Immunology, 7*(7), 50–56.

Shokri, Z., Khoshbin, M., Koohpayeh, A., et al. (2018). Thyroid diseases: Pathophysiology and new hopes in medicinal plants and natural antioxidants treatment. *International Journal of Green Pharmacy, 12*, S473–S482. https://doi.org/10.22377/ijgp.v12i03.2007 (accessed on 28th June 2025).

Singh, B., Singh, J. P., Singh, N., & Kaur, A. (2017). Saponins in pulses and their health promoting activities: A review. *Food Chemistry, 233*, 540–549. https://doi.org/10.1016/j.foodchem.2017.04.161 (accessed on 28th June 2025).

Singh, H. P., Singh, T. G., & Singh, R. (2020). Sinapic acid attenuates cisplatin-induced nephrotoxicity through peroxisome proliferator-activated receptor gamma agonism in rats. *Journal of Pharmacy & Bioallied Sciences, 12*(2), 146–154. https://doi.org/10.4103/jpbs.JPBS_220_19 (accessed on 28th June 2025).

Singh, M., Sharma, P., Singh, P. K., Singh, T. G., & Saini, B. (2020). Medicinal potential of heterocyclic compounds from diverse natural sources for the management of cancer. *Mini Reviews in Medicinal Chemistry, 20*(11), 942–957. https://doi.org/10.2174/1389557520666200212104742 (accessed on 28th June 2025).

Stansbury, N. J., Saunders, P. P., & Winston, R. A. (2012). Promoting healthy thyroid function with iodine, bladderwrack, guggul and iris. *Journal of Restorative Medicine, 1*, 83–90. https://doi.org/10.14200/jrm.2012.1.1008 (accessed on 28th June 2025).

Taddei, S., Caraccio, N., Virdis, A., Dardano, A., Versari, D., Ghiadoni, L., Ferrannini, E., Salvetti, A., & Monzani, F. (2006). Low-grade systemic inflammation causes endothelial dysfunction in patients with Hashimoto's thyroiditis. *The Journal of Clinical Endocrinology and Metabolism, 91*(12), 5076–5082. https://doi.org/10.1210/jc.2006-1075 (accessed on 28th June 2025).

Tsao, R., & Li, H. (2012). Antioxidant properties in vitro and in vivo: Realistic assessments of efficacy of plant extracts. *Plant Sciences Reviews, 7*(9), 11–13.

Valko, M., Leibfritz, D., Moncol, J., Cronin, M. T. D., Mazur, M., & Telser, J. (2007). Free radicals and antioxidants are used in normal physiological functions and in treating human disease. *International Journal of Biochemistry & Cell Biology, 39*(1), 44–84. https://doi.org/10.1016/j.biocel.2006.07.001 (accessed on 28th June 2025).

Vishwakarma, R. K., Kumari, U., & Khan, B. M. (2016). Memory booster plant *Bacopa monniera* (Brahmi): Biotechnology and molecular aspects of bacoside biosynthesis. In *Medicinal plants. Recent advances in research and development* (pp. 167–189). Springer Publication. https://doi.org/10.1007/978-981-10-1085-9_6 (accessed on 28th June 2025).

Vitale, M., Di Matola, T., D'Ascoli, F., Salzano, S., Bogazzi, F., Fenzi, G., Martino, E., & Rossi, G. (2000). Iodide excess induces apoptosis in thyroid cells through a p53-independent mechanism involving oxidative stress. *Endocrinology, 141*(2), 598–605. https://doi.org/10.1210/endo.141.2.7291 (accessed on 28th June 2025).

Wink, D. A., Hines, H. B., Cheng, R. Y., Switzer, C. H., Flores-Santana, W., Vitek, M. P., Ridnour, L. A., & Colton, C. A. (2011). Nitric oxide and redox mechanisms in the immune response. *Journal of Leukocyte Biology, 89*(6), 873–891. https://doi.org/10.1189/jlb.1010550 (accessed on 28th June 2025).

Wu, D., Liu, Z., Li, J., Zhang, Q., Zhong, P., Teng, T., Chen, M., Xie, Z., Ji, A., & Li, Y. (2019). Epigallocatechin-3-gallate inhibits the growth and increases the apoptosis of human thyroid carcinoma cells through suppression of EGFR/RAS/RAF/MEK/ERK signaling pathway. *Cancer Cell International, 19*, 43. https://doi.org/10.1186/s12935-019-0762-9 (accessed on 28th June 2025).

Wu, Y., & Koenig, R. J. (2000). Gene regulation by thyroid hormone. *Trends in Endocrinology and Metabolism, 11*, 207–211. https://doi.org/10.1016/S1043-2760(00)00263-0 (accessed on 28th June 2025).

Yang, Y., Chen, Q., Yu, W. Y., Zhang, H. H., Zhong, Y. S., Zhang, S. Z., Wang, J. F., & Yu, C. H. (2020). Herbal active ingredients: An emerging potential for the prevention and treatment of papillary thyroid carcinoma. *BioMed Research International, 2020*, 1340153. https://doi.org/10.1155/2020/1340153 (accessed on 28th June 2025).

Yao, X., Cheng, X., Zhang, L., Yu, H., Bao, J., Guan, H., & Lu, R. (2017). Punicalagin from pomegranate promotes human papillary thyroid carcinoma BCPAP cell death by triggering ATM-mediated DNA damage response. *Nutrition Research (New York, N.Y.), 47*, 63–71. https://doi.org/10.1016/j.nutres.2017.09.001 (accessed on 28th June 2025).

Ye, H., & Shaw, I. C. (2019). Food flavonoid ligand structure/estrogen receptor-α affinity relationships – Toxicity or food functionality? *Food and Chemical Toxicology, 129*, 328–336. https://doi.org/10.1016/j.fct.2019.04.008 (accessed on 28th June 2025).

Zhang, N., Wang, L., Duan, Q., Lin, L., Ahmed, M., Wang, T., & Yao, X. (2015). Metallothionein-I/II knockout mice aggravate mitochondrial superoxide production and peroxiredoxin 3 expression in thyroid after excessive iodide exposure. *Oxidative Medicine and Cellular Longevity, 2015*, 267027. https://doi.org/10.1155/2015/267027 (accessed on 28th June 2025).

Index

B

C

D

E

J

K

L

M

N

T

www.ingramcontent.com/pod-product-compliance
Lightning Source LLC
LaVergne TN
LVHW020627300926
849161LV00004B/633
* 9 7 8 1 9 9 8 5 1 1 8 6 0 *